REGENERATIVE MEDICINE IN SMALL ANIMAL MUSCULOSKELETAL CONDITIONS

Advance praise for *Regenerative Medicine in Small Animal Musculoskeletal Conditions*

'This book is a much needed resource for veterinary students, clinicians, and specialists alike. By focusing on practical applications it offers real-world insights and bridges the gap between research and clinical relevance, making it invaluable for implementing cutting-edge treatments in clinical practice.' – **Andy Armitage BSc BVM&S MRCVS, Clinical Director, Greenside Regenerative Therapies**

'I have been eagerly anticipating the release of this book. I would encourage all veterinarians to acquire their own copy and use it as their regenerative medicine bible.' – **Dr Joanna Miller, Cell Therapy Sciences**

'There is increasing interest in regenerative medicine and orthobiologics within companion animal practice; particularly within the areas of osteoarthritis management and musculoskeletal disease. This book provides a comprehensive yet accessible overview of current understanding for these technologies and products. Focusing particularly on mesenchymal stem cells and platelet rich plasma, the reader is provided an overview of their scientific history and development, as well as insight into their therapeutic benefits and evidence. With clear and concise notes outlining their effective preparation and administration, as well as clinical case examples, this book also provides the practical knowledge essential for those interested in developing their use in their own clinical practice.' – **Ross Allan BVMS PGCertSAS MRCVS, Clinical Director, Pets N Vets**

'Veterinary regenerative medicine is a rapidly growing medical branch seeking to develop disease modifying therapies for a number of chronic and degenerative animal diseases. Despite the vast body of published scientific literature, a challenge remains in transforming the science into efficient clinical decision-making.

In a direct answer to the needs of busy clinical practitioners, Dr Russell Chandler has consolidated the latest scientific findings on stem cell and platelet rich plasma therapies. His book *Regenerative Medicine in Small Animal Musculoskeletal Conditions* brings together knowledge from various disciplines reflecting accurately the multidisciplinary profile of veterinary regenerative medicine.

Dr Chandler provides a comprehensive overview of the current clinical applications integrated with practical know-how drawn from his own personal experience in small animal orthopaedics.

I highly recommend this book as a valuable resource for clinical practitioners looking to introduce, improve or refresh their knowledge on regenerative medicine treatments in their day-to-day clinical work.' – **Dr Ana Ivanovska, University of Galway**

REGENERATIVE MEDICINE IN SMALL ANIMAL MUSCULOSKELETAL CONDITIONS

A practical guide for veterinary professionals

Dr Russell Chandler

BVSc CertSAO MSc(OrthoEng) MSc(StemCells) MRCVS
Advanced Practitioner in Small Animal Orthopaedics

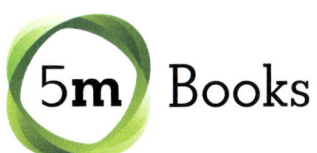

5m Books

First published 2025

Published by
5M Books Ltd,
Lings, Great Easton,
Essex CM6 2HH, UK
Tel: +44 (0)330 1333 580
www.5mbooks.com

EU GPSR Authorised Representative
LOGOS EUROPE, 9 rue Nicolas Poussin, 17000, LA ROCHELLE, France
E-mail: Contact@logoseurope.eu

A Catalogue record for this book is available from the British Library

ISBN 9781789183733
eISBN 9781789183795
DOI 10.52517/9781789183795

Important note

All opinions expressed in this book are solely those of the author and do not necessarily reflect or represent those of the publishers, editors, reviewers, or other affiliated organisations. Where generic, branded, licensed, or unlicensed medicinal products are cited, it is the responsibility of the clinician to use their professional judgement and consult appropriate published data sheets and other materials before choosing to administer these products. Manufacturer's claims are not guaranteed or endorsed by the author or publisher.

While every possible care has been taken in compiling the information presented in this volume, factual errors remain inevitable. Such inaccuracies, although made in good faith, are the sole responsibility of the author. Any clinician using this guide is advised to seek independent verification of any contestable proposition or suggestion. As with all matters of veterinary medicine and surgery, the onus rests firmly on the shoulders of the attending clinician to act in the patient's best interests at all times and to use only those therapies that they can support with relevant underpinning scientific information from multiple sources.

Neither the author nor the publisher accepts any liability for loss or damage resulting from clinicians using this book to undertake veterinary treatments for pets under their care.

Book layout by Cheshire Typesetting Ltd, Cuddington, Cheshire
Printed by Hobbs the Printers
Photos by the author unless otherwise indicated

Cover images: right: AdobeStock_253344507 Par Karoline Thalhofer; bottom left: AdobeStock_503731162 Par StockPhotoPro; top left: by the author

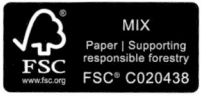

During the writing of this book, one of the giants of regenerative medicine, and in particular mesenchymal stem cell research, Dr Arnold Caplan, PhD (1942–2024), sadly passed away. The author humbly acknowledges and is grateful for the enormous contribution to this field made by Dr Caplan.

Contents

SECTION V

SECTION VI

Preface

The 21st century has witnessed major advances in the field of regenerative medicine. This has especially been the case in the veterinary context, where regenerative medicine therapies have been applied to horses, dogs and other species. Keeping up to date with the rapidly accelerating developments in these technologies is particularly challenging. One of the aims of this volume is to clarify the existing regenerative medicine therapies that are applicable in the small animal field so that practising veterinarians can incorporate these into their everyday medical offerings.

The two pre-eminent modes of delivering regenerative medicine in small animals are platelet-rich plasma and mesenchymal stem cell therapies. Either or both can be utilised to benefit veterinary patients where the goal is to promote healing and regeneration of tissues. These may be used alone or in combination.

The most common indication for the use of platelet-rich plasma (PRP) and/or mesenchymal stem cells (MSCs) is in the musculoskeletal system. Of the potential musculoskeletal system conditions that are amenable to regenerative medicine, by far the most common condition in which this is used is osteoarthritis (OA). The rationale for the use of regenerative medicine, its mechanism of action, the methodology associated with its administration, and the likely outcomes will be discussed in subsequent sections.

In common with all publications of this kind, it is only possible to produce a 'snapshot' of the current state of the art in any given field. Inevitably, with such a rapidly progressing discipline as regenerative medicine, the material presented may quickly become outdated. Since the information cannot be future-proofed, readers should always be aware that ongoing developments may advance our understanding, leading to the abandonment of certain practices and their replacement by newer innovations.

The focus of this book is on regenerative medicine (RM) in musculoskeletal (MSK) conditions as they affect small animal (canine and feline) patients. Despite this relatively narrow focus, it is impossible to exclude comparative aspects of regenerative medicine in other species, most notably in humans. The rationale for citing human studies and procedures is that these serve to greatly support and underpin many of the assertions proposed in veterinary regenerative medicine (VRM).

Who this book is for

Veterinary regenerative medicine is a relatively recent development that has appeared over the last few decades. This is especially the case in pet animals, in which the discipline has hitherto somewhat lagged behind its equine counterpart. This volume aims to provide a readily accessible guide for veterinarians in practice. It is hoped that practitioners, armed with this book, will be able to rapidly acquire sufficient knowledge and understanding of small animal regenerative medicine to get started in applying this exciting therapeutic modality. The literature on this area is enormous and daunting. Only sufficient scientific details that are essential to illustrate the principles underpinning the subject are included. Specific nomenclature, as in all medical sub-specialities, is plentiful in the regenerative medicine realm. For example, the various bioactive molecules involved in cell biology in health and disease represent a daunting list of abbreviated names and acronyms. It is not necessary to have detailed knowledge of each and every molecule; it is more important to get some overall understanding of the biological principles involved. The author has sought to minimise the use of jargon while explaining unfamiliar or esoteric terms that are unavoidable. Most of the acronyms are listed in the glossary.

This book should also be a useful resource for veterinary undergraduates. At the current pace of development of small animal regenerative medicine, it seems likely that a working knowledge of the subject would be of enormous benefit to anyone embarking on a veterinary career. Indeed, it seems possible that regenerative therapies will play a greater role in clinical practice in the foreseeable future.

Veterinary musculoskeletal regenerative medicine occupies a position at the intersection of several other veterinary sub-specialities, including veterinary internal medicine, veterinary orthopaedics, and sports medicine. Accordingly, clinicians from all of these fields may be involved in the use of orthobiologics, with the common aim of advancing the recovery and welfare of patients under their care. Collaboration between practitioners from these related disciplines as well as veterinary physiotherapists, veterinary nurses and veterinary technicians, is to be encouraged for optimal patient outcomes.

How to use this book

The intention is that this book will provide a practical guide about regenerative medicine in small animal musculoskeletal conditions. In so doing, it is hoped that veterinarians, regardless of their experience in this field, may be able to pick up this guide and become proficient in the basics of veterinary regenerative medicine. This book was not envisaged as a work on the science of regenerative medicine, since it would be easy to overwhelm readers with the colossal amount of published work in this area.

Throughout the chapters, key points of practical relevance are listed to give context to the information provided. A reference section is included at the end of each chapter, which contains the sources that have been referred to in that chapter. A reference may appear at the end of more than one chapter. The further reading section at the end of the book, which contains all the references and additional sources, will allow readers to take a deeper dive into the subject areas should they wish to. One caveat is that where digital sources are referred to, such as websites, these are inevitably changed, updated, or may become unavailable with time. Another consideration is that websites are not, as a rule,

peer-reviewed. The information imparted by these sources must therefore be viewed with appropriate circumspection.

The chapters follow a logical progression so they can be read sequentially in a meaningful way. It is also possible to dip in at any chapter should the need arise. In essence, the author has endeavoured to write this book to form a suitable stepping-off point for small animal veterinary regenerative medicine. The author is primarily a clinician, and the information is presented in a way that should be practically applicable.

Explaining the complex concepts of regenerative medicine clearly to readers who may not have any background in the subject is a challenge. Wherever possible, diagrammatic and graphical summaries of the principles introduced are presented. These are deliberately kept as simple as possible without losing the underlying essence of what is being addressed.

The appendices contain some of the written client communication materials, which may assist clinicians in managing owner expectations as well as educating them on veterinary regenerative medicine in general.

Abbreviations

5-HT 5-hydroxytryptamine, serotonin

AD-MSCs adipose-derived mesenchymal stem cells

AE adverse event

B-cells B-lymphocytes

BCS body condition score

BID twice daily (Latin: bis in die)

BM bone marrow

BMMSC bone marrow-derived mesenchymal stem cell

CAD-CAM computer-assisted design/computer-assisted manufacture

CBD cannabidiol

CCL cranial cruciate ligament

CD cluster of differentiation

CGPE caregiver placebo effect

CM clinical metrology

CMI clinical metrology instrument

CT computed tomography

DMARD disease-modifying antirheumatic drug

DMOAT disease-modifying osteoarthritis therapy

DMSO dimethyl sulphoxide

EBVM evidence-based veterinary medicine

EGF epidermal growth factor

ESC embryonic stem cell

FCP fragmented coronoid process

FGF fibroblast growth factor

FOX3p Forkhead box 3p (also known as scurfin)

GMP Good Manufacturing Process

GVHD graft versus host disease

HA hyaluronic acid

Hb haemoglobin

hBMMSCs human bone marrow-derived mesenchymal stem cell

HCS haemopoietic stem cell

hESC human embryonic stem cell

HGF hepatocyte growth factor

hMSC human mesenchymal stem cell

IA intra-articular

IDO indolamine 2,3-dioxygenase

IGF insulin-like growth factor

IL-n interleukin-n (where n is the designated number of the interleukin in question)

MCP-1 monocyte chemoattractant protein-1

MetHb methaemoglobin

MHC major histocompatibility complex

miRNA microRNA

MMOAM multimodal osteoarthritis management

MMP-1 matrix metalloproteinase-1

MMP-3 matrix metalloproteinase-3

MMP-9 matrix metalloproteinase-9

mRNA messenger RNA

MSC mesenchymal stem cell, mesenchymal stromal cell, medicine signalling cell

MSK musculoskeletal

MSK-US musculoskeletal ultrasonography

NK cells natural killer cells

NSAID nonsteroidal anti-inflammatory drug

OA osteoarthritis

OCD osteochondritis dissecans

PA polyarthritis

PBMC peripheral blood mononuclear cells

PBMT photobiomodulation therapy by laser application

PDGF platelet derived growth factor

PGE2 prostaglandin-E2

PMN polymorph neutrophil

PRGF platelets rich in growth factors

PRP platelet rich plasma
ROM range of motion
SID once daily (Latin: semel in die)
TB trypan blue
T cells T-lymphocytes
TBG- α transforming growth factor-α
TGB-β transforming growth factor-β
TID three times daily (Latin: ter in die)

TIMP1 tissue inhibitor of metalloproteinases 1
TNF-α tumour necrosis factor α
TPLO tibial plateau levelling osteotomy
Treg cells regulatory T-lymphocytes
VAS visual analogue scale
VEGF vascular endothelial growth factor
WOMAC Western Ontario and McMaster Universities Arthritis Index

Definitions

Allogeneic
Cells and tissues derived from a different individual of the same species as the recipient patient.

Apoptosis
A process of programmed cell death.

Apoptotic bodies
A subset of apoptosis derived extracellular vesicles formed by apoptotic cell disassembly, these have important paracrine functions when they arise from mesenchymal stem cells.

Autocrine
Cell signalling that occurs when a cell releases bioactive molecules that subsequently engage with receptors on the cell's own surface, initiating a biochemical cascade of processes within the cell.

Autologous
Cells and tissues derived from the patient in question and re-transplanted back into the same individual.

Cell signalling
The chemical processes by which cells interact and communicate with each other using molecular messengers.

Conditioned medium
An orthobiologic produced from the soluble components of the cell secretome.

Confluency
The density of the cell population on the plastic surface in the laboratory, expressed as a percentage of the available area occupied by cells.

Developmental plasticity
The ability of cells with the same genotype to produce different phenotypes according to the proximate environmental influences.

Differentiation
The process by which stem cells and progenitor cells alter their phenotype and gene expression to become more specialised and ultimately fully mature adult cells.

Endocrine
Cell signalling that occurs remotely from one hormone-secreting cell to a distant target cell.

Epigenetics
A mechanism by which gene-expression is controlled and regulated by reversible modifications of the DNA such as acetylation and methylation.

Epigenome
The collection of chemical modifications superimposed on the genome and histone proteins that regulate gene expression.

Extracellular vesicles
Membrane bound 'packets' of bioactive molecules that are released from a cell.

Hypoimmunogenicity
Cells may be referred to as hypoimmunogenic if they have characteristics that make them unlikely to provoke a host immune reaction after transplant. An important feature of MSCs that contributes to their hypoimmunogenicity is the lack of MHC II surface marker.

Immunophenotype
This refers to the identity of a cell type based on antigens that are mostly expressed on the cell surface.

'Licensing'
This refers to a maturation process that occurs in cells such as mesenchymal stem cells, in which environmental molecular influences, such as those present in inflamed tissues, induce the cells to adopt a different phenotype (and therefore function).

Lyosecretome
A freeze-dried product derived from the secreted extra-cellular bioactive protein molecules, largely contained within vesicles.

Mesenchymal stem cell (or mesenchymal stromal cell)
A stem cell category that is found in mesoderm-derived tissues. Mesenchymal stem cells are by definition multipotent.

Multipotency
The ability of a stem cell to give rise to multiple different adult differentiated cell types of that particular embryonal tissue layer. In the case of mesenchymal stem cells, these can differentiate, into osteoblasts, chondrocytes, or adipocytes.

Orthobiologic
A biological product that is transplanted or injected into a musculoskeletal tissue with the intention of producing a beneficial biological effect.

Paracrine
A category of cell to cell signalling that occurs over short distances requiring cells to be in close proximity.

Passage
Cell passage occurs when cells are harvested from a cell culture and used to start new cultures in separate vessels with fresh culture medium.

Photobiomodulation
A therapeutic modality that uses laser light to influence the biochemical and physiological processes of a target tissue or organ.

Platelet-rich plasma
An orthobiologic derived from (usually autologous) blood, in which the platelet concentration is increased and the red blood cell and white blood cell concentrations are typically reduced.

Pluripotency
The ability of a stem cell to give rise to any of the adult differentiated cells of the body, from any of the embryonal cell layers (ectoderm, mesoderm, or endoderm).

Regenerative medicine
A medical sub-discipline that aims to restore, replace, or recreate cells, tissues, or organs to treat or mitigate human and animal diseases.

Secretome
The collection of secreted bioactive molecules that are released from a cell.

Stem cell
An undifferentiated eukaryotic cell that has the latent capability of dividing symmetrically to replace itself, or asymmetrically along a path of differentiation ultimately leading to the production of fully mature adult tissue cells.

Totipotency

The ability that embryonic stem cells have to give rise to any and all of the cells within the body as well as those of the extra-embryonic tissues.

Transcriptome

The collective sum of mRNA that is transcribed from the DNA, that is the gene expression profile.

Xenogeneic

Cells and tissues for transplant that originate in another mammalian species than the recipient animal.

Section I

Chapter 1

Introduction

Introduction

A new paradigm in veterinary medicine and surgery has emerged over the last decade or so in the shape of veterinary regenerative medicine (VRM). This assemblage of innovative developments is especially applicable in the field of musculoskeletal (MSK) conditions, and in particular joint diseases. It is noteworthy and encouraging that the possible novel treatment modalities available for conditions such as osteoarthritis (OA) have expanded markedly over this time.

Take OA as the most obvious example of a condition in which regenerative medicine (RM) may be applicable. The current framework for OA management is multimodal (Fox, 2017) and multidisciplinary in nature. There is no single modality that can be applied on its own and be expected to give optimal OA outcomes in all cases. Instead, combinations of different modalities are applied together for their synergistic effects. For example, analgesic medication such as non-steroidal anti-inflammatory drugs (NSAIDs), which have long been the cornerstone of OA therapy, are typically used in combination with other treatments such as physical therapy, photobiomodulation, and adiposity management. Delivering effective multimodal OA management frequently requires a team approach where allied professionals, including veterinarians, veterinary nurses, veterinary technicians, and veterinary physiotherapists collaborate.

To date, despite all the modes of therapy that are available, including RM, OA in all species (including humans, horses, and small animals) remains an incurable and progressive disease. Pharmaceutical treatments for this condition, hitherto, have remained symptom-modifying only. The quest for a genuinely disease-modifying OA therapy has been and continues to be a major challenge.

The advent of RM in the form of platelet-rich plasma (PRP) and **mesenchymal stem cells** (MSCs) has, for the first time, offered the promise of some genuinely disease-modifying treatments. The potential of RM to impact the underlying disease pathology is an attractive proposition. If rather than simply reducing the pain associated with, for example, an osteoarthritic joint, it could be possible to influence the underlying cellular mechanisms and tilt these towards tissue regeneration rather than attrition or catabolism, then markedly improved patient outcomes could be expected.

Considerable progress has been made in the understanding of the cellular, subcellular, and molecular changes occurring in diseased tissues in recent decades; it is beyond the scope of this book to rehearse the minutiae of what is known.

It will sometimes be necessary, however, to describe certain aspects of the relevant cell biology and molecular mechanisms to explain both the pathological process and the actions of RM.

Overview of stem cell biology, terminology, and origins

From the organism's development standpoint, all cells in the body can be traced back to their ancestral origin, which is a stem cell. Natural cell replacement within the mammalian body is also within the purview of stem cells. The presence of sufficient reserves of functioning stem cells is essential to maintain life. Certain cells, such as circulating blood corpuscles, have a relatively short lifespan. The haemopoietic stem cells (HSCs) in the bone marrow (BM), through their descendant cell lines, perform the function of constantly replenishing the circulating erythrocytes, leukocytes, and platelets. This is an essential system that needs to be extremely efficient. Animals do not survive for long in the absence of functioning BM.

Stem cells of various kinds are widespread within most, though not all, tissues and organs of the body. For example, in the brain, there are only a few areas in which stem cells reside. Where stem cells derive from is briefly discussed below.

In mammals, fertilisation occurs when male and female gametes join, leading to the formation of a single-celled conceptus designated a zygote (Fig. 1.1). This single cell subsequently divides mitotically (cleaves) to produce cells called blastomeres. When the sixteen-cell stage is reached, the conceptus is referred to as a morula. The cells of the morula are **totipotent** since they give rise to all cells in the organism, both of the body and those of the extra-embryonic (and later extra-fetal) tissues. After further cell division and compaction, the conceptus

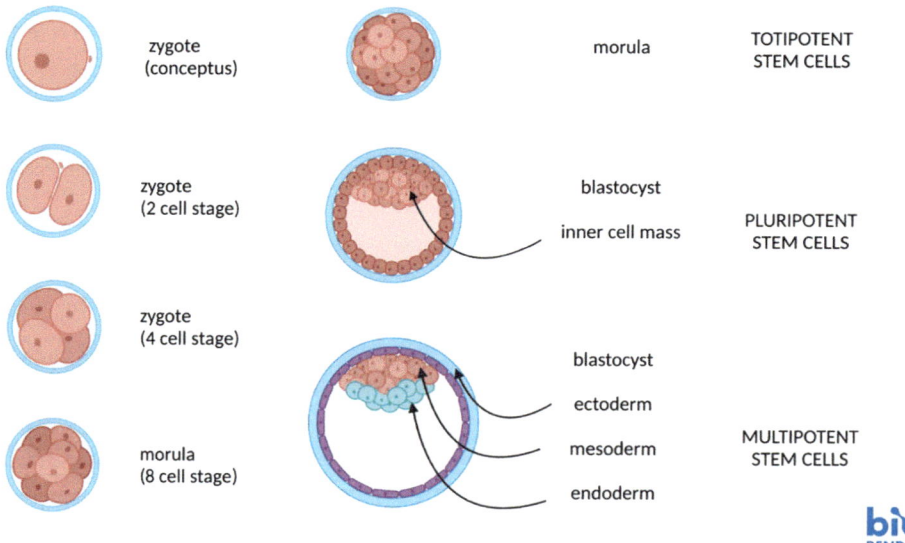

Fig. 1.1 Early embryonic mammalian development. Before the inner cell mass develops within the embryo, all the cells are totipotent since they can potentially give rise to any cell type, including those of the extra-embryonic tissues. Once the inner cell mass is established, its cells become pluripotent, meaning they can differentiate into cells of any embryonic germ layer (ectoderm, mesoderm, or endoderm). Once the three embryonic cell layers have formed, the range of cell types that can subsequently arise is limited to that cell layer.

develops into a blastocyst by the formation of a fluid-filled central cavity lined by cells. One part of the blastocyst lining thickens and becomes the inner cell mass. The inner cell mass can give rise to any adult differentiated cells in the body; hence, they are referred to as **pluripotent**. The blastocyst may implant into the maternal endometrium.

The next stage of development is the formation of the embryo. The embryo has three classical layers of cells that have different 'cell fates' to which they are committed. On the outside is the ectodermal layer. Ectoderm gives rise to skin and adnexal structures, as well as the central nervous system and pigment cells. The middle layer is the mesoderm. The cells, tissues, and structures derived from mesodermal cells include muscle (cardiac, skeletal, and smooth), connective tissues, bone, cartilage, adipose tissue, blood cells, and blood vessels. The pertinent stem cell of the mesodermal lineage is the MSC. MSCs are differentiated sufficiently that they do not ordinarily differentiate along non-mesodermal lineages. They retain the ability to self-renew by symmetrical division. MSCs can also divide asymmetrically, giving rise to daughter cells that may differentiate into any of the multiple cell lineages within the mesodermal group. For this reason, MSCs are referred to as **multipotent**. As we will discuss later at some length, MSCs are the most relevant stem cells we currently have at our disposal for VRM. The endodermal embryonic cell layer is the source of, for example, the alveolar cells of the lungs, the thyroid cells, and the pancreas cells.

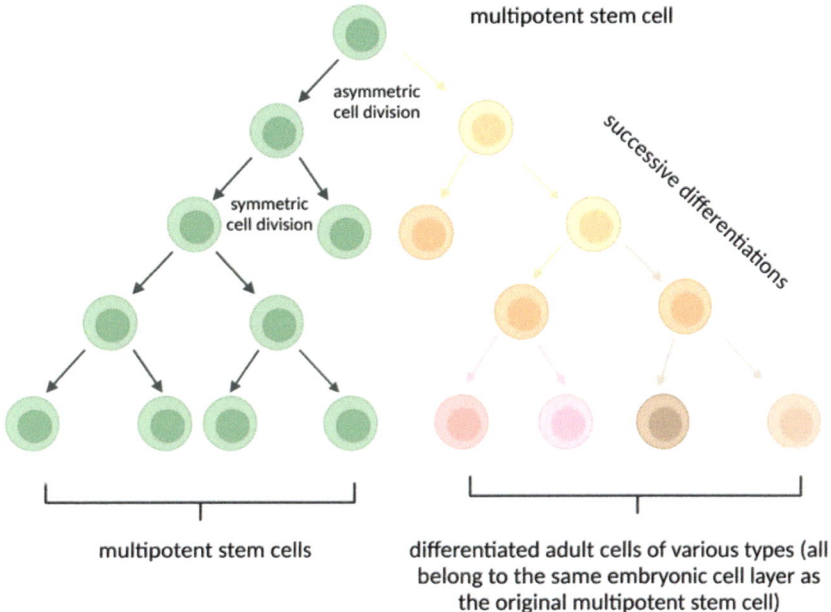

Fig. 1.2 Multipotent stem cell division and daughter cell fates. The green cells (on the left of the diagram) represent the symmetrical cell division of the starting multipotent stem cell to replenish the stem cell reservoir. The other coloured cells (on the right side) represent the process of differentiation, which results in the formation of adult cells of the same embryonic cell layer as the parent multipotent stem cell. This graphic is to illustrate the principle; no attempt has been made to represent the actual relative quantities of each of these theoretical cell categories.

The use of human embryonic stem cells in the laboratory is the subject of ethical concern. It is important to note that there is a strict legislative framework concerning the use of human embryonic stem cells in scientific research. While many countries permit the use of these stem cells, most restrict this to a certain age. In the United Kingdom, embryos being used in experiments, under licence from the government, must be destroyed before they are 14 days old. (Human Fertilisation and Embryology Act 1990, Schedule 2). Fortunately, there are now alternatives to using embryonic stem cells for laboratory experimentation, such as induced pluripotent stem cells (iPSCs).

Over recent decades, stem cells have become indispensable in scientific and biomedical research. Some of the uses of stem cells include *in vitro* disease modelling, *in vitro* drug testing, and cell transplantation. For the purposes of this book, most of the discussions will centre around cell transplantation as a therapy for MSK disorders in companion animal species.

The process by which adult somatic cells are produced and replenished from an originating stem cell, whose daughter cells undergo successive differentiations, represents a readily understood scheme of the natural process. This clearly oversimplifies the complexity of the subcellular mechanisms that make this possible. For veterinary clinicians in practice, however, this is a convenient framework in which to perceive the role of stem cells.

A revolution in our understanding of the process of cell differentiation occurred in the 2000s. Before this time, our understanding was that pluripotent stem cells, once they had differentiated, thereby losing their pluripotency (or stemness), had undertaken a one-way journey to the adult cell of a particular kind (myocyte, neuron, fibroblast, etc). Differentiated adult cells could not retrace their steps and dedifferentiate back to pluripotency and resume the characteristics (phenotype) of a stem cell. Takahashi and Yamanaka (2006) proved that, at least in the laboratory, mouse fibroblasts may be induced to do exactly this and become what is now known as iPSCs. Soon after this monumental achievement, for which Shinya Yamanaka would later receive a share of a Nobel Prize (with Sir John Gurdon), Thompson's laboratory (Yu et al., 2007) achieved similar results by manufacturing human iPSCs. The ground-breaking methods used by these pioneering scientists are beyond the scope of this book; interested readers should consult the landmark papers cited (Takahashi & Yamanaka, 2006; Yu et al., 2007). In the relatively short period of time that iPSCs have been available to cell scientists, they have become firmly embedded as a tool for disease modelling and drug testing research. While they are potentially suitable for cell transplantation, there remain considerable hurdles to overcome before this becomes a reality. The greatest of these is the tumorigenic potential of iPSCs (Doss et al., 2019). One defining property of undifferentiated iPSCs is their pluripotency, which is demonstrable by their ability to form teratomas when injected into mice (Gunaseeli et al., 2010). There is an obvious risk that transplanting cells that contain undifferentiated iPSCs into patients could result in teratoma formation. The potential tumorigenesis of iPSCs is not limited to teratomas; other malignant neoplasms may also form (Gunaseeli et al., 2010).

Chapter 1 key points

- Most tissues have resident stem cells.
- Stem cells are essential for tissue maintenance and repair.
- Embryonic stem cells have the widest range of potential cell types in their offspring. When they originate from the inner cell mass of the blastocyst, they are pluripotent.
- Cells with very similar properties to embryonic stem cells, namely induced pluripotent stem cells (iPSCs), can be produced in the laboratory by the dedifferentiation of adult cells.
- Mesodermal tissues contain MSCs. MSCs are multipotent, meaning that they can only generate cells of mesodermal origin.
- Uses of stem cells include *in vitro* disease modelling, *in vitro* drug testing, and cell transplantation.

Chapter 1 references

Doss, M. X., & Sachinidis, A. (2019). Current challenges of iPSC-based disease modeling and therapeutic implications. *Cells*, *8*(5), 403. https://doi.org/10.3390/cells8050403

Fox, S. M. (2017). *Multimodal management of canine osteoarthritis*. CRC Press. ISBN 9781840761832.

Gunaseeli, I., Doss, M. X., Antzelevitch, C., Hescheler, J., & Sachinidis, A. (2010). Induced pluripotent stem cells as a model for accelerated patient- and disease-specific drug discovery. *Current Medicinal Chemistry*, *17*(8), 759–766. https://doi.org/10.2174/092986710790514480

Human Fertilisation and Embryology Act 1990. (2008) (Remedial) Order. The human fertilisation and embryology act p. 2018. https://www.legislation.gov.uk/ukpga/1990/37/contents. https://www.legislation.gov.uk/ukpga/2008/22/contents, Schedule 2.

Takahashi, K., & Yamanaka, S. (2006). Induction of pluripotent stem cells from mouse embryonic and adult fibroblast cultures by defined factors. *Cell*, *126*(4), 663–676. https://doi.org/10.1016/j.cell.2006.07.024

Yu, J., Vodyanik, M. A., Smuga-Otto, K., Antosiewicz-Bourget, J., Frane, J. L., Tian, S., Nie, J., Jonsdottir, G. A., Ruotti, V., Stewart, R., Slukvin, I. I., & Thomson, J. A. (2007). Induced pluripotent stem cell lines derived from human somatic cells. *Science*, *318*(5858), 1917–1920. https://doi.org/10.1126/science.1151526

Chapter 2

History of veterinary regenerative medicine (VRM)

Definition of regenerative medicine (RM)

Regenerative Medicine is an emerging inter-disciplinary field of research and clinical applications focused on the repair, replacement or regeneration of cells, tissues, or organs to restore impaired function resulting from any cause, including congenital defects, disease, trauma, and ageing. It uses a combination of several technological approaches that moves it beyond traditional transplantation and replacement therapies. These approaches may include, but are not limited to, the use of soluble molecules, gene therapy, stem cell transplantation, tissue engineering and the reprogramming of cell and tissue types. (Greenwood et al., 2006, pp. 60–77)

For decades, the tantalising prospect of effective RMs for the treatment of various intractable human conditions has been bandied around. Despite enormous resources, not least financial, being expended in this endeavour, the translation of RM from bench to bedside has been disappointing (Jacques & Suuronen, 2020). To date, the mainstream medical offering has yet to include the significant use of cell-based therapies. The obvious exception to this statement is the field of BM transplantation. HSCs are the crucial multipotent stem cell type in this instance.

The existence of a reservoir of progenitor cells that constantly replenish the circulating erythrocytes, leukocytes, and platelets had long been postulated despite such stem cells remaining elusive (Weissman & Shizuru, 2008). Somewhat ironically, allogeneic BM transplantation in humans, first pioneered by Dr E Donnall Thomas in 1956 (Thomas et al., 1957; Henig & Zuckerman, 2014), preceded the actual discovery and description of BM HSCs. In fact, it was not until 1988 when the first HSCs were definitively isolated, and even then, it was only in mice (Spangrude et al., 1988). The success of BM transplantation is exemplified by the report in 2012 (Gratwohl et al., 2015), where it was estimated that over one million transplants had been performed in humans worldwide.

Interestingly, HSCs found a crucial human clinical application long before the actual HSCs themselves had been precisely described and their features elucidated. Other examples of similar attempts at achieving a therapeutic effect from mixed cell transplants in VRM include the concept of stromal vascular fraction (SVF) injection. SVF is a mixed concentration of various kinds of cells that derive from adipose tissue or BM. It is prepared as a point-of-care product by in-house enzymatic or physical processing and is thus minimally manipulated. A wide range of viable cell types may be present (Astor et al., 2013), and these will be heterogeneous. It cannot be known what fraction of these cells are stem cells, which would be the theoretically desired cell type for achieving a therapeutic result.

Timeline of mesenchymal stem cells (MSCs)

Selected events in the development of stem cell science are depicted in Fig. 2.1. Ernst Haeckel

is credited with coining the term 'stem cell' in 1868 (Ramalho-Santos & Willenbring, 2007). The foundation for the science of MSCs was laid down in the late 20th century. In 1974, Alexander Friedenstein published findings on the discovery of fibroblast precursor cells (Friedenstein et al., 1974). These cells were found to be a reservoir for mesenchymal (mesodermal) tissues. By 1988, these 'stromal cells' were shown to have several interesting properties (Owen, 1988). They were capable of self-renewal; they showed multipotentiality (they could differentiate into different mature cell types) and could give rise to osteogenic (bone-forming) cells.

It was Arnold Caplan (Caplan, 1991) who coined the term 'mesenchymal stem cell' (MSC). [Note: mesenchymal stem cell is a widely used term. Caplan (2017) subsequently suggested

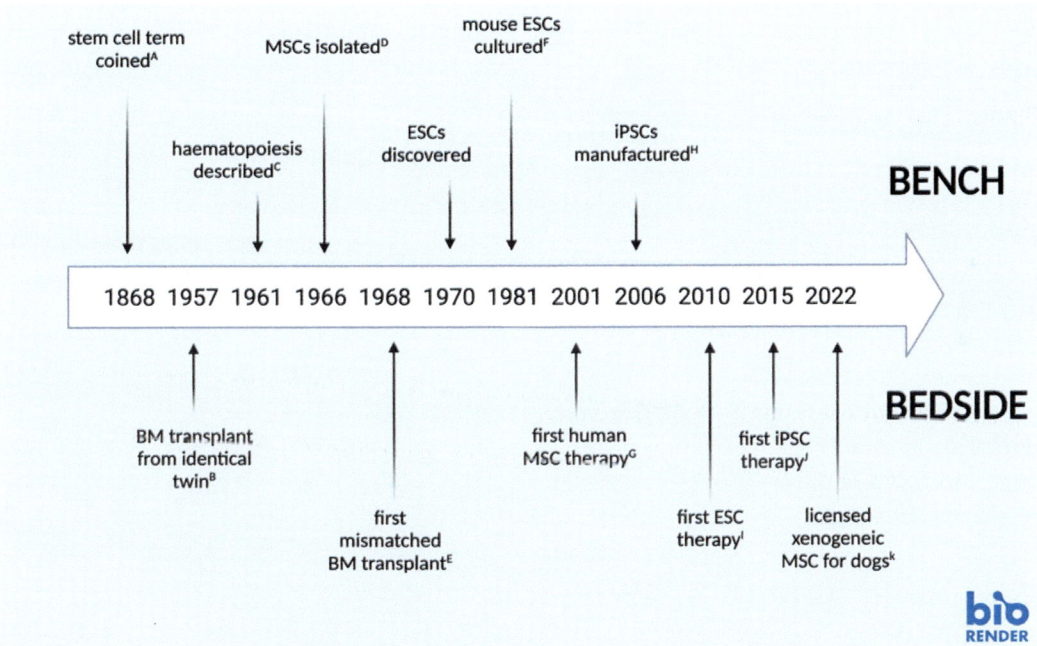

Fig. 2.1 Timeline of mesenchymal stem cell developments. Some of the landmark events in stem cell research (BENCH) and stem cell therapy (BEDSIDE). Image inspired by a lecture by Prof Frank Barry as part of the Second International Meeting on Veterinary Regenerative Medicine, Skopje, Northern Macedonia (2023). [A] Ramalho-Santos & Willenbring, 2007; [B] Thomas et al. 1957; [C] Till & McCulloch, 1961; [D] Friedenstein et al. 1966; [E] Perry & Linch, 1996; [F] Martin, 1981; [G] Koc & Lazarus, 2001; [H] Takahashi & Yamanaka, 2006; [I] Lebowski, 2011; [J] Garber, 2015; [K] Punzón et al. 2022.

that the acronym MSC should be kept while 'medicine signalling cell' could be a more accurate term for these cells. The term 'mesenchymal stem cell' has persisted in the literature, which is why it has been adopted in this book]. Caplan described the multilineage potential for MSC differentiation, particularly in the formation of bone and cartilage (Fig. 2.5). In 1995, the first human Phase I clinical safety trial using injected allogeneic MSCs was reported (Lazarus et al., 1995). Pittenger et al. (1999) isolated human BM-derived MSCs and demonstrated their tri-lineage capacity for forming adipose tissue, cartilage, and bone. They noted that MSCs in the laboratory assume and remain in a monolayer in culture. Their morphology resembled that of fibroblasts. The cell surface markers that determine the immunophenotype of the MSCs were also reported.

In 2006, the International Society for Cellular Therapy proposed minimal criteria to define human MSCs (Dominici et al., 2006). These criteria are as follows:

1 Adherence of the cells to plastic under standard laboratory cell culture conditions.
2 Expression of a set of surface molecules 'without' expressing any of a second set.
3 The capacity to differentiate *in vitro* into adipocytes, osteoblasts, and chondroblasts.

Despite decades of research, there is no single test or marker that can identify *bona fide* MSCs *in vitro*. This is even more frustrating in the *in vivo* situation, where observations of MSCs are extremely troublesome.

Mesenchymal stem cell (MSC) characteristics

In 2022, an equivalent set of characteristics for veterinary MSCs was proposed by Guest et al. (2022). They stated that in order to qualify as MSCs, cells must:

- Be tissue-derived.
- Exhibit plastic adherence in the laboratory.
- Possess spindle-shaped morphology.
- Demonstrate proliferative capacity.
- Show multipotent differentiation capacity *in vitro*.
- Have the property of immunomodulation.

MSC plastic adherence

Native MSCs in the tissues reside in certain MSC niches. These locations provide a three-dimensional physical environment in which the MSC is 'attached'. Such physical adherence appears to be necessary for the survival and maintenance of the MSC. In the laboratory, this propensity for adherence to surfaces is advantageous since it provides a method of 'extracting' MSCs from a heterogeneous sample where there are multiple other cell types. Lavage of the mixture removes the unwanted cells, leaving an enriched population of MSCs adherent to the surface of the plastic laboratory cell-culture dish.

Morphology of MSCs

Under light microscopy, MSCs are long and spindle-shaped and have an appearance that is reminiscent of fibroblast morphology (Fig. 2.2).

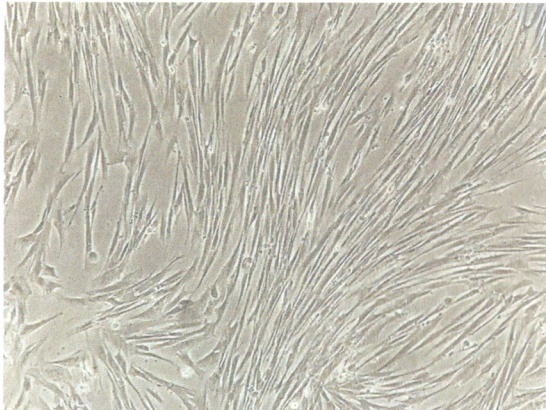

Fig. 2.2 Microscopic image of MSCs in laboratory culture showing typical spindle-shaped morphology. Image courtesy of Dr Ana Ivanovska.

MSC immunophenotype

The surface protein markers expressed at the cell membrane provide a means of determining the kind of cell (that is, the phenotype) that any given cell has assumed as a consequence of the processes of differentiation. In different species, the combination of these immunophenotypic markers varies. There are certain markers that the MSC must express, while others that they must not. For canine MSCs, the combination that has been found to define the immunophenotype is depicted in Fig. 2.3 (Guest et al., 2022) and graphically in Fig. 2.4. Ideally, it would be preferable if a given cell line could be demonstrated to express all five clusters of differentiation (CD) markers and none of the markers that should be negative. In addition, the absence of major histocompatibility complex II (MHC-II) on the MSC surface is critical for this cell. MHC-II is the predominant means that the recipient patient's innate immune system recognises a transplanted cell as 'foreign'. The absence of the MHC-II antigen on the surface

Defining characteristics of canine MSCs	Minimum	Optimal
Plastic adherence	•	•
Tri-lineage differentiation	•	•
Surface antigen expression Markers commonly positive CD 90 CD 73 CD 105 CD 29 CD 44	Two positive markers	All markers
Surface antigen expression Markers commonly negative CD79alpha/CD19 CD14/CD11b CD 34 CD 45	Two negative markers	All markers
Negative MHC-II expression Important in allogeneic and xenogeneic transplants	•	•
In vitro immune suppression		•
Other analytic methods of potency		•

Fig. 2.3 The defining characteristics of canine MSCs (modified from Guest et al., 2022)

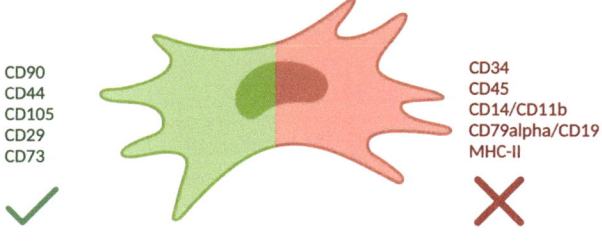

CD90
CD44
CD105
CD29
CD73

CD34
CD45
CD14/CD11b
CD79alpha/CD19
MHC-II

Fig. 2.4 Surface markers of canine mesenchymal stromal cells. The immunophenotype of the MSC is determined by the cell surface proteins (CD markers and MHC). The positive markers defining the MSC are shown in green on the left of the diagram, while the markers that must be absent are shown in red on the right side. MSC = mesenchymal stem cell; CD = cluster of differentiation; MHC = major histocompatibility complex.

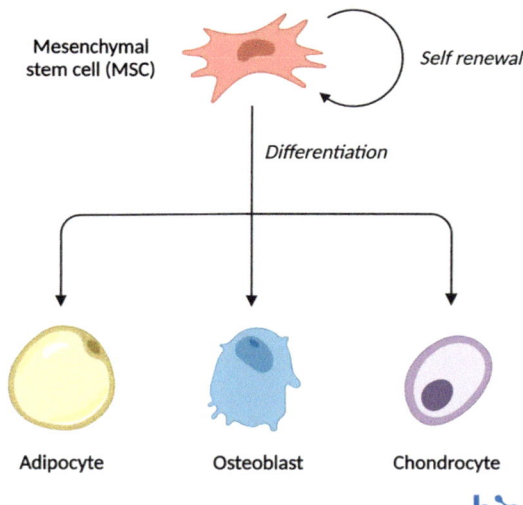

Fig. 2.5 Tri-lineage differentiation of MSCs in the laboratory demonstrates that they are multipotent for the mesenchymal lineages of cells.

of the MSC permits it to largely evade the host immune surveillance and go undetected after transplantation.

Tri-lineage differentiation of MSCs

A further essential defining characteristic of MSCs is related to their multipotency. *In vitro*, it is imperative that MSCs can be demonstrated to be capable of tri-lineage differentiation. Under suitable culture conditions with the appropriate 'cocktail' of biochemical molecular factors, MSCs must be shown to be able to differentiate into mature cells of each and all the adipocyte (albeit that this may be a challenge with canine MSCs – Dr Jo Miller, 2023, personal communication), osteoblast, and chondrocyte lineages (Fig. 2.5). This is over and above the MSC's ability to self-renew. This differentiation that can be induced *in vitro* is not generally what can be expected after the transplant of MSCs *in vivo*. The current paradigm of MSCs used as an orthobiologic (a biological product that is transplanted or injected into MSK tissue with the intention of producing a beneficial biological effect) emanates from the paracrine signal-

ling that transplanted MSCs provide and the downstream profound impact this has on the recipient cells and tissues.

Mesenchymal stem cells (MSCs) and the recipient immune system

When transplanted, MSCs are hypoimmunogenic (Ryan et al., 2005). Several features and mechanisms are involved in rendering MSCs unlikely to provoke immune rejection. These include:

- The absence of the cell surface glycoprotein MCH-II (major histocompatibility complex class II).
- Immunomodulation by effects on dendritic cells, natural killer cells, and T-cells.
- Actions of prostaglandins, IL-10, and indoleamine 2,3-dioxygenase.

For clarity and to avoid doubt, the current use of MSC transplants in small animals has its actions via paracrine mechanisms

(Caplan, 2017). That is to say that the MSC secretome (the mixture of released molecules) interacts with the adjacent cells present within the injected tissue. The MSCs are capable of differentiating into various mesodermal cell lineages *in vitro*; however, when injected, the MSCs do not engraft and do not directly give rise to daughter cells such as chondrocytes or osteoblasts (Caplan, 2017).

Timeline of platelet-rich plasma (PRP) development

Thus far the discussion has centred solely on the development of MSCs for RM. Apart from MSC therapy, the other major RM in common use is PRP therapy. Any discussion of the history of RM would not be complete without mentioning PRP.

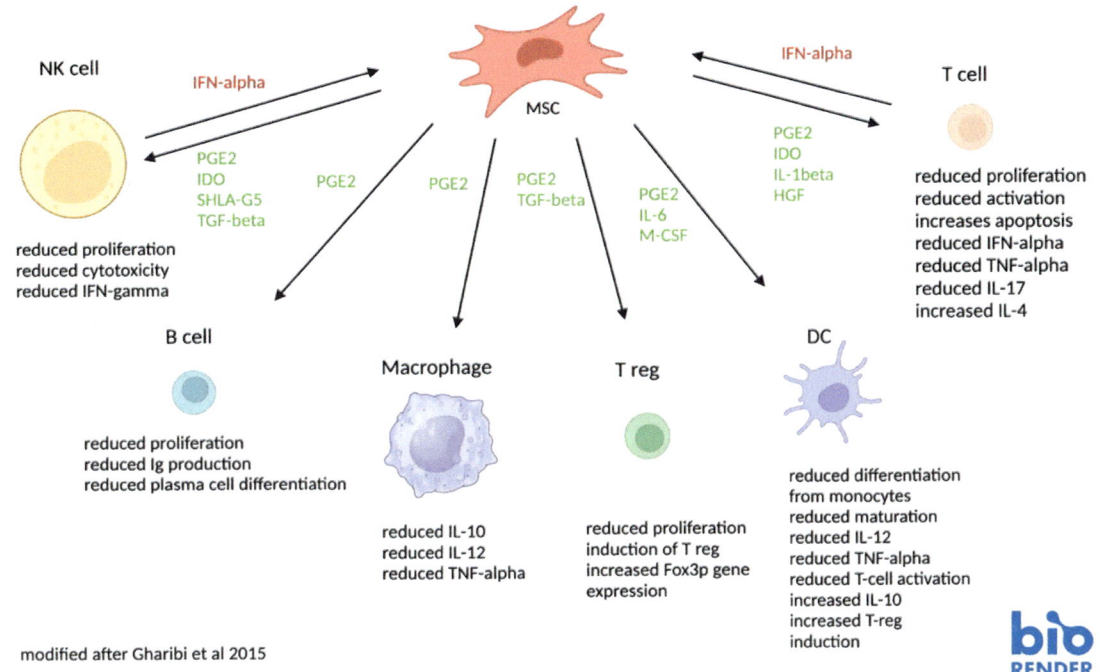

modified after Gharibi et al 2015

Fig. 2.6 The effects of MSCs on immune cells and some of the mediators involved.
NK = natural killer cell, B-cell = B-lymphocyte, T-reg = regulatory T-lymphocyte, DC = dendritic cell, T-cell = T-lymphocyte.
IFN = interferon, PGE2 = prostaglandin E, IDO = indolamine, SHLA-G5 = soluble human leukocyte antigen G5, TGF = transforming growth factor, M-CSF = granulocyte macrophage colony-stimulating factor, HGF = hepatocyte growth factor, Fox3p = Forkhead Box P3.
The various kinds of immune cells are influenced by the MSC secretome, which exerts its paracrine effects via different signalling molecules (Gharibi et al., 2015). Overall, the activities of inflammatory cells, including NK cells, DC, T-cells, and B-cells are downregulated. Conversely, regulatory T-cells and B-cells are recruited, and their activity is induced. Macrophages, under the influence of PGE2, TSG-6, IL-6, IDO, and TGF-beta-1 from the MSCs, tend to be polarised from an inflammatory M1 phenotype to an anti-inflammatory M2 phenotype (see Fig. 2.7).

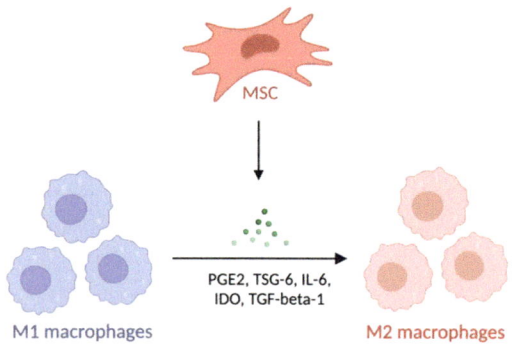

modified from Zheng et al 2015

Fig. 2.7 The polarisation from M1 to M2 macrophage phenotype by the secreted bioactive molecules from MSCs.
PGE2 = prostaglandin E2, TSG-6 = tumour necrosis factor-stimulated gene-6, IL-6 = interleukin-6, IDO = indolamine, TGF-beta-1 = transforming growth factor beta-1. Modified by Zheng et al., (2015).

The details of what PRP is, how it is produced, and its applications are discussed in detail in Chapters 4–6. For the time being, it is sufficient to report that over the last several decades, PRP has become an indispensable part of orthopaedics and sports medicine in human, equine, and canine patients. The development of PRP in the various human medical specialities is summarised in Fig. 2.8.

The 'third blood corpuscle' was first described around 1842 (Cooper, 2005), though Giulio Bizzozero, working in 1882, is generally credited with their discovery (Ribatti & Crivellato, 2007). In the 1980s, initial reports of PRP use for indications other than platelet transfusion emerged (Knighton et al., 1982; Marx et al., 1998; Monteleone et al., 2000). A concise review of the development of autologous PRP in human medicine is provided by Mościcka and Przylipiak (2021).

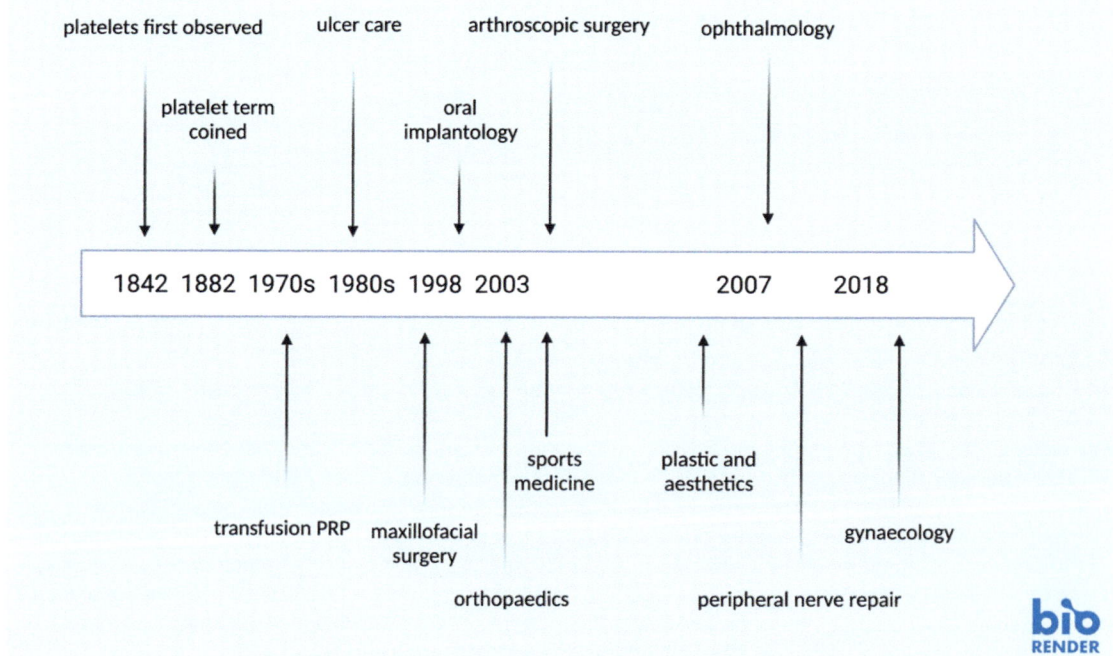

Fig. 2.8 The history of PRP development in various human medical fields (expanded after the publication by the Biobridge Foundation: Standardised Platelet-rich Plasma for Musculoskeletal Disorders, 2020).

Chapter 2 key points

- MSCs are derived from the biopsy of living tissue.
- MSCs exhibit plastic adherence in the laboratory.
- MSCs have a fibroblast-like, spindle-shaped morphology *in vitro*.
- MSCs are strongly proliferative.
- MSCs exhibit multipotent differentiation capacity *in vitro*.
- MSCs have anti-inflammatory properties. For example, they promote the polarisation of M1 macrophages to an M2 phenotype.
- MSCs are able to modulate the local immune system in the milieu into which they are injected.
- MSCs lack the MCH II surface antigen, which assists them in evading immune detection and immune rejection.
- Transplanted MSCs do not engraft into host tissues. Their effects are instead mediated by their paracrine influences on existing host cells at the injection site.
- PRP has several decades of use in various medical and veterinary applications.
- PRP can be used alone or added to MSC therapy.

Chapter 2 references

Astor, D. E., Hoelzler, M. G., Harman, R., & Bastian, R. P. (2013). Patient factors influencing the concentration of stromal vascular fraction (SVF) for adipose-derived stromal cell (ASC) therapy in dogs. *Canadian Journal of Veterinary Research*, *77*(3), 177–182.

Barry, F. (2023). *Lecture from second international regenerative medicine, Skopje, Northern Macedonia*.

Biobridge Foundation. (2020). Standardized Platelet-rich Plasma for musculoskeletal disorders. http://www.biobridge-event.com/knowledge

Caplan, A. I. (1991). Mesenchymal stem cells. *Journal of Orthopaedic Research*, *9*(5), 641–650. https://doi.org/10.1002/jor.1100090504

Caplan, A. I. (2017). Mesenchymal stem cells: Time to change the name! *Stem Cells Translational Medicine*, *6*(6), 1445–1451. https://doi.org/10.1002/sctm.17-0051

Cooper, B. (2005, October). Osler's role in defining the third corpuscle, or "blood plates". In *University Medical Centre Proceedings* (Vol. 18, No. 4, pp. 376–378). Taylor & Francis, 18(4), 376–378. https://doi.org/10.1080/08998280.2005.11928097

Dominici, M. L. B. K., Le Blanc, K., Mueller, I., Slaper-Cortenbach, I., Marini, F. C., Krause, D. S., Deans, R., Keating, A., Prockop, DJ., & Horwitz, E. M. (2006). Minimal criteria for defining multipotent mesenchymal stromal cells. The International Society for Cellular Therapy position statement. *Cytotherapy*, *8*(4), 315–317. https://doi.org/10.1080/14653240600855905

Friedenstein, A. J., Chailakhyan, R. K., Latsinik, N. V., Panasyuk, A. F., & Keiliss-Borok, I. V. (1974). Stromal cells responsible for transferring the microenvironment of the hemopoietic tissues: Cloning in vitro and retransplantation in vivo. *Transplantation*, *17*(4), 331–340. https://doi.org/10.1097/00007890-197404000-00001

Friedenstein, A. J., Piatetzky-Shapiro, I. I., & Petrakova, K. V. (1966). Osteogenesis in transplants of bone marrow cells. *Journal of Embryology and Experimental Morphology*, *16*(3), 381–390. https://doi.org/10.1242/dev.16.3.381

Garber, K. (2015). RIKEN suspends first clinical trial involving induced pluripotent stem cells. *Nature Biotechnology*, *33*(9), 890–891. https://doi.org/10.1038/nbt0915-890

Gharibi, T., Ahmadi, M., Seyfizadeh, N., Jadidi-Niaragh, F., & Yousefi, M. (2015). Immunomodulatory characteristics of mesenchymal stem cells and their role in the treatment of multiple sclerosis. *Cellular Immunology*, *293*(2), 113–121. https://doi.org/10.1016/j.cellimm.2015.01.002

Gratwohl, A., Pasquini, M. C., Aljurf, M., Atsuta, Y., Baldomero, H., Foeken, L., Gratwohl, M., Bouzas, L. F., Confer, D., Frauendorfer, K., Gluckman, E., Greinix, H., Horowitz, M., Iida, M., Lipton, J., Madrigal, A., Mohty, M., Noel, L., Novitzky, N., . . . & Worldwide Network for Blood and Marrow Transplantation (WBMT). (2015). One million haemopoietic stem-cell transplants: A retrospective observational study. *The Lancet. Haematology*,

2(3), e91–e100. https://doi.org/10.1016/S2352-3026 (15)00028-9

Greenwood, H. L., Thorsteinsdóttir, H., Perry, G., Renihan, J., Singer, P. A., & Daar, A. S. (2006). Regenerative medicine: New opportunities for developing countries. *International Journal of Biotechnology*, *8*(1/2), 60–77. https://doi.org/10.1 504/IJBT.2006.008964

Guest, D. J., Dudhia, J., Smith, R. K. W., Roberts, S. J., Conzemius, M., Innes, J. F., Fortier, L. A., & Meeson, R. L. (2022). Position statement: Minimal criteria for reporting veterinary and animal medicine research for mesenchymal stromal/stem cells in orthopaedic applications. *Frontiers in Veterinary Science*, 9, 817041. https://doi.org/10.3389/fvets.2022.817041

Henig, I., & Zuckerman, T. (2014). Hematopoietic stem cell transplantation-50 years of evolution and future perspectives. *Rambam Maimonides Medical Journal*, *5*(4), e0028. https://doi.org/10.5041/RMMJ. 10162

Jacques, E., & Suuronen, E. J. (2020). The progression of regenerative medicine and its impact on therapy translation. *Clinical and Translational Science*, *13*(3), 440–450. https://doi.org/10.1111/cts.12736

Knighton, D. R., Hunt, T. K., Thakral, K. K., & Goodson 3rd, W. H. (1982). Role of platelets and fibrin in the healing sequence: An in vivo study of angiogenesis and collagen synthesis. *Annals of Surgery*, *196*(4), 379–388. https://doi.org/10.1097/00000658-198210000-00001

Koç, O. N., & Lazarus, H. M. (2001). Mesenchymal stem cells: Heading into the clinic. *Bone Marrow Transplantation*, *27*(3), 235–239. https://doi.org/ 10.1038/sj.bmt.1702791

Lazarus, H. M., Haynesworth, S. E., Gerson, S. L., Rosenthal, N. S., & Caplan, A. I. (1995). Ex vivo expansion and subsequent infusion of human bone marrow-derived stromal progenitor cells (mesenchymal progenitor cells): Implications for therapeutic use. *Bone Marrow Transplantation*, *16*(4), 557–564.

Lebkowski, J. (2011). GRNOPC1: The world's first embryonic stem cell-derived therapy. Interview with Jane Lebkowski. *Regenerative Medicine*, *6*(6) Suppl., 11–13. https://doi.org/10.2217/rme.11.77

Martin, G. R. (1981). Isolation of a pluripotent cell line from early mouse embryos cultured in medium conditioned by teratocarcinoma stem cells.

Proceedings of the National Academy of Sciences of the United States of America, *78*(12), 7634–7638. https:// doi.org/10.1073/pnas.78.12.7634

Marx, R. E., Carlson, E. R., Eichstaedt, R. M., Schimmele, S. R., Strauss, J. E., & Georgeff, K. R. (1998). Platelet-rich plasma: Growth factor enhancement for bone grafts. *Oral Surgery, Oral Medicine, Oral Pathology, Oral Radiology, and Endodontics*, *85*(6), 638–646. https://doi.org/10.1016/s1079-210 4(98)90029-4

Monteleone, K., Marx, R., & Ghurani, R. (2000, September). Wound repair/cosmetic surgery healing enhancement of skin graft donor sites with platelet-rich plasma. In 82nd Annual Meeting of the American Association of Oral and Maxillofacial Surgeons, San Francisco, CA.

Mościcka, P., & Przylipiak, A. (2021). History of autologous platelet-rich plasma: A short review. *Journal of Cosmetic Dermatology*, *20*(9), 2712–2714. https:// doi.org/10.1111/jocd.14326

Owen, M. (1988). Marrow stromal stem cells. *Journal of Cell Science. Supplement* (Supplement_10), 10, 63–76. https://doi.org/10.1242/jcs.1988.supplement_10.5

Perry, A. R., & Linch, D. C. (1996). The history of bone-marrow transplantation. *Blood Reviews*, *10*(4), 215–219. https://doi.org/10.1016/s0268-960x(96)90 004-1

Pittenger, M. F., Mackay, A. M., Beck, S. C., Jaiswal, R. K., Douglas, R., Mosca, J. D., Moorman, M. A., Simonetti, D. W., Craig, S., & Marshak, D. R. (1999). Multilineage potential of adult human mesenchymal stem cells. *Science*, *284*(5411), 143–147. https:// doi.org/10.1126/science.284.5411.143

Punzón, E., Salgüero, R., Totusaus, X., Mesa-Sánchez, C., Badiella, L., García-Castillo, M., & Pradera, A. (2022). Equine umbilical cord mesenchymal stem cells demonstrate safety and efficacy in the treatment of canine osteoarthritis: A randomized placebo-controlled trial. Journal of the American Veterinary Medical Association, 260(15), 1947–1955. https://doi.org/10.2460/javma.22.06.0237

Ramalho-Santos, M., & Willenbring, H. (2007). On the origin of the term "stem cell". *Cell Stem Cell*, *1*(1), 35–38. https://doi.org/10.1016/j.stem.2007.05.013

Ribatti, D., & Crivellato, E. (2007). Giulio Bizzozero and the discovery of platelets. *Leukemia Research*, *31*(10), 1339–1341. https://doi.org/10.1016/j.leukr es.2007.02.008

Ryan, J. M., Barry, F. P., Murphy, J. M., & Mahon, B. P. (2005). Mesenchymal stem cells avoid allogeneic rejection. *Journal of Inflammation*, *2*, 8. https://doi.org/10.1186/1476-9255-2-8

Spangrude, G. J., Heimfeld, S., & Weissman, I. L. (1988). Purification and characterization of mouse hematopoietic stem cells. *Science*, *241*(4861), 58–62. https://doi.org/10.1126/science.2898810

Takahashi, K., & Yamanaka, S. (2006). Induction of pluripotent stem cells from mouse embryonic and adult fibroblast cultures by defined factors. *Cell*, *126*(4), 663–676. https://doi.org/10.1016/j.cell.2006.07.024

Thomas, E. D., Lochte, Jr., H. L., Lu, W. C., & Ferrebee, J. W. (1957). Intravenous infusion of bone marrow in patients receiving radiation and chemotherapy. *The New England Journal of Medicine*, *257*(11), 491–496. https://doi.org/10.1056/NEJM195709122571102

Till, J. E., & McCulloch, E. A. (2011). A direct measurement of the radiation sensitivity of normal mouse bone marrow cells 1. *Radiation Research*, *175*(2), 145–149. https://doi.org/10.1667/RRXX28.1

Weissman, I. L., & Shizuru, J. A. (2008). The origins of the identification and isolation of hematopoietic stem cells, and their capability to induce donor-specific transplantation tolerance and treat autoimmune diseases, *The Journal of the American Society of Hematology*. *Blood*, *112*(9), 3543–3553. https://doi.org/10.1182/blood-2008-08-078220

Zheng, G., Ge, M., Qiu, G., Shu, Q., & Xu, J. (2015). Mesenchymal stromal cells affect disease outcomes via macrophage polarization. *Stem Cells International*, *2015*, 989473. https://doi.org/10.1155/2015/989473

Chapter 3

Administration of veterinary regenerative medicine (VRM) in musculoskeletal (MSK) conditions

This chapter addresses the when, where, and how of VRMs. By 'when' to use VRM, we are referring to the indications for this therapeutic approach. The 'where' alludes to the anatomical location of the injury, lesion, or disease being managed. The methodology of administration is covered by the 'how'.

Indications for veterinary regenerative medicine (VRM)

For the purposes of this book, discussion of VRM indications is confined to those conditions that affect the MSK system of pet animals, namely dogs and cats. The author acknowledges that VRM is a broad subject and has potential indications in multiple additional body systems, such as the nervous system, the urinary system, and the digestive system, to name only a few. It is also recognised that the discipline of VRM is well-developed in other veterinary species, notably in horses. Again, these body systems and species are not the focus of this book.

Turning to canine and feline VRM for MSK conditions, the two principal categories of pathological conditions that are described here are joint diseases that lead to OA and sports medicine-type conditions affecting muscles, tendons, ligaments, and so forth.

VRM for joint diseases

In the United Kingdom at least, the presence of clinically significant OA is the most frequent reason to consider the use of VRM. In humans, OA is typically viewed as a disease of advanced age in which chronic attrition through decades of wear and tear results in the irreversible, progressive degeneration of the tissues of the joint (Meeson et al., 2019). While there are parallels in the canine patient, it is now accepted that OA in dogs can and does instantiate from a much earlier age in many cases (Enomoto et al., 2024). The condition of canine OA represents a common disease manifestation that can have a variety of precipitating aetiologies. Broadly speaking, these are conditions that cause either joint incongruency, joint instability, or both.

Examples of conditions causing joint incongruence:

- Elbow dysplasia
- Osteochondritis dissecans (OCD)
- Hip dysplasia

Examples of conditions causing joint instability:

- Medial shoulder instability
- Cranial cruciate ligament (CCL) dysfunction
- Patellar luxation

The relatively young age at which dogs are affected by OA following developmental joint conditions such as elbow dysplasia and hip dysplasia means that early veterinary intervention is advisable. Where a problem justifies and is amenable to surgical correction, it is likely to be the preferable option. Examples of this would be surgery for CCL disruption, stabilisation of luxating patella, and total hip replacement for severe hip dysplasia. Many conditions will not be surgically amenable for a variety of reasons, such as there not yet being a reliable surgical procedure for the condition, there are multiple joints affected, or there are constraints of facilities, expertise, or finance. It may also be the case that the surgical management of an MSK condition may be augmented by the preceding, concurrent, or subsequent administration of orthobiologic products.

Thus, we have a situation in which a significant proportion of the pet population is severely affected by developmental joint diseases that directly cause OA at a young age. This may be seen as an opportunity for the veterinary community to embrace VRM in these patients to harness the disease-modifying potential of such therapies.

The major limb joints that are readily accessible to IA injections are depicted in Figure 3.1:

- Shoulder
- Elbow
- Carpus
- Hip
- Stifle
- Tarsus (hock)

VRM for sports medicine conditions

A detailed treatise on the domain of veterinary sports medicine is outside the scope of this book. Instead, readers are referred to other sources for more comprehensive and in-depth information on this subject (e.g., Markley, 2023). It suffices to say that many of the conditions that are encountered within this discipline of veterinary medicine are potentially treatable using VRM. These include but are not limited to those depicted in Figure 3.2:

- Biceps tendon injury, bicipital tenosynovitis (Aleksiewicz et al., 2023)
- Medial shoulder ligament pathologies
- Supraspinatus tendinopathy (McDougall et al., 2018)
- Infraspinatus tendinopathy
- Elbow medial flexor tendinopathy

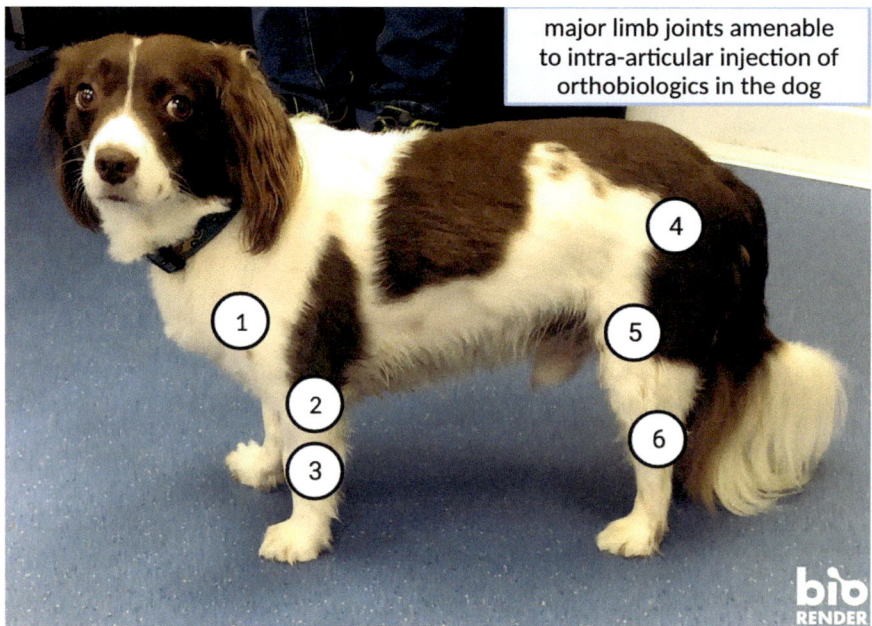

Fig. 3.1 Major limb joints amenable to intra-articular (IA) injection of orthobiologics in the dog.
1. shoulder (glenohumeral) joint; 2. elbow (humeroulnar) joint; 3. carpal (radiocarpal) joint; 4. hip (coxofemoral) joint; 5. stifle (femorotibial and patellofemoral) joint; 6. hock (tibiotarsal) joint.

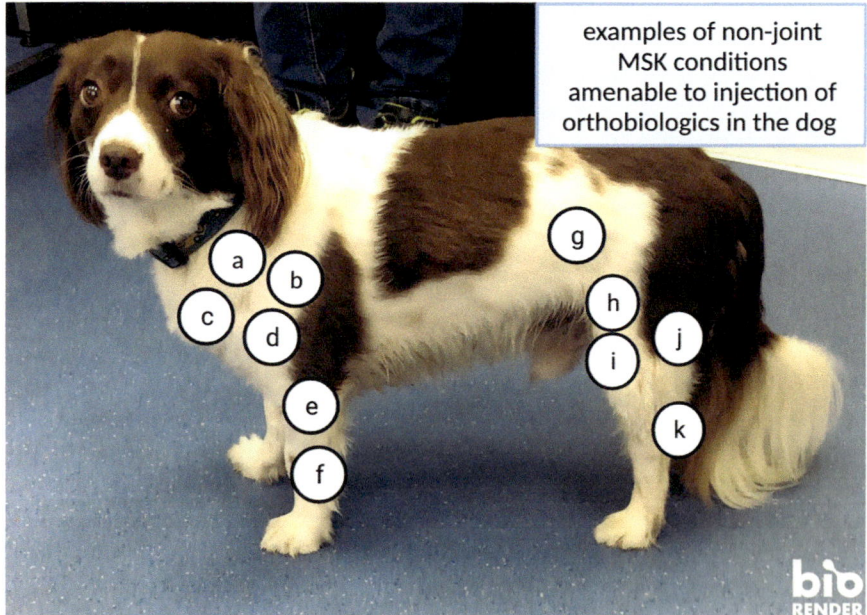

Fig. 3.2 Examples of non-joint MSK conditions amenable to injection of orthobiologics in the dog.
a. supraspinatus tendon; b. infraspinatus tendon; c. medial glenohumeral ligaments; d. biceps tendon; e. medial elbow flexor tendons; f. ulnaris lateralis tendon; g. iliopsoas tendon; h. cranial cruciate ligament (CCL); i. patellar tendon; j. proximal gastrocnemius tendon; k. calcaneal (Achilles) tendon.

- Flexor carpi ulnaris tendon injury (Franini et al., 2023)
- Calcaneal (Achilles) tendon damage or degeneration
- CCL degeneration
- Pathology of the head of gastrocnemius muscle
- Patellar tendinitis
- Iliopsoas muscle damage (Sack et al., 2023)

How to inject veterinary regenerative medicine (VRM)

Currently, most joint injections in practice are performed 'blind'. This means that the surgeon uses visible, and more importantly, palpable anatomical landmarks to navigate the optimal location for needle entry into the joint. Where the requisite skills and equipment are available, the use of MSK ultrasound-guided needle placement may greatly improve accuracy. Similarly, though perhaps less conveniently, fluoroscopic guiding is also a theoretical possibility.

Which joints can be injected? The major joints of the appendicular skeleton are all, as a rule, amenable to IA injection. These include the shoulder, elbow, carpus, hip, stifle, and hock (see Fig. 3.1).

Equipment list for arthrocentesis and intra-articular (IA) injection

Clinicians who are inexperienced with joint injections may be initially daunted by the concept of inserting very sharp metal needles into the articular tissues. This is understandable since a cavalier approach to IA injections will increase the risk of iatrogenic damage. Despite this obvious caveat, in essence, joint injection is a straightforward technique that is readily learned. The ability to collect fluid from, and to inject orthobiologics into joints is an essential skill in VRM.

The principles and methods for joint fluid collection and joint injection are almost identical.

The following is a suggested equipment list and inventory of disposable items (acknowledgement for equipment list: Dr Ross Allan). It includes sterile vessels for the collection of synovial fluid for subsequent laboratory analysis, including bacterial culture, as indicated.

- 2 × 2ml syringes
- 2 × 5ml syringes
- 2 × 10ml syringes
- 2 × 21-gauge × 50mm needles
- 2 × 22-gauge × 50mm needles
- 2 × 23-gauge × 50mm needles
- 2 × 18-gauge × 90mm spinal needles
- 2 × 20-gauge × 90mm spinal needles
- 2 × EDTA blood tubes
- 2 × plain blood tubes
- 1 × blood culture bottle
- Skin preparation swabs
- Skin preparation solutions
- 2 × pair of sterile surgeon's gloves
- Hair clippers
- Drape for instruments
- Fenestrated drape for patient

General principles of joint injection

The goal of the synovial joint injection is to administer the orthobiologic suspension safely and effectively. Safe injection implies no iatrogenic damage to the joint structures, especially the articular cartilage. The latter is known for being slow to repair itself, and since it has no sensory innervation, it may not be immediately apparent that needle damage has occurred. Attention to detail and using an approach, where possible, that avoids the weight-bearing surfaces of the articular cartilage may be preferable. Safety also means minimising the risk of introducing bacterial infection into the joint by using a strict aseptic technique.

Effective joint injection requires the orthobiologic to be delivered accurately into the synovial 'space'. This is crucial when MSCs are used since these cells influence the host tissues by

A

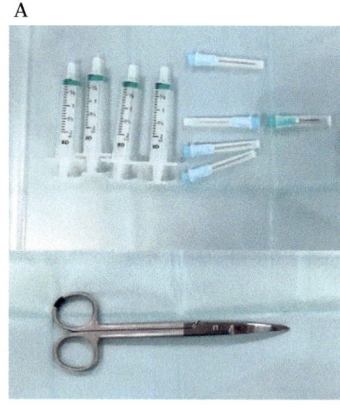

Sterile equipment

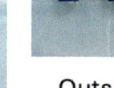

Outside of
vials are
non-sterile

C Unscrubbed assistant
holds MSC vial

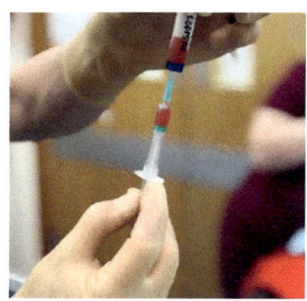

Scrubbed veterinarian
Withdraws MSCs from vial

B Unscrubbed assistant
holds MSC vial

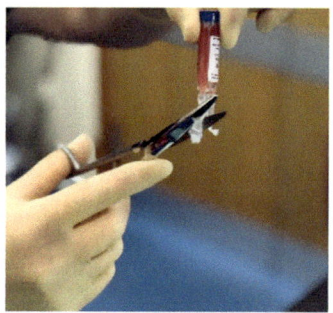

Scrubbed veterinarian
opens filter on MSC vial

D

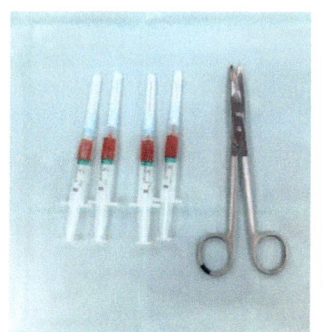

Syringes containing
MSCs
aseptically collected
from vials

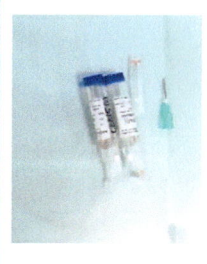

Empty
MSC
vials

Fig. 3.3 (a–d) Sequence of photographs outlining the preparation of autologous culture-expanded adipose-derived mesenchymal stem cells (AD-MSCs) for IA injection. (a) The frozen cell vials are gradually allowed to thaw at ambient temperature. The tray contains syringes, needles, sterile scissors, and an alcohol swab. (b) The operator dons sterile surgical gloves. The lower seal of the vial is peeled away, and the port is swabbed with alcohol and allowed to dry for sixty seconds. The filter port is opened by cutting. It should be noted that the outside of the vial containing the MSCs may not be sterile (depending on the laboratory protocol used). If there is any doubt, then it is better to have the vial held by an 'unscrubbed' assistant while the surgeon aseptically withdraws the cell product. (c) Using a later discarded needle, the contents of the vial (MSCs in the vehicle) is drawn up into the syringes. Care is taken to preserve aseptic technique and to avoid spillage. (d) The MSCs are ready for IA injection.

cell-to-cell paracrine communication. Missing the target will not produce optimal results. The appearance of synovial fluid in the needle hub confirms correct intrasynovial needle placement. The phenomenon of a 'dry synovial tap' occurs occasionally. Reasons for this may be a relative lack of synovial fluid. Normal joints have only a thin film of fluid between the opposing articular surfaces. This can be difficult to collect in any quantity, especially in small joints. One response of the pathological processes that affect the joint is the increase in fluid volume, known as synovial effusion. Effused joints typically yield a larger volume of synovial fluid. This can be reassuring in practice, as collecting 0.25ml to 3ml generally suggests significant IA pathology and that we are about to inject the correct (that is, diseased) joint. It is possible that during the latter stages of degeneration by osteoarthritic processes that any synovial fluid may be difficult to collect. In such cases, confirmation of correct needle placement may require a different method. Assuming that we have correctly identified the landmarks, then testing for resistance to injection may be effective. A small volume (say 1ml) of sterile isotonic saline can be injected. If the saline injects easily, then this is good evidence for correct needle placement. Resistance requiring excessive force on the syringe plunger is consistent with the needle tip not being intrasynovial.

An alternative technique, which can be considered if available, is ultrasound-guided IA injection. As more clinicians become equipped with high-frequency (15–18MHz) linear transducers and acquire the requisite skills and experience, these assisted IA injections will become commonplace. By way of comparison, ultrasound-guided IA injection of orthobiologics is considered the standard of care in human sports medicine.

Sequence of steps for joint injection

The veterinary surgeon follows the sequence below.

Review of technique

A few anatomical approaches are possible in most joints. Practising one of these for each of the joints will allow the veterinarian to perfect the technique. It is always worthwhile having alternatives since the chosen method may be precluded by variations in anatomy and/or pathology that obscure or restrict the preferred injection site. An example of the latter could be pronounced osteophytosis, which could prevent needle entry in the standard location. Having diagrams of the method at hand for reference is also recommended so that these can be referred to during the procedure. These may be digitally displayed and/or printed and laminated.

Revision of anatomy

There is no substitute for anatomical knowledge of the main limb joints. Revising the pertinent

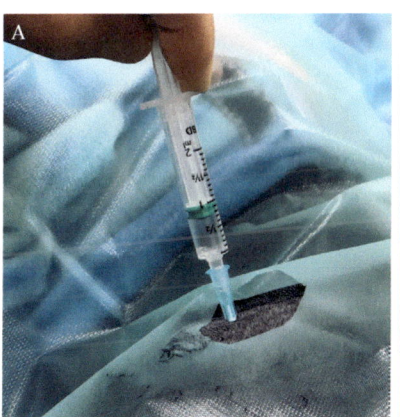
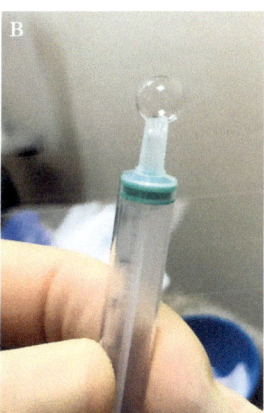
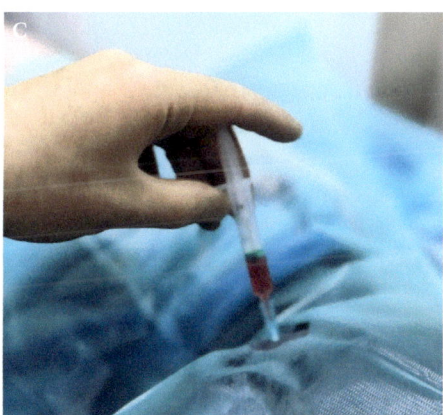

Fig. 3.4 (a) Aseptic aspiration of a canine shoulder joint. The typical appearance of synovial fluid in the syringe hub following needle aspiration of a joint. Often only small volumes are collected. (b) The synovial fluid is viscous, forming a bubble on the syringe tip. (c) Subsequent IA shoulder injection.

osseous and soft tissue structures associated with the joint is advisable. In particular, neurovascular elements need to be considered and avoided. It is always worth bearing in mind that joints are three-dimensional structures, and that the operator will need to mentally visualise the internal structures based on the palpation of surface landmarks. Fortunately, this is a skill veterinarians will have honed during their lengthy training since it is a prerequisite for becoming competent in veterinary surgery.

Display imaging

As we all know, pet dogs and cats vary widely in size and conformation. Giant breed dogs have rather different elbow joint morphology than miniature, chondrodystrophoid breeds for example. Considering the anatomy of the joint the clinician is injecting is essential. One useful adjunct to this is diagnostic images produced in advance. Radiographs are the most ubiquitous modality. Orthogonal radiographs may be displayed to give extra confidence to the clinician on the correct placement of the needle.

Anaesthesia and analgesia

IA injection is associated with pain, which must be prevented. Humane joint injection in companion animals mandates either deep sedation or general anaesthesia. Even with good technique, joint distension by the orthobiologic is painful *per se*. The smaller the volume used, the less stretching of the synovial membrane and periarticular tissues. Figure 3.13 tabulates the suggested maximum volumes of orthobiologic to be injected. If aspiration of the joint before injection can be done, this is advantageous, as it may be possible in effused joints to remove a volume of fluid and 'replace' it with the orthobiologic without any net additional joint distension. Narcotic analgesics are incorporated into the sedation or anaesthesia cocktail to prevent any procedure-induced pain. Sufficient provision of appropriate and potent enough analgesic medication during and after the procedure is, in the author's opinion, non-negotiable.

Asepsis

The joint is a sterile environment unless the patient has a type of bacterial infective arthritis, and clinicians should aim to prevent or at least minimise the risk of bacteria entering the joint. Iatrogenic infections, if they occur, are severely damaging to the joint and may be challenging to eliminate.

The environment chosen for the joint injection should be as clean as possible. An operating room is preferred. Personnel should respect the procedure, from the viewpoint of aseptic technique, as they would a surgical operation. Aseptic skin preparation commences with wide and careful clipping of the skin. In this way, clipper rashes should be avoided or minimised. While skin cannot be sterilised as the commensal bacteria will not be eliminated completely, 'surgical standard' skin preparation is undertaken. Making the clipped area wide enough to maintain asepsis is necessary. The author recommends the use of both surgical gloves and sterile drapes (see Figs 3.3 & 3.4).

Needle selection

Hypodermic needles need to be long enough to penetrate through the skin and tissues into the joint. A range of lengths should be available. Very 'deep' joints, such as the hip, may require the longest needles, and spinal needles may be a good choice in this instance since they are stiffer due to the presence of a stylet. As a rule, the smallest gauge needle that will allow the joint injection or synovial fluid collection is chosen. This may be as small as 23-gauge in many joints. Having extra needles of different lengths and gauges to hand is advisable, in case the first attempt proves challenging.

Avoiding articular cartilage damage

Articular cartilage is not innervated, so the sedated patient may not react to having a needle inadvertently scrape or plough into it. Since a needle can cause considerable damage to this tissue, the selection of an injection site where the risk is minimised is desirable. Aiming for the pouch of a joint rather than the 'space' between weight-bearing cartilage surfaces, where possible, should be attempted.

Injection sites

Standard injection sites are described in this section. Having a secondary injection site as an alternative option can be useful to fall back on if the first choice proves unworkable.

Synovial fluid collection

To collect synovial fluid for analysis, a needle is placed into the joint until a drop of the former appears in the needle hub. A syringe is then attached, and a sample is gently drawn out. Patience at this stage may avoid iatrogenic blood contamination of the synovial fluid collected. The range of tests requested will depend on the suspected conditions based on the clinical picture and the fluid volume available. As a minimum, cytology is desirable. Spreading a drop of fluid between microscope slides and air drying them will provide a means of performing microscopic examination and differential cell count. If more fluid is collected, then plain and EDTA tubes may be filled. Injecting the remainder into a medium blood culture bottle will enhance the likelihood that bacteria will be cultured in cases where joint infection is suspected.

Joint injection

Once synovial fluid has been collected, the joint may be injected. With the needle still *in situ* in the joint, the pre-prepared injection is slowly injected into the joint. The level of resistance to the injection is related to the size of the joint and the volume of the product being injected. Chronically diseased joints may present in a grossly distended state since they may be associated with large synovial effusions. Such joints may offer little resistance to injection. Smaller joints, such as hocks, may offer much more resistance to injection into a relatively confined space. In general, stretching the joint tissues by forcing in a larger volume of orthobiologics that can be comfortably accommodated will increase post-injection pain. After the needle is withdrawn, gentle pressure is applied with a digit to limit the backflow of injected fluid.

Aftercare

The incidence of complications following IA injections is low (Armitage et al., 2023). In cases where adverse events occur, these are typically mild and of short duration. Owners are routinely warned that following IA injection, the joint may be more painful than its pre-injection state. For this reason, pre-emptive analgesic administration is routine to minimise or preferably prevent any exacerbation of the discomfort. A minority of cases, especially after PRP injection, experience a 'joint flare' in which there is inflammation and perhaps swelling of the joint. This typically occurs after 8–12 hours (after the patient has returned home) and will generally be self-limiting, subsiding after several days. A short course of analgesic medication may be required. The use of NSAIDs after PRP injection is controversial. It has long been argued that the temporary inflammation that may follow the PRP administration is beneficial to the joint, and therefore NSAIDs are contra-indicated; hence in human sports medicine, it is probable that NSAIDs will be withheld before and after PRP administration. However, this assertion has recently been found to be unsupported by scientific evidence (Magruder & Rodeo, 2021; Armitage et al., 2023). Exercise should be moderated for five days or so after IA injection before a gradual return to normal activity.

Arthrocentesis and joint injection of the main canine limb joints are described in the following section.

Shoulder

The canine glenohumeral joint is relatively large and, with practice, lends itself well to IA injection (Fig. 3.5). The sedated or anaesthetised animal is placed in lateral recumbency with the affected limb uppermost. The joint is partially flexed. An assistant may apply slight external rotation and distal traction to 'open' the joint space. A 22g × 50mm needle is sufficient to penetrate the joint in most large breed dogs. The insertion site is between the distal extremity of the acromion and the greater tubercle of the humerus. When the needle punctures the synovial membrane, a 'pop' is often felt. Releasing the traction on the limb may 'lock' the needle in position. If there is significant pathology in the joint (such as OCD, joint infection, or biceps brachii tenosynovitis), a large volume (4ml or so) of effused synovial fluid is often collected.

Elbow

The canine elbow is frequently affected by developmental conditions collectively termed elbow dysplasia. Dysplastic joints, as a rule, become osteoarthritic. This makes the elbow a frequent source of pain and disability, which can be an indication for IA injection of RM products.

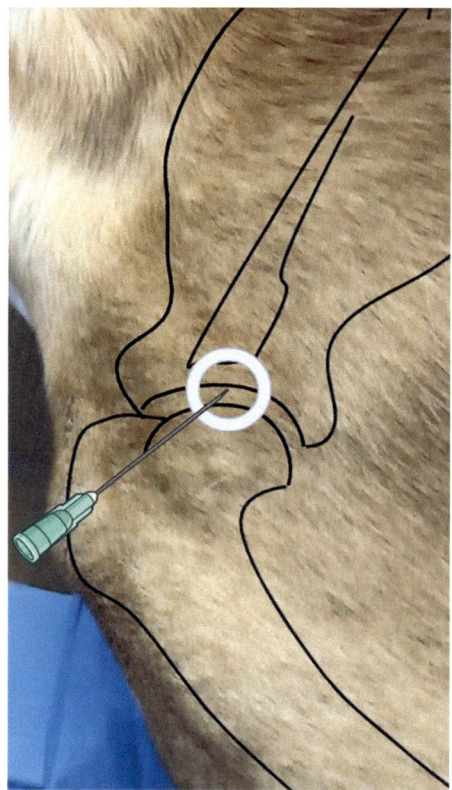

Fig. 3.5 Canine glenohumeral joint injection. The landmarks are the distal extremity of the acromion and the greater tubercle of the humerus.

The caudolateral approach to elbow injection

This is a convenient target for needle placement. The sedated or anaesthetised patient is placed in lateral recumbency with the affected limb uppermost. The joint is fully flexed by an assistant, and the limb is abducted. A 23-gauge needle of suitable length is chosen. The landmarks are the lateral humeral epicondyle, the lateral condylar ridge, the anconeal process (if palpable), and the triceps tendon (Fig. 3.6). Advancing the needle between the lateral condylar ridge and the triceps tendon is performed, aiming for the (non-palpable) supracondylar foramen. The appearance of synovial fluid in the needle hub signals correct needle placement. The fluid can be collected by gentle syringe aspiration as

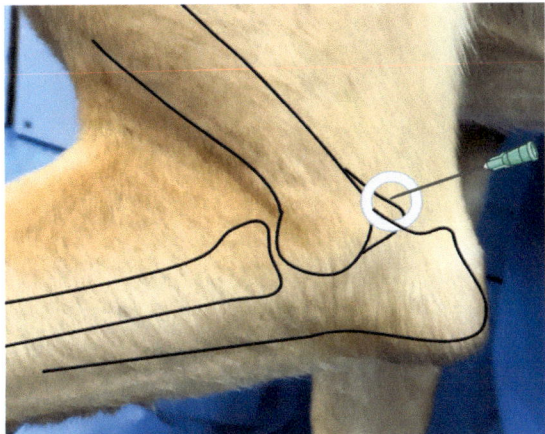

Fig. 3.6 The caudolateral approach to elbow injection. The landmarks are the lateral humeral epicondyle, the lateral condylar ridge, the anconeal process (if palpable), and the triceps tendon.

required for analysis, and the syringe exchanged for one containing PRP and/or MSCs for injection. There should be relatively little resistance to injection in most joints as long as the volume injected is appropriate.

The medial approach to elbow injection

The patient is placed in dorsal recumbency, with the affected limb abducted by an assistant. A padded fulcrum can be used under the humerus so that the medial joint compartment may be 'opened'. The elbow and carpus are flexed by around 90°, and the latter may also be externally rotated. This injection location is the same as that for portal placement in arthroscopy cases. The major palpable landmark is the medial epicondylar prominence. The injection needle is inserted approximately 1.5cm (in medium-sized dogs) distal to this point, perpendicular to the skin. Again, synovial fluid is expected to appear when the joint is penetrated.

Carpus

Injection into the radiocarpal joint is relatively easily achieved (Fig. 3.7). Sternal or lateral

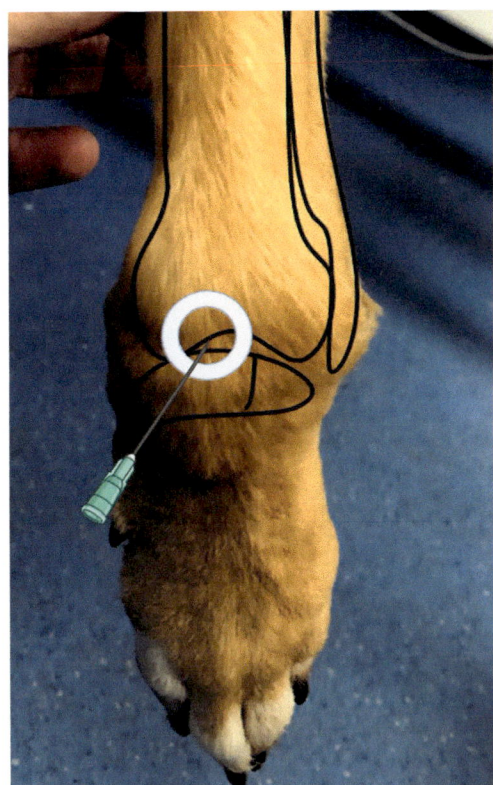

Fig. 3.7 Radiocarpal joint injection.

recumbency is acceptable. The carpus is flexed by about 90°; this 'opens' the radiocarpal joint widely. The joint is readily palpated, in most cases between the distal radius and the radial carpal bone. Long needles are rarely needed as there is minimal soft tissue between the skin and the synovial 'joint space'. Insert the needle medial to the cephalic vein and common digital extensor tendon, just lateral to the tendon of the extensor carpi radialis. In smaller joints, temporary traction applied by an assistant may allow larger volumes of fluid to be injected with less resistance.

Hip

Coxofemoral joint injection may be challenging. Various needle locations have been described. The author prefers a lateral approach, as depicted in Figure 3.8. The difficulty in navigating to the

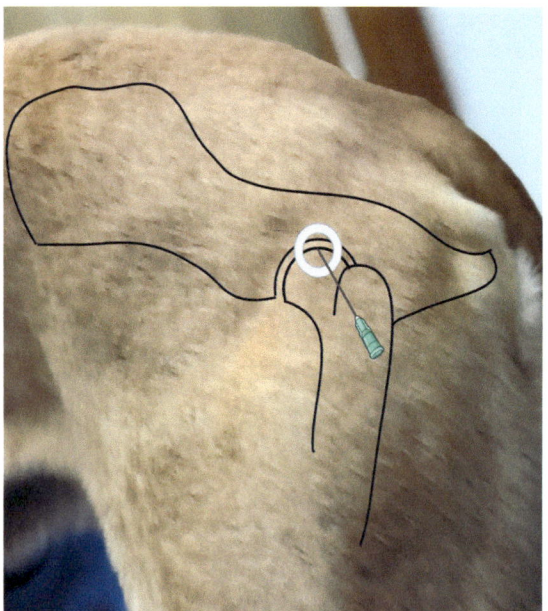

Fig. 3.8 Lateral approach to coxofemoral joint injection. See text below for description.

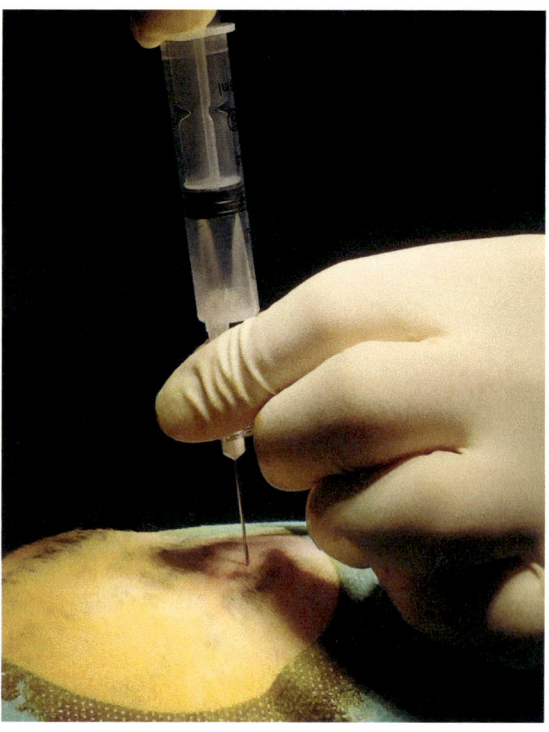

Fig. 3.9 Aspiration of synovial fluid prior to IA injection of PRP into the right hip joint of a dog. Photograph courtesy of Associate Professor Ksenjia Ilieska.

correct location is because the joint is relatively 'deep' within the body, and the acetabular rim and femoral head are usually not palpable. The patient is placed in lateral recumbency with the affected limb uppermost. The stifle is flexed to a 90° angle by an assistant. The limb is then externally rotated, and distal traction is applied to 'open' the joint. Long enough needles are essential to reach the joint. The target, aimed at blindly, is between twelve o'clock and ten o'clock on the acetabular arc of the left hip, or between twelve o'clock and two o'clock on the acetabular arc of the right hip. The main palpable bony landmark is the greater trochanter. The needle is placed just cranial to this structure and advanced in a vertical direction (horizontal if the dog was standing), aiming for the joint. Often the needle tip is felt to come into contact with either the femoral neck or the acetabular rim. In either case, the direction is slightly adjusted to 'walk off' the bone so that the needle point then 'drops' into the joint. Synovial fluid in the needle hub confirms correct placement (see Fig. 3.9).

Stifle

Several different approaches can be used for stifle injection. These are lateral femorotibial, medial femorotibial, and lateral parapatellar. The latter has the advantage that the needle does not risk violating the articular cartilage of the weight-bearing femoral and tibial joint surfaces or the IA soft tissue structures, such as the cruciate ligaments and menisci. Stifle injection is readily achieved in most cases. The sedated patient is positioned in dorsal recumbency or lateral recumbency with the affected limb uppermost.

Lateral stifle injection

The stifle joint is held in mid-flexion. Landmarks are the patella, patellar tendon, and tibial tuberosity. The needle is inserted midway between the

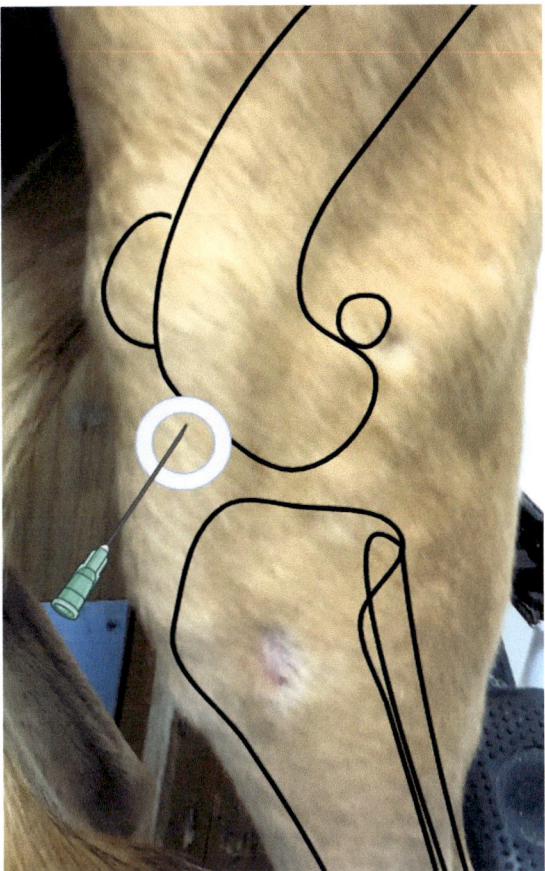

Fig. 3.10 The location for IA injection of the left stifle. See text below for description.

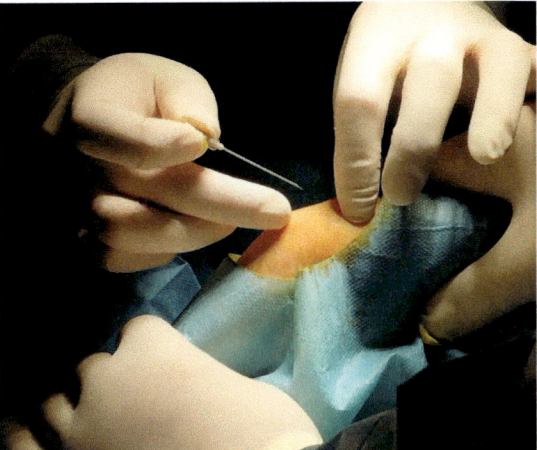

Fig. 3.11 The location for IA injection via a lateral approach to the right stifle of a dog. Digital palpation identifies the patella (left hand) and tibial tuberosity (right hand). Photograph courtesy of Associate Professor Ksenjia Ilieska.

Lateral parapatellar stifle injection

A further alternative IA injection site for the stifle is the lateral pouch of the patellofemoral joint. This is somewhat more superficially located. Joint distension may be apparent in cases of synovial effusion, which facilitates the procedure. The needle should be aimed from distal to proximal just beneath to the lateral parapatellar cartilage.

Hock

The hock joint has a relatively small articular compartment. This often necessitates smaller, more concentrated volumes of the chosen orthobiologic. The 22g × 25mm needle can be inserted from craniomedial, craniolateral, or caudolateral aspects (Fig. 3.12).

Injecting other musculoskeletal (MSK) structures

Orthobiologics are frequently injected into sites other than joints. Accurate diagnosis of the pathology and location within the

patella and tibial tuberosity, about 1cm lateral to the tendon. The direction of the needle aim is toward the femorotibial joint in the midline (Figs 3.10 & 3.11). After traversing the infrapatellar fat pad, synovial fluid is typically detected. Excessively 'deep' needle penetration and rotation or other manipulations of the needle are to be kept to a minimum to avoid violating the cruciate ligaments.

Medial stifle injection

This method is similar to that described for the lateral technique, except that the needle enters midway between the patella and tibial tuberosity, 1cm medial to the tendon.

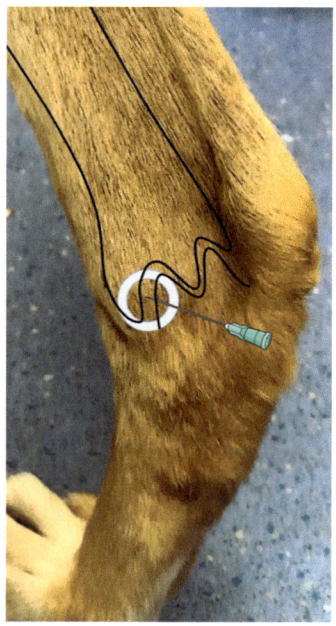

Fig. 3.12 Location of caudomedial injection into right hock.

affected structure is crucial. To this end, MSK ultrasonography may be indispensable for ultrasound-guided injection. Where this equipment or expertise is not available, injecting 'blindly' is possible, though this is obviously less likely to yield optimal results. A detailed description of MSK ultrasound is beyond the scope of this current book.

Some of the MSK structures that are amenable to intra-lesional injection are the following:

- Biceps tendon (Aleksiewicz et al., 2023)
- Medial shoulder ligaments
- Supraspinatus tendon (McDougall et al., 2018)
- Infraspinatus tendon
- Elbow medial flexor tendons

	Shoulder	Elbow	Carpus	Hip	Stifle	Tarsus
Needle	22-gauge 38mm	22-gauge 38mm	22-gauge 25mm	22-gauge 75mm or 60-75mm spinal needle	22-gauge 38mm	22-gauge 25mm
Weight						
Miniature <5kg	0.5ml	0.25–0.5ml	<0.25ml	0.5ml	0.5ml	<0.25ml
Small 5–12kg	0.5–1ml	0.5–1ml	0.25–0.5ml	0.5-1ml	0.5–1ml	0.25–0.5ml
Medium 12–25kg	1–1.5ml	1-1.5ml	0.5–1ml	1–1.5ml	1–1.5ml	0.5–1ml
Large 25–50kg	1.5–2ml	1.5–2ml	0.75–1ml	1.5–2ml	1.5–2ml	0.75–1ml
Giant >50kg	2–3ml	2–2.5ml	1ml	2–3ml	2–3ml	1ml

Fig. 3.13 Chart for injection volumes for dogs (adapted from www.nupsala.com).

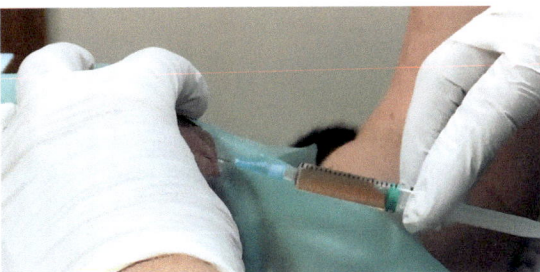

Fig. 3.14 Injection of 8.2 million autologous MSCs into site of patellar tendon injury.

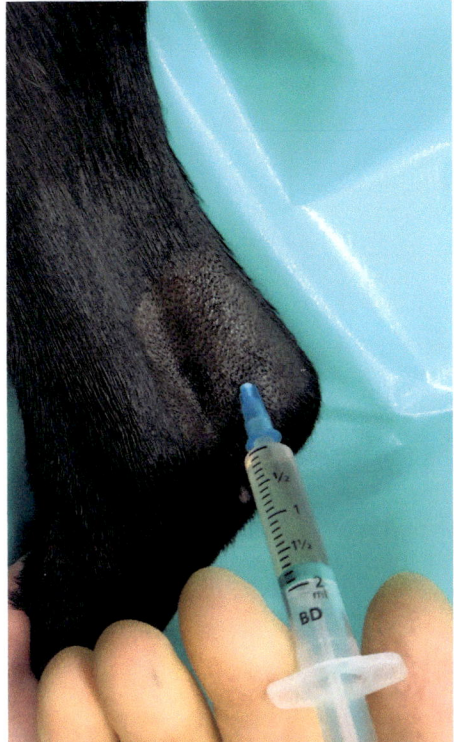

Fig. 3.15 Injection of autologous MSCs into site of calcaneal tendon injury. MSK ultrasound will significantly increase the accuracy of the delivery of cells to the relevant locations in the damaged tissue.

- Flexor carpi ulnaris tendon (Franini et al., 2023)
- Calcaneal tendon (Fig. 3.15)
- CCL
- Head of gastrocnemius muscle
- Patellar tendon (Fig. 3.14)
- Iliopsoas muscle and tendon

Chapter 3 key points

- In broad terms, VRMs can be injected into joints via IA injection techniques and/or into MSK soft-tissue structures other than the joints.
- VRM in small animals requires the clinician to be skilled in IA injections.
- IA injections are readily learnt, as long as the clinician uses their basic knowledge of anatomy and follows the described approaches.
- The risk of joint damage and infection is minimised by careful technique and attention to asepsis.
- Ultrasonography is effective in guiding joint injections and identifying MSK soft tissue structures for injection.

Chapter 3 references

Aleksiewicz, R., Lutnicki, K., & Marcinek, T. (2023). Ultrasound monitoring of the regenerative treatment of biceps tendonitis and tenosynovitis in dogs by stem cells injections. *Medycyna Weterynaryjna*, *79*(10), 525–529.

Armitage, A. J., Miller, J. M., Sparks, T. H., Georgiou, A. E., & Reid, J. (2023). Efficacy of autologous mesenchymal stromal cell treatment for chronic degenerative musculoskeletal conditions in dogs: A retrospective study. *Frontiers in Veterinary Science*, 9, 1014687. https://doi.org/10.3389/fvets.2022.1014687

Enomoto, M., de Castro, N., Hash, J., Thomson, A., Nakanishi-Hester, A., Perry, E., Aker, S., Haupt, E., Opperman, L., Roe, S., Cole, T., Thompson, N. A., Innes, J. F., & Lascelles, B. D. X. (2024). Prevalence of radiographic appendicular osteoarthritis and associated clinical signs in young dogs. *Scientific Reports*, *14*(1), 2827. https://doi.org/10.1038/s41598-024-52324-9

Franini, A., Entani, M. G., Colosio, E., Melotti, L., & Patruno, M. (2023). Case report: Flexor carpi ulnaris tendinopathy in a lure-coursing dog treated with three platelet-rich plasma and platelet lysate injections. *Frontiers in Veterinary Science*, 10, 1003993. https://doi.org/10.3389/fvets.2023.1003993

Magruder, M., & Rodeo, S. A. (2021). Is antiplatelet therapy contraindicated after platelet-rich plasma treatment? A narrative review. *Orthopaedic Journal of Sports Medicine*, *9*(6), 23259671211010510. https://doi.org/10.1177/23259671211010510

Pechette Markley, A. (2023). Management of Injuries in Agility Dogs. The Veterinary Clinics of North America. Small Animal Practice, 53(4), 829–844. https://doi.org/10.1016/j.cvsm.2023.02.012

McDougall, R. A., Canapp, S. O., & Canapp, D. A. (2018). Ultrasonographic findings in 41 dogs treated with bone marrow aspirate concentrate and platelet-rich plasma for a supraspinatus tendinopathy: A retrospective study. *Frontiers in Veterinary Science*, *5*, 98. https://doi.org/10.3389/fvets.2018.00098

Meeson, R. L., Todhunter, R. J., Blunn, G., Nuki, G., & Pitsillides, A. A. (2019). Spontaneous dog osteoarthritis—A One Medicine vision. *Nature Reviews. Rheumatology*, *15*(5), 273–287. https://doi.org/10.1038/s41584-019-0202-1

Sack, D., Canapp, D., Canapp, S., Majeski, S., Curry, J., Sutton, A., & Cullen, R. (2023). Iliopsoas strain demographics, concurrent injuries, and grade determined by musculoskeletal ultrasound in 72 agility dogs. *Canadian Journal of Veterinary Research*, *87*(3), 196–201.

Chapter 3 further resources

British Small Animal Veterinary Association (BSAVA) (A Montesinos 2018) on joint injections. www.bsavalibrary.com

Dogstem®. www.dogstem.co.uk

Nupsala website www.nupsala.com

Veterinary Osteoarthritis Alliance website www.vet-oa.com

Section II

Chapter 4

Platelet-rich plasma (PRP) therapy

Why consider platelet-rich plasma (PRP) therapy?

When choosing a VRM, PRP has several features that make it an attractive option. These are that PRP is (typically) autologous, it is simple to prepare patient-side, it can be used in several anatomical sites simultaneously, it can be repeated multiple times, and it is easy to inject. Since the PRP is prepared immediately before it is injected into the target tissue, it is available at once and without delay. Therefore, *prima facie*, PRP would appear to be an excellent choice for an orthobiologic for VRM in small animals.

Definition of platelet-rich plasma (PRP)

PRP is a biological product that is derived from peripheral blood. It is usually autologous. PRP contains plasma and a concentration of platelets and molecules such as growth factors and cytokines that are higher than those of the original blood. The actual ideal concentration of platelets in PRP has yet to have achieved consensus, though it is usual to aim for four to six times that of the starting peripheral blood (Carr, 2022). In human PRP medicine, it is considered standard best practice to analyse the PRP before injection so that the platelet and cellular formulation is known and recorded. This may require calibration of the haematology analyser in question to measure PRP parameters. In some cases, dilution of the sample is needed to determine an accurate platelet count. In other cases, platelet clumping may affect the validity of the results. Recently, in VRM, there has been a trend to determine the actual platelet concentration in the PRP before injection as a more accurate means of describing a product, which is to be encouraged.

What are the sources of platelet-rich plasma (PRP)?

Up until very recently, PRP therapy was almost invariably referred to as autologous PRP. This means that autologous peripheral blood is collected, and the PRP is produced by concentrating the platelets. This is done patient-side using either centrifugation or filtration (see Chapter 5). Pooled allogeneic PRP is available 'off-the-shelf' in the United States, at the time of writing, and this is likely to become available elsewhere in the world in the future.

Properties of platelets

Platelets were discovered in 1882 by Giulio Bizzozero (Ribatti & Crivellato, 2007). Bizzozero observed moving platelets within the blood vessels of living animals and described their role in blood coagulation. Also known as thrombocytes, platelets are anucleate particles or cell fragments, approximately 2–3μm in diameter, found in the circulating blood. Their parent cell is the megakaryocyte found in the BM. Platelet functions broadly consist of two categories: haemostasis and tissue repair. It is the reparative functions that are most relevant to VRM.

Reparative functions, processes, and other properties of platelets:

- Secreting of proteins, cytokines, and other mediators.
- Promoting cell migration.
- Promoting cell proliferation.
- Promoting angiogenesis.
- Promoting tissue repair.
- Anti-inflammatory.
- Immunomodulatory.
- Analgesic (Everts et al., 2020).

Platelet structure and function

As already stated, platelets originate from megakaryocytes in the BM. They enter the circulation and may be stored in the spleen. Tissue damage involving haemorrhage or extravasation of blood results in the release of platelets into the tissues (Fig. 4.1).

Resting platelets are discoid 'cells' (by definition, cells must have a nucleus, so by this criterion, platelets are not cells in the conventional sense) measuring 2–3μm. Relevant organelles include α-granules, dense granules, and lysosomes. A complex network of canaliculi permeates the platelet and connects the interior to the exterior. Secretion of the granules, it is suggested, can occur by fusion with the granule membranes with either the plasma membrane or the open canalicular system (Fitch-Tewfik & Flaumenhaft, 2013). The dense granules contain the molecules involved in haemostasis, while the function of the lysosomes has not been well studied.

The contact with the damaged tissue environment, including type I collagen, activates the platelets. Activation involves the release of α-granule contents, that is, the combination of cytokines and growth factors, including PDGF, VEGF, TGFβ-1, TGFβ-2, IGF-1, EGF, and FGF.

Cell signalling, growth factors, and cytokines

The nomenclature of the various biological molecules that are involved in the regulation of cell growth and the proliferation of cells is confusing and not completely logical. This is because their discovery did not occur in a linear manner, and as more becomes known about each of the signalling molecules, more biochemical effects may be elucidated. Protein signalling molecules attach to (meaning that they are ligands for) transmembrane receptors. The binding of these ligands to the receptors triggers downstream intracellular cascades along biochemical pathways resulting in changes in the target cell. Some of these require alterations in gene transcription, while others are independent of this.

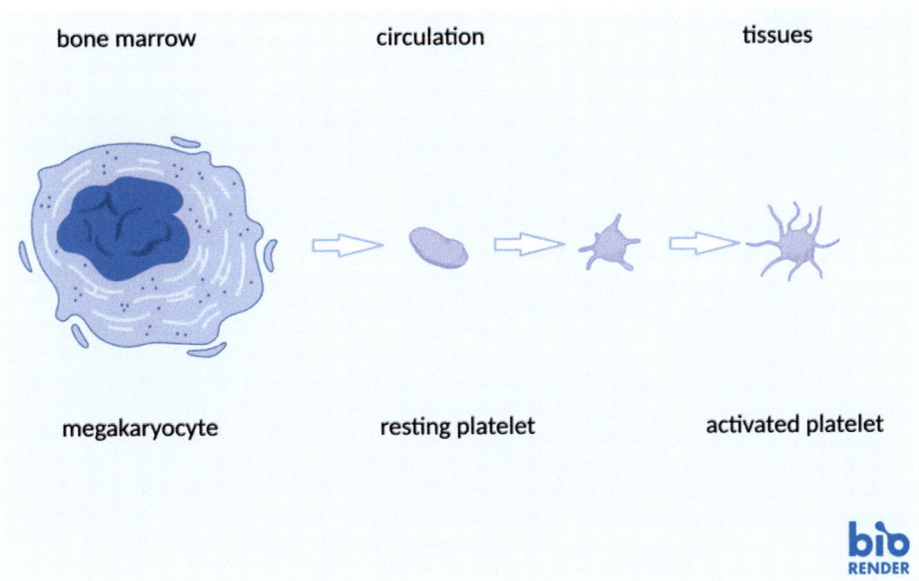

Fig. 4.1 Simplified natural history of platelets from their origin from the BM megakaryocyte to the activated tissue platelet.

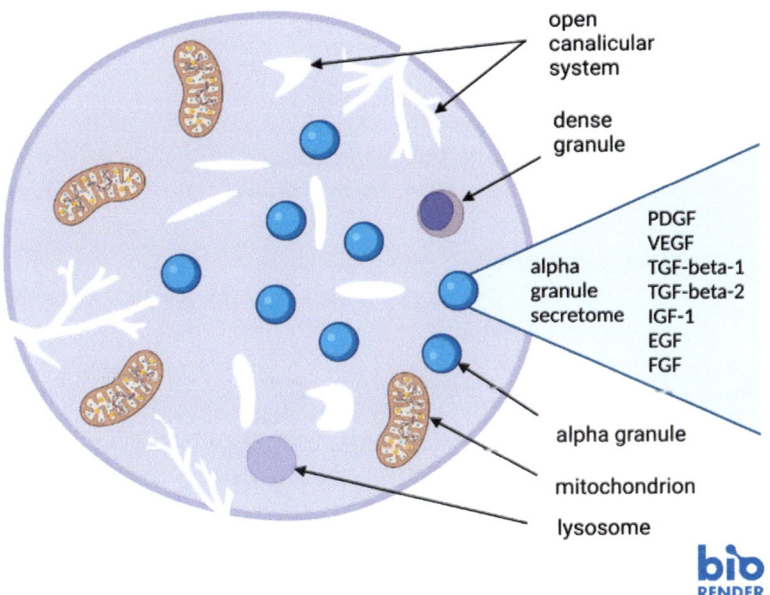

Fig. 4.2 Schematic diagram of a resting platelet. PDGF = platelet-derived growth factor; VEGF = vascular endothelial growth factor; TGFβ-1 = transforming growth factor beta-1; TGFβ-2 = transforming growth factor beta-2; IGF-1 = insulin-like growth factor-1; EGF = epidermal growth factor; FGF = fibroblast growth factor.

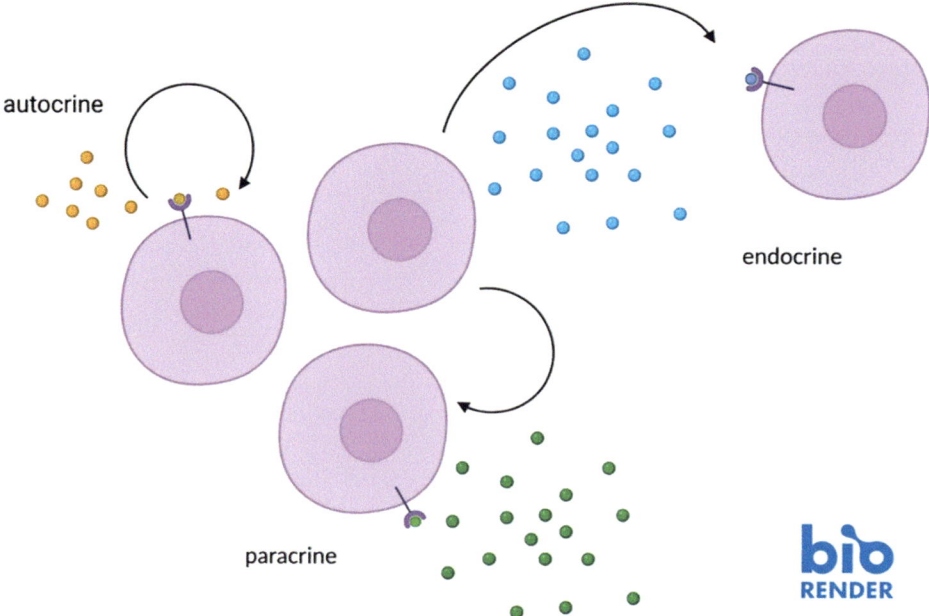

Fig. 4.3 Cell signalling may be autocrine, paracrine, or endocrine. In autocrine signalling, the bioactive molecule (orange circles) is released by the same cell that receives the receptor binding. Paracrine signalling occurs between different but locally neighbouring cells (green circles). Endocrine signalling occurs when the molecule (a hormone) reaches a distant cell after being transported in the circulation and binds to its receptor (blue circles). Redrawn from Elton (2022) (or https://qkine.com/2022/05/27/growth-factors-vs-cytokines/).

Cell-to-cell communication may be paracrine or endocrine. Paracrine signalling means that the secreting cell and the target cell are neighbouring each other; that is, it occurs over small distances. This is the predominant means by which VRM functions. The target cell may also be the cell that has released the signalling molecule, in which case, this is referred to as autocrine signalling (see Fig. 4.3).

There are three broad divisions in the classification of protein signalling molecules. These are the commonly referred to growth factors, cytokines, and hormones (see Fig. 4.4). The latter have their effects on distant cells (by endocrine signalling) and are of no concern to the current discussion. Cytokines are a subset of the growth factor family and are typically those molecules involved in the regulation of cells of the blood and immune system. The most common families of cytokines are interleukins (ILs), interferons (INFs), and tumour necrosis factors (TNFs).

The platelet secretome

The biologically active protein molecules, namely growth factors and cytokines that are known to be released by platelets, are numerous, to say the least. Those relevant to VRM are listed in Table 4.1.

The potential for a three-dimensional fibrin scaffold after platelet-rich plasma (PRP) administration

A detailed discussion of three-dimensional scaffolds in bioengineering is beyond the scope of this book. However, it is worth noting that the future applications of scaffolds with orthobiologics in human and VRM are likely to be wide-ranging and significant. The use of platelet-rich fibrin as an implantable orthobiologic has received attention in human medicine

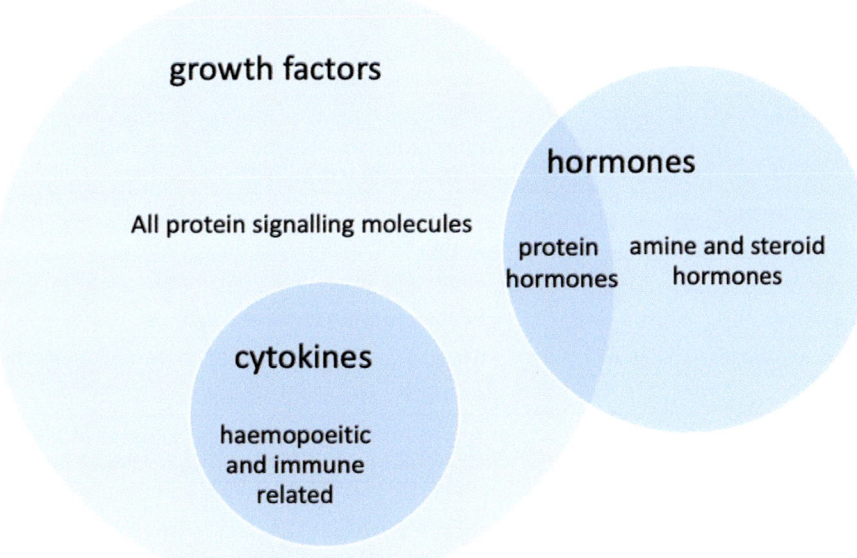

Fig. 4.4 Graphical representation of the relationship between growth factors, cytokines, and hormones. Redrawn from Elton (2022) (https://qkine.com/2022/05/27/growth-factors-vs-cytokines/).

(Narayanaswamy et al., 2023), and these products continue to evolve and improve.

PRP preparation protocols typically involve the use of an anticoagulant, which is usually acid-citrate dextrose-A (ACD-A). This prevents the formation of a clot since it chelates calcium, temporarily interfering with the clotting cascade. Once the PRP is injected into the body, where the ACD-A can diffuse away and physiological calcium concentrations are found, a fibrin aggregate clot may form. This has the potential to act as a scaffold for the injected platelets as well as for the tissue-regenerating cells that are attracted to the site by chemotaxis (Dr J Miller, Cell Therapy Sciences, 2023, personal communication). This phenomenon is also important to be aware of when combining PRP with any orthobiologic such as MSCs. It is observed that PRP mixed with MSCs, such as AdiShot® (which contains autologous serum and therefore calcium and fibrinogen), will clot within a few minutes in the syringe if the mixture is not immediately injected (Dr Andrew Armitage, Greenside Veterinary Clinic, 2023, personal communication).

Platelet function in tissue damage

Platelets have multiple physiological functions. After tissue injury, platelets are broadly described as being integral to haemostasis and the tissue healing cascade.

PRP has recently been demonstrated to have marked beneficial effects in human osteoarthritic knees (Lin, 2023). The researchers compared IA-PRP to IA hyaluronic acid for naturally occurring symptomatic patients with knee OA. The outcome measures were visual analogue scale (VAS) and Western Ontario and McMaster Osteoarthritis Index (WOMAC) scores, subchondral bone oedema measured using MRI, and synovial fluid biomarkers (TNFα, IL-6, MCP-1, MMP-1, MMP-3, and MMP-9). Across all these measures, the PRP group showed significant improvements ($P < 0.05$) compared to the hyaluronic acid group.

Table 4.1 List of some of the known PRP-derived growth factors and cytokines (modified after Carr, 2022).

Name (in alphabetical order)	Abbreviation	Functions (selected)
Angiopoeitin-1	Ang-1	Promotes angiogenesis and endothelial cell proliferation.
Basic fibroblast growth factor	bFGF	Promotes mitosis of fibroblasts, osteoblasts, and chondrocytes. Also favours chondrogenic and osteogenic differentiation of stem cells.
Connective tissue growth factor	CTGF	Stimulates cartilage regeneration, angiogenesis, fibrosis, and platelet adhesion.
Epidermal growth factor	EGF	Promotes proliferation of keratinocytes and fibroblasts. Promotes endothelial cell mitosis.
Hepatocyte growth factor	HGF	Stimulates neovascularisation during wound healing. Promotes repair of epithelia.
Insulin-like growth factor	IGF-1	Anabolic effects such as promotion of protein synthesis. Chemotactic effects towards fibroblasts. Stimulatory effects on osteoblast multiplication and differentiation.
Keratinocyte growth factor	KGF	Involved in wound healing by promoting migration and proliferation of epithelial cells.
Platelet-derived growth factor	PDGF	Promotes mitosis in osteoblasts and fibroblasts. Chemotaxis is stimulated in various cell types. Collagen metabolism regulation.
Transforming growth factor	TGF-alpha, TGF-beta	Promotes the proliferation of undifferentiated mesenchymal cells. Regulates mitosis in various cells. Collagen metabolism regulation. Stimulation of endothelial chemotaxis and angiogenesis. Inhibition of macrophage and lymphocyte proliferation.
Tumour necrosis factor	TNF	Regulation of monocyte migration, fibroblast proliferation, macrophage activation, and angiogenesis.
Vascular endothelial growth factor	VEGF	Promotes mitosis of endothelial cells and angiogenesis.

One means by which tissue healing may be facilitated by platelets is by their positive effects on resident MSCs (Levoux et al., 2021). It has been shown that platelets may donate mitochondria to MSCs. This can, in turn, increase the pro-angiogenic activity of the MSCs (Levoux et al., 2021).

Analgesic effects of platelet-rich plasma (PRP)

A key benefit of using an orthobiologic like PRP is the reduction in pain perceived by the patient. This effect is thought to arise from the immuno-modulatory and anti-inflammatory effects of the PRP, as well as the promotion of tissue healing. Additionally, it has been postulated that PRP may exert direct analgesic effects through other mechanisms. In laboratory animals and humans, PRP has been shown to have these effects (Everts et al., 2020), with evidence suggesting this is likely to be mediated via the 5-hydroxytryptamine, (also known as serotonin) system. PRP at standard concentrations of 4–6 times the platelet concentration of peripheral blood contains very high levels of 5-hydroxytryptamine. Therefore, it is likely that PRP can have direct analgesic properties independent, though synergistic with, PRP's ability to reduce inflammation.

Non-platelet components of platelet-rich plasma (PRP)

Discussions about PRP tend to centre on the platelets themselves. This is understandable since these remarkable bodies have such wide-ranging and complex effects in the orchestration of healing processes. It is also important, however, to consider the other constituents of the PRP. These components include the plasma itself, and the soluble molecules contained therein, leukocytes (of various kinds), red blood corpuscles (RBCs), and fibrinogen. Controversy has long characterised the discourse on the leukocyte contingent of PRP; this subject is discussed further in Chapter 5.

Contra-indications for platelet-rich plasma (PRP)

Broadly speaking, conditions that affect the healthy composition and/or function of the blood, involving infection, or neoplasia, usually preclude PRP therapy. The main contra-indications are listed below (modified from Carr, 2022).

Anaemia

Harvesting large volumes of blood is obviously not appropriate in patients with anaemia. If possible, the cause of the anaemia should be determined and managed appropriately.

Anticoagulant medication

This is less common in veterinary patients than in human medicine. Blood drawing is better avoided where there is a haemorrhage risk, and the anticoagulants will interfere with platelet function.

Antiplatelet therapy

This is mainly a concern in human patients. It is possible, however, that aspirin may occasionally be used in veterinary patients. This is known to affect platelet function.

Coagulopathy

Coagulopathies will contra-indicate the harvesting of autologous blood.

Dermatitis

Avoiding IA injections where the overlying skin is infected is the best practice to minimise the risk of iatrogenic joint infection. Similarly, the location of the harvested tissue required for MSC culture, such as adipose tissue or BM, should not be overlain by infected skin, lest the risk of bacterial contamination of the sample would become unacceptably high.

Immune-mediated disease

While MSCs may in time find indications in the management of a variety of autoimmune diseases, too little information currently exists, to the author's knowledge, to make recommendations to use PRP in pet animal autoimmune MSK diseases.

Neoplasia

The interaction of PRP with the plethora of different cancer disorders that are possible is difficult to predict. Since PRP is replete with growth factors that can stimulate angiogenesis, PRP could, at least theoretically promote tumour growth. Concentrating on oncological management of the neoplastic disease seems a sensible priority.

Septic arthritis

Where joint infection is diagnosed, treatment involves culture and sensitivity-informed antibiosis, and perhaps wound lavage. PRP is not appropriate in this acute situation.

Thrombocytopenia

Since the circulating platelet concentration is important, as is the ability to further concentrate it to produce PRP, thrombocytopenia will hamper this. Additionally, avoiding venepuncture is desirable where clotting is likely to be compromised. Instead, identifying the cause of the thrombocytopenia and managing it appropriately is recommended.

Chapter 4 key points

- Platelets play critical roles in both haemostasis and tissue repair and regeneration.
- The substances, growth factors, and cytokines present within the α-granules are essential in the regenerative processes.
- PRP is in widespread clinical use.
- PRP is readily prepared patient-side, facilitating rapid autologous injection.
- Allogeneic pooled PRP is also available for dogs in certain locations.
- PRP once injected may produce a three-dimensional fibrin biological scaffold.
- PRP can be co-injected with MSCs.
- It is important to be aware of the contraindications of PRP.

Chapter 4 references

Carr, B. J. (2022). Platelet-rich plasma as an orthobiologic: Clinically relevant considerations. *The Veterinary Clinics of North America. Small Animal Practice*, *52*(4), 977–995. https://doi.org/10.1016/j.cvsm.2022.02.005

Elton. (2022) (orhttps://qkine.com/2022/05/27/growth-factors-vs-cytokines/).

Everts, P., Onishi, K., Jayaram, P., Lana, J. F., & Mautner, K. (2020). Platelet-rich plasma: New performance understandings and therapeutic considerations in 2020. *International Journal of Molecular Sciences*, *21*(20), 7794. https://doi.org/10.3390/ijms21207794

Fitch-Tewfik, J. L., & Flaumenhaft, R. (2013). Platelet granule exocytosis: A comparison with chromaffin cells. *Frontiers in Endocrinology*, *4*, 77. https://doi.org/10.3389/fendo.2013.00077

Levoux, J., Prola, A., Lafuste, P., Gervais, M., Chevallier, N., Koumaiha, Z., Kefi, K., Braud, L., Schmitt, A., Yacia, A., Schirmann, A., Hersant, B., Sid-Ahmed, M., Ben Larbi, S., Komrskova, K., Rohlena, J., Relaix, F., Neuzil, J., & Rodriguez, A.-M. (2021). Platelets facilitate the wound-healing capability of mesenchymal stem cells by mitochondrial transfer and metabolic reprogramming. *Cell Metabolism*, *33*(2), 283–299.e9. https://doi.org/10.1016/j.cmet.2020.12.006

Lin, W., Xie, L., Zhou, L., Zheng, J., Zhai, W., & Lin, D. (2023). Effects of platelet-rich plasma on subchondral bone marrow edema and biomarkers in synovial fluid of knee osteoarthritis. *The Knee*, *42*, 161–169. https://doi.org/10.1016/j.knee.2023.03.002

Narayanaswamy, R., Patro, B. P., Jeyaraman, N., Gangadaran, P., Rajendran, R. L., Nallakumarasamy, A., Jeyaraman, M., Ramani, P., & Ahn, B.-C. (2023). Evolution and clinical advances of platelet-rich fibrin in musculoskeletal regeneration. *Bioengineering*, *10*(1), 58. https://doi.org/10.3390/bioengineering10010058

Ribatti, D., & Crivellato, E. (2007). Giulio Bizzozero and the discovery of platelets. *Leukemia Research*, *31*(10), 1339–1341. https://doi.org/10.1016/j.leukres.2007.02.008

Chapter 4 further reading

Arnoczky, S. P., & Sheibani-Rad, S. (2013). The basic science of platelet-rich plasma (PRP): What clinicians need to know. *Sports Medicine and Arthroscopy Review*, *21*(4), 180–185. https://doi.org/10.1097/JSA.0b013e3182999712

Catarino, J., Carvalho, P., Santos, S., Martins, Â., & Requicha, J. (2020). Treatment of canine osteoarthritis with allogeneic platelet-rich plasma: Review of five cases. *Open Veterinary Journal*, *10*(2), 226–231. https://doi.org/10.4314/ovj.v10i2.12

Dos Santos, R. G., Santos, G. S., Alkass, N., Chiesa, T. L., Azzini, G. O., da Fonseca, L. F., Dos Santos, A. F., Rodrigues, B. L., Mosaner, T., & Lana, J. F. (2021). The regenerative mechanisms of platelet-rich plasma: A review. *Cytokine*, *144*, 155560. https://doi.org/10.1016/j.cyto.2021.155560

Opneja, A., Kapoor, S., & Stavrou, E. X. (2019). Contribution of platelets, the coagulation, and fibrinolytic systems to cutaneous wound healing. *Thrombosis Research*, *179*, 56–63. https://doi.org/10.1016/j.thromres.2019.05.001

Chapter 5

Platelet-rich plasma (PRP) apparatus and PRP composition

Principle of platelet-rich plasma (PRP) therapy

The fundamental principle in PRP therapy is to selectively concentrate the platelet fraction of peripheral blood to produce a plasma-based suspension of the platelets. This PRP can then be activated either artificially before injection or naturally upon injection. The activated platelets release an alpha-granule secretome rich in cytokines and growth factors. This process is summarised in Figure 5.1.

Autologous versus allogeneic platelet-rich plasma (PRP)

PRP is traditionally autologous-derived and produced patient-side. Recently pooled, allogeneic canine PRP products have been studied (Catarino et al., 2020). At the time of writing, to the author's knowledge, one such freeze-dried product is commercially available in the United States (Precise PRP™ Canine, VetStem Biopharma Inc., Poway, California). The availability of an off-the-shelf PRP product, where this exists, obviates the need for any patient-side PRP preparation apparatus. The current situation, however, is that the vast majority of small animal PRP formulations are prepared individually and autologously using some form of apparatus.

Platelet-rich plasma (PRP) apparatus

Blood collection

The starting point for any PRP processing is to collect patient blood, usually via jugular venepuncture. The volume collected is between 5ml and 60ml, and a syringe primed with an anticoagulant is used. The author prefers a butterfly cannula for the venepuncture.

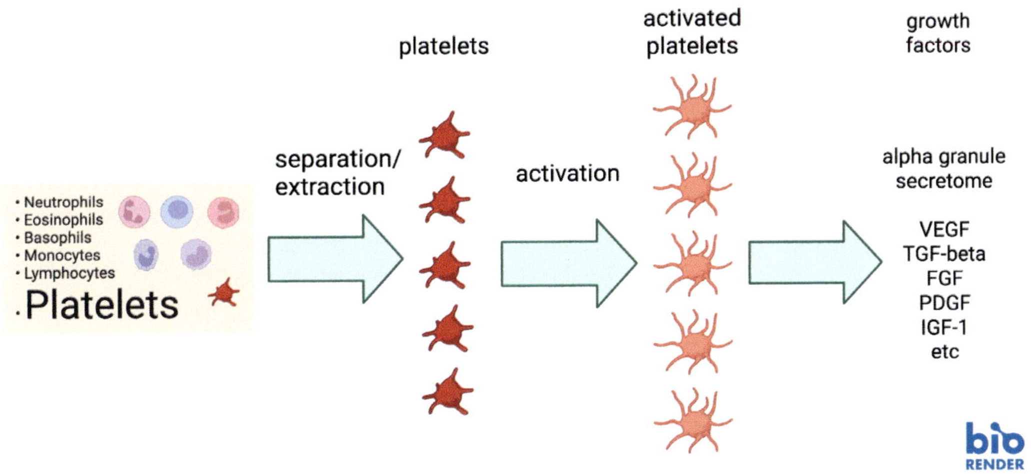

Fig. 5.1 Flow diagram of PRP therapy from blood collection to release of secreted factors into the tissues. VEGF = vascular endothelial growth factor; TGF-beta = transforming growth factor-beta; FGF = fibroblast growth factor; PDGF = platelet derived growth factor; IGF-1 = insulin like growth factor-1.

PRP production by filtration

An autologous platelet-rich suspension may be produced by gravity filtration. This process is exemplified by the V-PET™ system (Pall Corporation, Port Washington, New York). In essence, a closed system to which citrated blood is added is equipped with a filter that is intended to permit the passage of RBCs and white blood cells (WBCs) while causing adherence of platelets. The platelets captured on the filter are subsequently back-flushed using saline, producing a product similar to PRP. This is not actually, by definition, PRP since it does not contain plasma. Instead, the platelets are suspended in sterile isotonic saline. Furthermore, the 'V-PET™ PRP' tends to be leukocyte-rich and RBC-rich. This was a very popular choice of 'PRP' system since the capital investment in a centrifuge for PRP production was unnecessary. To the author's knowledge, this product has been discontinued and is no longer available.

PRP production by centrifugation

The different components of whole blood have different densities (specific gravities). This means that when centrifuged, these different elements divide into fractions that may then be amenable to separation (Fig. 5.2). To date, no consensus has been reached for the optimal methodology of centrifugation to produce PRP (Collins et al., 2021).

Blood may undergo a single or double spin. The latter is believed to concentrate platelets better. In the double spin situation, the first 'soft spin' separates the RBCs. The second 'hard spin' of the plasma supernatant, which is faster and/or longer in duration, concentrates the platelets into the final PRP product (Carr, 2022).

It is commonplace for clinicians to purchase a complete 'PRP system', which includes the centrifuge, separating devices, and disposables (Fig. 5.3). This is convenient, albeit it may be relatively expensive. An alternative is to use a lower-cost centrifuge and inexpensive sterile disposables to achieve a similar result. One should be cautious when using a 'home-made' PRP process that the following points are followed. Sterility is of paramount importance and is a non-negotiable principle in PRP production. If this cannot be guaranteed, a commercial closed system is a preferable choice. The formulation of the final PRP should be known

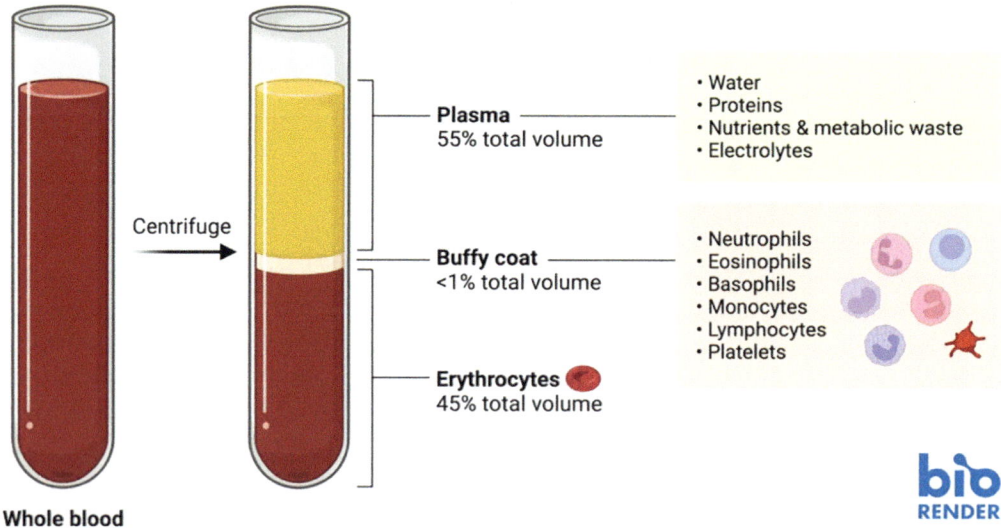

Fig. 5.2 Haematocrit, blood, and its components. Centrifugation of whole anticoagulated blood separates the plasma from the buffy coat and the packed cell fraction of RBCs (haematocrit).

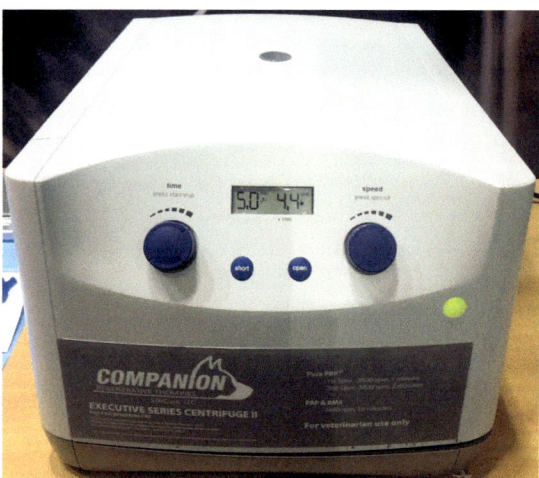

Fig. 5.3 An example of a commercially available centrifuge that is supplied with consumables for a standard leukocyte-poor PRP of relatively consistent formulation.

In the human PRP field, a multiplicity of different PRP centrifuge systems are available. Several commercial centrifuge systems similarly exist in the veterinary market. Many of these may have been adapted from the human

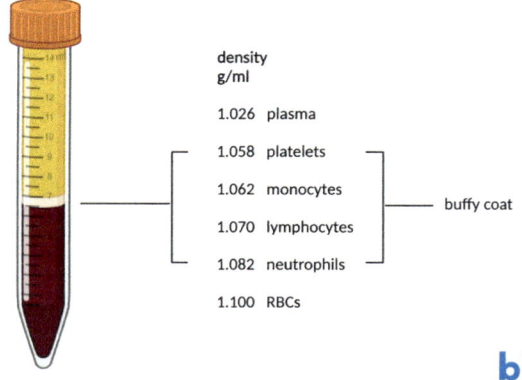

Fig. 5.4 Redrawn after Alves and Grimalt (2018). Centrifugation separates blood components according to density. The buffy coat may be approximately divided into platelets (least dense), monocytes, lymphocytes, and neutrophils (progressively denser). RBCs are the densest, hence they occupy the lower part of the tube.

so that the clinician is clear on exactly what is injected. Taking an aliquot of the PRP intended for injection and subjecting this to haematological analysis (bearing in mind that haematology machines may need recalibrating for PRP) before administration is a reasonable means of quality control.

Table 5.1 Canine PRP preparation. Reproduced after lecture slide by Professor Stefano Grolli, University of Parma, 2023. g = gravitational acceleration (9.8m/s/s).

	First centrifugation		Second centrifugation	
	Time (minutes)	g	Time (minutes)	g
Kim et al. 2009	10	629	15	1233
Tambella, 2014	20	180	15	650
Zubin et al. 2015	30	150	15	800
Canapp et al. 2016	10	800	10	4000
Upchurch et al. 2016	4	978	8	978
Farghali et al. 2017	10	250	10	2000
Shin et al. 2017	5	1000	15	1500

field, and as such, the principle of caveat emptor (buyer beware) comes into play. It is ultimately the responsibility of the clinician to ensure that whatever is injected can stand up to the rigours of evidence-based veterinary medicine. Referring to studies such as Carr et al. (2015), in which several different systems were studied, and using this to inform choices, should put the clinician's feet on firmer ground vis-à-vis ensuring that the PRP meets the requirements for the patient.

G-force and duration of centrifugation

For the 'double spin' method of PRP production, different authors have reported that widely varying g-force (while the common term is g-force, this is terminologically inexact as 'g' indicates the constant of gravitational acceleration) and duration of centrifugation have been applied (Table 5.1).

As will be appreciated from Table 5.1, there is wide variation in both the multiple of 'g' applied to the blood to produce PRP, and the duration of the centrifugation. Such heterogeneity of methodology is commonly encountered in VRM. This inconsistency tends to hamper comparison of different studies.

Platelet-rich plasma (PRP) constituents

The majority of PRP therapies performed in small animals to date are autologous. By their very nature, autologous PRPs are individual so no two PRP doses will be identical in composition. The heterogeneity of this biological – rather than pharmaceutical – product continues to hamper scientific studies on the efficacy of PRP. In this respect, the advent of a more uniformly constituted, off-the-shelf, pooled allogeneic PRP, such as the aforementioned Precise PRP™ Canine, is likely to provide a more suitable PRP for clinical studies.

The main 'active ingredient' of PRP is the platelets themselves. It is also important to consider what other constituents are present in any particular PRP and in what concentrations. The non-platelet components of the PRP, in particular the RBCs and WBCs, may have a significant influence (positive or negative) on the performance of the PRP. The main components of PRP are:

- Plasma
- Platelets
- RBCs
- Granulocyte leukocytes
- Agranulocyte leukocytes
- Plasma proteins (albumin, globulin, and fibrinogen)

Red blood corpuscles (RBCs)

RBCs are present to varying degrees in PRP. Laboratory studies have demonstrated that human synoviocyte death significantly increased in the presence of RBC concentrate (in this case, the RBC concentration was double that of the original blood) (Braun et al., 2014). The known mechanisms by which RBCs can promote damage to joint tissues (synovium and articular cartilage) are via reactive oxygen species and inflammatory cytokines such as IL-1 and transforming growth factor-alpha (TGF-alpha) (Sundman et al., 2011). Regarding the mechanism by which toxic radicals are generated, it is the haemoglobin-coupled iron liberated by haemolysis that initiates the process. A chemical process known as the Fenton reaction involves oxidation of haemoglobin to methaemoglobin (MetHb), with the formation of highly damaging hydroxyl radicals (Caviglia et al., 2020). This process, unfortunately, occurs naturally in human haemophilia patients affected by spontaneous IA haemorrhage, resulting in profound cartilage damage. Interestingly, IA PRP can reduce the Fenton reaction, presumably the mechanism involves the albumin present within the PRP (Caviglia et al., 2020).

In summary, efforts to reduce the concentration of RBCs in the PRP are advisable, and choosing a commercially available system to do this is recommended (Carr, 2022).

Granulocyte leukocytes

The inclusion of polymorph neutrophils in PRP is controversial (Carr, 2022). One perspective is that they release a plethora of pro-inflammatory mediators, and leukocyte-rich PRP increases the rate of synoviocyte death *in vitro* (Braun et al., 2014). Therefore, it may be reasonably concluded that leukocyte-poor PRP would be preferable for IA administration. As with many aspects of VRM, even this hypothesis is subject to challenge. For example, Yaradilmis et al. (2020) found that leukocyte-rich PRP outperformed leukocyte-poor PRP in human male patients with knee OA.

Alternatively, when administering PRP for tendon injuries, different considerations may apply. To promote the healing process, an initial inflammatory phase may be necessary. In such cases, leukocyte-rich PRP may arguably be a more logical choice than leukocyte-poor PRP; there is evidence from the human field that this is efficacious in human tendinopathies (Fitzpatrick et al., 2016). Additionally, scar tissue formation, which is typically undesirable, may be greater if leukocyte-poor PRP is used (Zhou et al., 2015).

In summary, leukocyte-poor PRP is suggested for IA injection, while both leukocyte-poor PRP and leukocyte-rich PRP may have a place in tendon regeneration. However, controversy remains regarding the optimal granulocytic leukocyte concentrations in PRP for veterinary applications (Carr, 2022).

Agranulocyte leukocytes

Agranulocytes are theoretically less likely to have detrimental effects on recipient tissues and are more likely to have beneficial effects, particularly through their interaction with synovial fibroblasts. For example, monocytes influence these cells by reducing the expression of IFN-gamma and IL-12 (both of which are anti-angiogenic) and by IL-6-mediated collagen synthesis stimulation (Naldini et al., 2008; Yoshida & Murray, 2013).

In conclusion, fractionation of PRP, where possible, to reduce polymorph neutrophil concentration preferentially while retaining relatively greater concentrations of monocytes appears appropriate for optimal PRP formulation. Some commercially available PRP systems claim to have sufficient flexibility in the processing method that varying the composition of the leukocytes in this way may be possible on a case-by-case basis. This can be verified before PRP injection by haematological measurements.

Platelet activation in platelet-rich plasma (PRP)

The beneficial effects of PRP in the tissues result from the release of the substances contained within the alpha-granules from the 'activated' platelet. In VRM, it is not usual to add an *ex vivo* platelet activation stage to the processing of the PRP. Instead, it is assumed that sufficient and appropriate platelet activation occurs following injection into the recipient tissue at the site of tissue damage. It is the tissue damage that signals the platelets to activate.

Tissue damage and the thrombin cascade are the pathophysiological factors that ordinarily activate platelets in the body. In human PRP therapy, artificial platelet activation prior to PRP injection can be produced by the following:

- Bovine or human thrombin.
  The enzyme thrombin converts soluble plasma fibrinogen into insoluble fibrin as part of the haemostatic cascade. The polymerised fibrin forms a dense matrix that may inhibit cell migration to the detriment of the healing process. Xenogeneic bovine thrombin could have immunoreactivity, so allogeneic or autologous thrombin sources may be preferable.
- Calcium chloride or calcium gluconate.
  10% calcium chloride added to PRP also stimulates coagulation by the formation of a fibrin aggregate, albeit that this is initially softer than the thrombin-activated equivalent product.
- Type 1 collagen.
  Endogenous type I collagen is a weak platelet activator, so a lower yield of growth factors can be expected. On the plus side, the fibrin does not form a dense matrix.
- Photoactivation.
  A different method of activation is to expose the PRP for ten minutes to polychromatic light. This has been demonstrated to improve the release of growth factors.

Once again it is worth stating that while platelet activation is possible by thrombin, calcium chloride or calcium gluconate, and photoactivation, the most usual practice in small animal VRM is to rely on the tissue damage, including the exposed type I collagen, to activate the platelets in the PRP.

Controversies in platelet-rich plasma (PRP) therapy

The following questions regarding PRP formulation remain.

- Is there an optimal single PRP formulation and process for small animal VRM?
- What is the optimal platelet concentration in PRP for VRM?
- When and where should leukocyte-poor PRP be used?
- When and where should leukocyte-rich PRP be used?

As already stated, a large stumbling block in VRM is the heterogeneity of the product, and this is obviously the case in autologous PRP. To attempt to overcome this limitation, the practice of accurately measuring and recording the analysis of every PRP dose administered is recommended. In so doing, relevant and reliable conclusions may be drawn from a series of cases managed in practice. Alternatively, as mentioned above, using a pooled allogeneic PRP product may go a long way to removing many of the variables and unknowns about the PRP being injected.

The versatility afforded by the process of PRP production may be advantageous. Experienced clinicians and their technicians may become skilled in tailoring the PRP product to the condition being managed. In this way, PRP therapy may have elements of art as well as science. While this may seem like the antithesis of evidence-based veterinary medicine, it should nevertheless be borne in mind that the clinician does not have to accept a standardised ortho-biologic formulation and that adjustments can be made that could influence, and hopefully enhance, its biological activity. Where deviations from standard protocols are considered, precise recording of the analysis of the PRP before injection is advised.

Chapter 5 key points

- PRP in VRM is typically autologous, though an allogeneic product may become more widely available.
- Some form of PRP apparatus is required to produce autologous PRP.
- Filter systems have been used to concentrate platelets, though the product produced is not strictly speaking a PRP.
- Not all centrifuge systems produce equivalent PRP.
- The concentration of platelets in the PRP is important.
- The non-platelet constituents of PRP, including RBCs and various WBCs, need to be considered.
- Platelet activation prior to injection is possible.

Chapter 5 references

Alves, R., & Grimalt, R. (2018). A review of platelet-rich plasma: History, biology, mechanism of action, and classification. *Skin Appendage Disorders*, *4*(1), 18–24. https://doi.org/10.1159/000477353

Braun, H. J., Kim, H. J., Chu, C. R., & Dragoo, J. L. (2014). The effect of platelet-rich plasma formulations and blood products on human synoviocytes: Implications for intra-articular injury and therapy. *The American Journal of Sports Medicine*, *42*(5), 1204–1210. https://doi.org/10.1177/0363546514525593

Canapp, Jr., S. O., Canapp, D. A., Ibrahim, V., Carr, B. J., Cox, C., & Barrett, J. G. (2016). The use of adipose-derived progenitor cells and platelet-rich plasma combination for the treatment of supraspinatus tendinopathy in 55 dogs: A retrospective study. *Frontiers in Veterinary Science*, 3, 61. https://doi.org/10.3389/fvets.2016.00061

Carr, B. J. (2022). Platelet-rich plasma as an orthobiologic: Clinically relevant considerations. *The Veterinary Clinics of North America. Small Animal Practice*, *52*(4), 977–995. https://doi.org/10.1016/j.cvsm.2022.02.005

Carr, B. J., Canapp, Jr., S. O., Mason, D. R., Cox, C., & Hess, T. (2015). Canine platelet-rich plasma systems: A prospective analysis. *Frontiers in Veterinary Science*, 2, 73. https://doi.org/10.3389/fvets.2015.00073

Catarino, J., Carvalho, P., Santos, S., Martins, Â., & Requicha, J. (2020, August). Treatment of canine osteoarthritis with allogeneic platelet-rich plasma: Review of five cases. *Open Veterinary Journal*, *10*(2), 226–231. https://doi.org/10.4314/ovj.v10i2.12

Caviglia, H., Daffunchio, C., Galatro, G., Cambiaggi, G., Oneto, P., Douglas Price, A. L., Landro, M. E., & Etulain, J. (2020). Inhibition of Fenton reaction is a novel mechanism to explain the therapeutic effect of intra-articular injection of PRP in patients with chronic haemophilic synovitis. *Haemophilia*, *26*(4), e187–e193. https://doi.org/10.1111/hae.14075

Collins, T., Alexander, D., & Barkatali, B. (2021). Platelet-rich plasma: A narrative review. *EFORT Open Reviews*, *6*(4), 225–235. https://doi.org/10.1302/2058-5241.6.200017

Farghali, H. A., AbdElKader, N. A., Khattab, M. S., & AbuBakr, H. O. (2017). Evaluation of subcutaneous infiltration of autologous platelet-rich plasma on skin-wound healing in dogs. *Bioscience Reports*, *37*(2). https://doi.org/10.1042/BSR20160503

Fitzpatrick, J., Bulsara, M., & Zheng, M. H. (2016). The effectiveness of platelet-rich plasma in the treatment of tendinopathy: A meta-analysis of randomized controlled clinical trials. *The American Journal of Sports Medicine*, *45*(1), 226–233. https://doi.org/10.1177/0363546516643716

Kim, J.-H., Park, C., & Park, H.-M. (2009). Curative effect of autologous platelet-rich plasma on a large cutaneous lesion in a dog. *Veterinary Dermatology*, *20*(2), 123–126. https://doi.org/10.1111/j.1365-3164.2008.00711.x

Naldini, A., Morena, E., Fimiani, M., Campoccia, G., Fossombroni, V., & Carraro, F. (2008). The effects of autologous platelet gel on inflammatory cytokine response in human peripheral blood mononuclear cells. *Platelets*, *19*(4), 268–274. https://doi.org/10.1080/09537100801947426

Shin, H.-S., Woo, H.-M., & Kang, B.-J. (2017). Optimisation of a double-centrifugation method for preparation of canine platelet-rich plasma. *BMC Veterinary Research*, *13*(1), 198. https://doi.org/10.1186/s12917-017-1123-3

Sundman, E. A., Cole, B. J., & Fortier, L. A. (2011). Growth factor and catabolic cytokine concentrations are influenced by the cellular composition of platelet-rich plasma. *The American Journal of Sports Medicine*, *39*(10), 2135–2140. https://doi.org/10.1177/0363546511417792

Tambella, A. M., Attili, A. R., Dini, F., Palumbo Piccionello, A., Vullo, C., Serri, E., Scrollavezza, P., & Dupré, G. (2014). Autologous platelet gel to treat chronic decubital ulcers: A randomized, blind controlled clinical trial in dogs. *Veterinary Surgery*, *43*(6), 726–733. https://doi.org/10.1111/j.1532-950X.2014.12148.x

Upchurch, D. A., Renberg, W. C., Roush, J. K., Milliken, G. A., & Weiss, M. L. (2016). Effects of administration of adipose-derived stromal vascular fraction and platelet-rich plasma to dogs with osteoarthritis of the hip joints. *American Journal of Veterinary Research*, *77*(9), 940–951. https://doi.org/10.2460/ajvr.77.9.940

Yaradilmis, Y. U., Demirkale, I., Safa Tagral, A., Caner Okkaoglu, M., Ates, A., & Altay, M. (2020). Comparison of two platelet-rich plasma formulations with viscosupplementation in treatment of moderate grade gonarthrosis: A prospective randomized controlled study. *Journal of Orthopaedics*, *20*, 240–246. https://doi.org/10.1016/j.jor.2020.01.041

Yoshida, R., & Murray, M. M. (2013). Peripheral blood mononuclear cells enhance the anabolic effects of platelet-rich plasma on anterior cruciate ligament fibroblasts. *Journal of Orthopaedic Research*, *31*(1), 29–34. https://doi.org/10.1002/jor.22183

Zhou, Y., Zhang, J., Wu, H., Hogan, M. V., & Wang, J. H.-C. (2015, September 15). The differential effects of leukocyte-containing and pure platelet-rich plasma (PRP) on tendon stem/progenitor cells – Implications of PRP application for the clinical treatment of tendon injuries. *Stem Cell Research and Therapy*, *6*(1), 173. https://doi.org/10.1186/s13287-015-0172-4

Zubin, E., Conti, V., Leonardi, F., Zanichelli, S., Ramoni, R., & Grolli, S. (2015). Regenerative therapy for the management of a large skin wound in a dog. *Clinical Case Reports*, *3*(7), 598–603. https://doi.org/10.1002/ccr3.253

Chapter 6

Clinical platelet-rich plasma (PRP) applications

- Acute MSK injuries
  - muscle strains
  - ligament sprains
  - tendon injuries
- Chronic MSK conditions
  - partial CCL tears
  - OA
  - calcaneal tendon degeneration

Which tissues to inject?

Joints

IA injection is probably the most common site for PRP administration. Several of the techniques for IA injection were discussed in Chapter 3.

Ligaments

Ligament injection is best performed under MSK-ultrasound guidance.

Tendons

Again, ultrasonography is preferable for guiding the injections. A pattern of multiple, low-volume deposits of PRP throughout the damaged tendon is preferred. The technique of fenestration can be performed alongside PRP injection (Chiavaras & Jacobson, 2013). This involves repeatedly passing the needle through

When and where should platelet-rich plasma (PRP) be considered?

PRP can be applied when there is acute or chronic MSK pathology. In the acute situation, PRP has anti-inflammatory and analgesic effects. The platelet-derived molecules are trophic and help to recruit various cell types to the site of damage, promoting healing. Chronic disease states, such as OA, can also be positively impacted by IA-PRP injection. PRP is indicated in MSK cases where a trophic stimulus to the damaged tissues would be beneficial. The MSK indications include examples such as:

the affected tissue, such as in a case of supraspinatus enthesopathy (McDougall et al., 2018). The rationale is to convert a chronic inflammatory lesion into an acute lesion, which is more likely to heal in the presence of PRP (Chiavaras & Jacobson, 2013).

Muscles

Muscle tears can be localised using ultrasound, and multiple PRP injections can be administered in a grid pattern.

How to inject platelet-rich plasma (PRP)

The volume and concentration of platelets in the PRP may be controlled in most centrifuge systems, which allows some flexibility when preparing PRP injections. PRP can be injected intra-articularly using standard techniques (see Chapter 3). Absolute sterility in PRP preparation and strict aseptic technique are imperative. The injection is commonly done 'blindly', although veterinary clinicians skilled in MSK ultrasonography may be capable of ultrasound-assisted injections. By comparison, in human sports and rehabilitation medicine, ultrasound-guided IA injections are the standard of care.

The 'dose' of platelet-rich plasma (PRP)

Canine blood contains between 175,000 and 500,000 platelets per microlitre. This is equivalent to 175–500 million platelets per millilitre. Since the usual IA 'dose' of PRP is 1–3ml and the PRP concentration of platelets is 4–7 times higher than in circulation, the actual 'dose' of platelets received by the patient is in the order of billions (0.7–3.5 billion in this example). In human RM, it is common to quote the dose of platelets injected in billions.

What is the evidence for the efficacy of platelet-rich plasma (PRP)?

Debate continues over the efficacy of PRP in the management of human OA. A weak endorsement of PRP emerges from certain systematic reviews, such as the one published by Gato-Calvo et al. (2019). Another review concluded that PRP was more efficacious than other non-surgical methods (oral NSAID or IA-hyaluronic acid) of OA management (Hong et al., 2021).

In dogs, the heterogeneity of experimental methodologies and the inconsistencies of PRP preparation confound the issue of proving efficacy (Pye et al., 2022). Relatively small numbers of dogs are included, which further limits the studies' usefulness.

Recent studies provide examples of PRP application. In 2020, Venator et al. used a single dose of PRP, injected into twelve unstable CCL-deficient canine stifles. Improvements in force plate data were measured, albeit no control group was available for comparison.

The safety and efficacy of allogeneic PRP were studied in five dogs that were refractory to other modalities of OA management (Catarino et al., 2020). Improvement was reported, yet once again, this is difficult to extrapolate to a larger dog population and is also limited by the lack of a control group.

A positive effect of two doses of IA PRP, two weeks apart, was objectively demonstrated in a study involving ten treated dogs, compared to ten controls. This effect was measured using four clinical metrology instruments (CMIs) and lasted about 130 days (Alves et al., 2021).

In summary, the study of the effectiveness of PRP in dogs requires a much more standardised approach to permit appropriate scientific rigour to be applied (Carr et al., 2016). Comparing 'like with like' is necessary with PRP preparation, experimental design, and methodology. If and when a standardised approach has been established, large-scale multicentre randomised controlled trials (RCTs) could be conducted.

Regarding PRP safety, IA injection of PRP in dogs is relatively free of adverse events. Where this does occur, there is a temporary joint flare, lasting two or three days. In one experimental study, the increased lameness in some PRP-treated dogs with hip OA resolved spontaneously without treatment (Alves et al., 2021). Since this exacerbation of the pain and lameness is likely to be due to an inflammatory response, it is the author's recommendation to manage this using standard analgesic administration. Other surgeons may add cryotherapy in these patients (Armitage, 2024, personal communication).

Allogeneic PRP

At the time of writing, commercially supplied, pooled canine PRP is available in the United States by VetStem Biopharma Inc., Poway, California (see Chapter 5). It would be useful if this could become available elsewhere in the world in future.

Post-platelet-rich plasma (PRP) management recommendations

It is usual to advise reduced patient activity immediately following PRP administration (Carr, 2022). Dogs may have their exercise reduced in line with the underlying condition that is being treated. This typically means running, jumping, and playing will be prevented for at least two weeks.

In both human and VRM, clinicians have tended to be cautious about the concurrent use of drugs that may inhibit platelet function with PRP, with many, if not most, recommending withdrawal of NSAIDs. This practice was reviewed by Magruder and Rodeo in 2021. These authors concluded that in human patients, there was no conclusive evidence that NSAIDs would diminish PRP effectiveness. It is therefore the opinion of the author that, where clinically

necessary, NSAIDs may be administered along with PRP. Furthermore, it may be argued that withholding analgesia from a veterinary patient with a painful MSK condition cannot be justified ethically. Since patients who require PRP invariably have pain associated with the underlying condition before the PRP is administered, the majority will already be receiving analgesic medication. Of these agents, the most frequently prescribed category of medication is NSAIDs. The author typically adds PRP to a multimodal approach for the condition, continuing with the pre-existing medication.

A significant minority of PRP patients who have IA PRP administered will experience a 'joint flare'. This is a temporary, aseptic, inflammatory response to the injection/injected PRP that occurs within hours of the injection. In this situation, pain is exacerbated, and there may be swelling of the joint and increased lameness. Rest, along with NSAID administration, invariably allows the situation to settle down comfortably. Such a joint flare should not be confused with the rare but nonetheless possible iatrogenic bacterial joint infection. The latter is much more serious and would be expected to manifest days rather than hours post-injection.

As already implied, PRP is one mode of therapy for the MSK condition in question and is rarely a stand-alone method of treatment. As such, rehabilitation by physical therapy is usually another integral part of the treatment plan. Combining rehabilitation with PRP, it is suggested, can enhance its effectiveness, such as the duration of the beneficial PRP effects. This was demonstrated by Cuervo et al. (2020), although this study used plasma rich in growth factors (PRGFs), not PRP. Accordingly, physical rehabilitation should be recommended whenever practicable before and after PRP administration.

Photobiomodulation therapy, also known as low-level laser therapy, is another well-established modality in veterinary MSK medicine. Its application with PRP appears logical since polychromatic light has been demonstrated to activate platelets *in vitro* (Irmak et al., 2020). In human medicine, the idea of using light to activate the platelets as part of the processing of the PRP before injection into the patient has been proposed, this is called photo-activated PRP (Paterson et al., 2016; Jeyaraman et al., 2022). In veterinary practices, Class IV lasers are relatively commonplace, so combining the effects of laser therapy after the injection of PRP seems logical.

The combined effects of PRP and laser therapy were demonstrated in a small series of cases of canine hip OA by Alves et al. (2023). Additionally, Armitage et al. (2023) reported a large series of cases where a combination of PRP, autologous MSCs, and laser therapy were administered to refractory MSK cases. This combined approach may be expected to produce synergistic benefits for the patient.

Complications of platelet-rich plasma (PRP) therapy

As outlined previously in this chapter, adverse effects of PRP injection are fortunately generally rare, mild, and short in duration. They include:

- Discomfort associated with the injection, especially if it is IA.
- Joint flare, which is an inflammatory response to the biological components of the PRP.
- Infection from bacterial organisms on the animal's skin. This risk is small and mini-mised by attention to aseptic technique (see Chapter 3).

The contra-indications of PRP therapy were dis-cussed in Chapter 5.

Platelet-rich plasma (PRP) gel

Formulating a solid PRP-containing gel is use-ful in many situations where it is desirable to maintain the PRP in its intended location, such as a healing tendon. If this is performed, an improved and more prolonged effect of PRP in the tissues may be achievable. Various methods of PRP gel production are possible (Mazzucco et al., 2009). A brief outline is detailed: Blood is centrifuged at 1,500-g for 15 minutes in a gel tube containing added calcium chloride. The mechanical stress of the spinning releases Ca^{2+} ions, which in turn allows the conversion of soluble fibrinogen into insoluble fibrin. The resulting clot includes platelets. Autologous thrombin is required, and this is extracted from the patient's blood before being added to autologous platelet-poor plasma and calcium gluconate. Finally, the addition of the throm-bin and PRP produces the formation of a gel (Fig. 6.1).

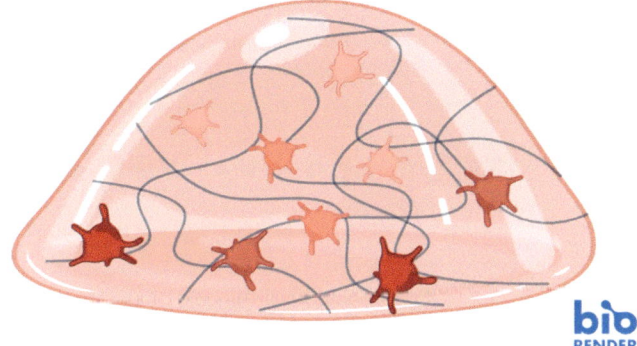

Fig. 6.1 A diagrammatic representation of PRP gel. The gel contains fibrin strands and suspended platelets.

Chapter 6 key points

- PRP is a versatile orthobiologic and is useful in both acute and chronic MSK conditions.
- PRP can be injected into joints, connective tissues (such as ligaments and tendons), and skeletal muscle.
- PRP can be injected blindly or, more preferably, with ultrasound guidance when targeting soft tissue lesions.
- There is a large literature on the efficacy of PRP in small animals.
- PRP can be integrated into a multimodal approach to conditions such as OA.
- Complications of PRP therapy are typically mild and short-lived.
- The contra-indications of PRP therapy should be known and adhered to.

Chapter 6 references

Alves, J. C., Santos, A., & Jorge, P. (2021). Platelet-rich plasma therapy in dogs with bilateral hip osteoarthritis. *BMC Veterinary Research*, *17*(1), 207. https://doi.org/10.1186/s12917-021-02913-x

Alves, J. C., Santos, A., & Carreira, L. M. (2023). A preliminary report on the combined effect of intra-articular platelet-rich plasma injections and photobiomodulation in canine osteoarthritis. *Animals: An Open Access Journal from MDPI*, *13*(20), 3247. https://doi.org/10.3390/ani13203247

Armitage, A. J., Miller, J. M., Sparks, T. H., Georgiou, A. E., & Reid, J. (2022). Efficacy of autologous mesenchymal stromal cell treatment for chronic degenerative musculoskeletal conditions in dogs: A retrospective study. *Frontiers in Veterinary Science*, *9*, 1014687. https://doi.org/10.3389/fvets.2022.1014687

Carr, B. J. (2022). Platelet-rich plasma as an orthobiologic: Clinically relevant considerations. *The Veterinary Clinics of North America. Small Animal Practice*, *52*(4), 977–995. https://doi.org/10.1016/j.cvsm.2022.02.005

Carr, B. J., Canapp, Jr., S. O., Mason, D. R., Cox, C., & Hess, T. (2016). Canine platelet-rich plasma systems: A prospective analysis. *Frontiers in Veterinary Science*, *2*, 73. https://doi.org/10.3389/fvets.2015.00073

Catarino, J., Carvalho, P., Santos, S., Martins, Â., & Requicha, J. (2020). Treatment of canine osteoarthritis with allogeneic platelet-rich plasma: Review of five cases. *Open Veterinary Journal*, *10*(2), 226–231. https://doi.org/10.4314/ovj.v10i2.12

Chiavaras, M. M., & Jacobson, J. A. (2013, February). Ultrasound-guided tendon fenestration. In *Seminars in Musculoskeletal Radiology* (Vol. 17, No. 01, pp. 085–090). Thieme Medical Publishers, 17(1), 85–90. https://doi.org/10.1055/s-0033-1333942

Cuervo, B., Rubio, M., Chicharro, D., Damiá, E., Santana, A., Carrillo, J. M., Romero, A. D., Vilar, J. M., Cerón, J. J., & Sopena, J. J. (2020). Objective comparison between platelet-rich plasma alone and in combination with physical therapy in dogs with osteoarthritis caused by hip dysplasia. *Animals: An Open Access Journal from MDPI*, *10*(2), 175. https://doi.org/10.3390/ani10020175

Gato-Calvo, L., Magalhaes, J., Ruiz-Romero, C., Blanco, F. J., & Burguera, E. F. (2019). Platelet-rich plasma in osteoarthritis treatment: Review of current evidence. *Therapeutic Advances in Chronic Disease*, *10*, 2040622319825567. https://doi.org/10.1177/2040622319825567

Hong, M., Cheng, C., Sun, X., Yan, Y., Zhang, Q., Wang, W., & Guo, W. (2021). Efficacy and safety of intra-articular platelet-rich plasma in osteoarthritis knee: A systematic review and meta-analysis. *BioMed Research International*, *2021*, 2191926. https://doi.org/10.1155/2021/2191926

Irmak, G., Demirtaş, T. T., & Gümüşderelioğlu, M. (2020). Sustained release of growth factors from photoactivated platelet-rich plasma (PRP). *European Journal of Pharmaceutics and Biopharmaceutics*, *148*, 67–76. https://doi.org/10.1016/j.ejpb.2019.11.011

Jeyaraman, M., Muthu, S., Jeyaraman, N., & Gupta, A. (2022). Photoactivated platelet-rich plasma: Is it the future of platelet-rich plasma? *Regenerative Medicine*, *17*(9), 607–609. https://doi.org/10.2217/rme-2022-0063

Magruder, M., & Rodeo, S. A. (2021). Is antiplatelet therapy contraindicated after platelet-rich treatment? A narrative review. *Orthopaedic Journal of Sports Medicine*, *9*(6), 23259671211010510. https://doi.org/10.1177/23259671211010510

Mazzucco, L., Balbo, V., Cattana, E., Guaschino, R., & Borzini, P. (2009). Not every PRP-gel is born equal Evaluation of growth factor availability for tissues through four PRP-gel preparations: Fibrinet®, RegenPRP-Kit®, Plateltex® and one manual procedure. *Vox Sanguinis*, *97*(2), 110–118. https://doi.org/10.1111/j.1423-0410.2009.01188.x

McDougall, R. A., Canapp, S. O., & Canapp, D. A. (2018). Ultrasonographic findings in 41 dogs treated with bone marrow aspirate concentrate and platelet-rich plasma for a supraspinatus tendinopathy: A retrospective study. *Frontiers in Veterinary Science*, *5*, 98. https://doi.org/10.3389/fvets.2018.00098

Paterson, K. L., Nicholls, M., Bennell, K. L., & Bates, D. (2016). Intra-articular injection of photo-activated platelet-rich plasma in patients with knee osteoarthritis: A double-blind, randomized controlled pilot study. *BMC Musculoskeletal Disorders*, *17*, 67. https://doi.org/10.1186/s12891-016-0920-3

Pye, C., Bruniges, N., Peffers, M., & Comerford, E. (2022). Advances in the pharmaceutical treatment options for canine osteoarthritis. *The Journal of Small Animal Practice*, *63*(10), 721–738. https://doi.org/10.1111/jsap.13495

Venator, K. P., Frye, C. W., Gamble, L.-J., & Wakshlag, J. J. (2020). Assessment of a single intra-articular stifle injection of pure platelet-rich plasma on symmetry indices in dogs with unilateral or bilateral stifle osteoarthritis from long-term medically managed cranial cruciate ligament disease. *Veterinary Medicine*, *11*, 31–38. https://doi.org/10.2147/VMRR.S238598

Section III

Chapter 7

Mesenchymal stem cells (MSCs)

All the cells of the body are descendants of stem cells. Stem cells are an essential component of the body's repair kit. Their functions include replacing cells and repairing damaged tissue. Without a functioning reserve of stem cells, animals cannot survive.

Stem cell classification by potency

Early embryos are composed of undifferentiated cells. These are capable of differentiating into any cell in the body or extra-embryonic tissues. These stem cells are referred to as **totipotent**.

Once the embryonic inner cell mass forms, it consists of cells that can become any cell type in the body but not the extra-embryonic tissues. These cells are referred to as **pluripotent**. Pluripotency means stem cells can give rise to cells of any of the three embryonic layers, namely ectoderm, mesoderm, or endoderm. As they develop into specialised adult cells, their potency becomes narrowed.

Cells may follow a haemopoietic path, giving rise to HSCs. These can differentiate down the erythrocyte, leukocyte, or myeloid lines. This ability is referred to as **multipotency**. Multipotent stem cells can differentiate into cell types of a particular embryonic cell layer. Examples of multipotent stem cells include neural stem cells and MSCs. Neural stem cells are ectodermal and can give rise to cells of the nervous system such as neurons and glial cells. MSCs, on the other hand, can differentiate into various cells of the mesodermal layer, such as adipocytes, chondrocytes, and osteoblasts. Notably, tri-lineage differentiation, in the laboratory, along the aforementioned three paths is one of the features that define MSCs in both humans and animals.

The further removed from the embryonic situation stem cells are found, the less 'potent' they become (potency describes the range of fully differentiated adult cells they can become). Hence, certain stem cells may also be described as **oligopotent** and **bipotent**.

An essential feature of all stem cells is their ability to self-renew. This prevents, under normal circumstances, the stem cell reserves from becoming exhausted, as such an eventuality would be catastrophic for the viability of the organism. Ageing is an enemy of stem cells, and older animals have depleted stem cell capabilities. This is of significance when considering the source of donor cells for a particular indication. For example, autologous adipose-derived MSCs (AD-MSCs) or bone marrow-derived MSCs may be considered for IA injection for OA. In the case of an elderly patient, one can predict that the MSCs acquired are likely to be less biologically active than those acquired from a younger patient. For this reason, an argument could be made for the use of younger MSCs being used to transplant into an older patient. This can be achieved by using either allogeneic or xenogeneic donor animals. The youngest adult MSCs are acquired from the fetal adnexa. Thus, umbilical cord MSCs such as DogStem® (Dômes Pharma) could theoretically be more efficacious.

The direction of travel of cells from pluripotent to multipotent, and so on, and becoming more specialised as they get closer to the fully differentiated adult somatic cells, was considered a compelling concept. It was believed that cells could become more specialised as successive rounds of asymmetrical division occurred, ultimately leading to a steady supply of specialist adult cells, while sufficient symmetrical division of stem cells maintained appropriate reserve populations in the various stem cell niches. This was until the discovery in 2006 by Yamanaka's and later Thompson's laboratories, who discovered that adult somatic cells could be reprogrammed back to a pluripotent state. The new branch of stem cell science relating to iPSCs was born. To date, the author is not aware of any clinically available iPSC product available for veterinary use. Nonetheless, some awareness of the technology that can effectively reverse the differentiation adult cells have undergone so they can be returned first to pluripotency and subsequently differentiated potentially into any type of cell does exist.

In summary, stem cells may be embryonic stem cells, adult stem cells, or iPSCs. Of these, it is only a member of the adult stem cell group, namely MSCs, that is currently available for VRM.

MSCs can be further classified by their source tissue (see Chapter 8).

What makes an MSC an MSC?

Mesenchymal stromal cells, or mesenchymal stem cells (MSCs), are the key cells used in orthobiologics. This term was coined by Arnold Caplan in 1991 to describe a multipotent precursor cell found in mesodermal tissues. MSCs have the following properties:

- Self-replication by symmetrical division.
- Multipotency such that they have tri-lineage differentiation capacity by asymmetrical division.
- Immunophenotype surface marker signature.
- Surface adherence.
- Spindle-shaped morphology.
- Gene expression profile.
- Paracrine effects.

Self-replication by symmetrical division

Stem cells are essential for life. Without continual replacement of cells that are lost, tissues and organs cannot be maintained, and repair will not be possible. Stem cells preserve their population numbers by mitotically dividing to produce identical daughter cells with the same gene-expression characteristics as the parent stem cell (Fig. 1.2). This is termed **symmetrical division**.

Stem cell senescence

It has been suggested that there may be a natural limit on the number of cell divisions that are possible throughout life. This is known as the 'Hayflick limit' (Hayflick & Moorhead, 1961). One determinant of chromosome longevity is the length of the telomeres. Telomeres are the non-coding nucleotide sequences at the chromosome ends. Their length is in inverse proportion to the cell's viability over successive divisions. Older cells have shorter telomeres. Eventually, the telomeres become too short to be compatible with effective chromosomal replication. MSCs are known to undergo senescence in both *in vivo* and *in vitro* situations (Liu et al., 2020).

Multipotency

MSCs, by definition, must be capable of multipotency, such that they have tri-lineage differentiation capacity by asymmetrical division. This is a prerequisite for a cell to be described as an MSC. It is important to note that while MSCs can be induced to differentiate *in vitro* by relevant laboratory conditions specific to each lineage, this may not necessarily be what occurs *in vivo*. As discussed elsewhere in this book, an implanted MSC is much more likely to rapidly undergo death by apoptosis than it is to survive, engraft, and differentiate. This apoptotic process, coun-ter-intuitively, appears to be an essential event in allowing the MSCs to have their therapeutic effects (Weiss & Dahlke, 2019).

Immunophenotype of mesenchymal stem cells (MSCs)

All cells have a surface marker expression, or cluster of differentiation (CD) signature, which is used to classify them according to their immunophenotype. Canine MSCs have a surface marker signature as depicted in Fig. 2.3 (Chapter 2). Positive markers found on canine MSCs include CD90, CD73, CD105, CD29, and CD44. A minimum of two of these is required for classification, though the expression of all five is ideal. Canine MSCs should not express the following: CD79alpha/CD19, CD14/CD11b, CD34, and CD45. Again, as a minimum, the absence of two of these is required, though the absence of expression of all four is ideal. Finally, and very importantly, MHC-II should be absent from the MSCs.

Surface adherence

The propensity of MSCs to adhere to surfaces, whether *in vitro* (e.g., laboratory plasticware) or *in vivo* (within the MSC niche), is an essential feature of these cells. This feature is highlighted by the International Society for Cellular Therapy in the human field (Dominici et al., 2006), with similar guidelines established in the veterinary field (Guest et al., 2022). The simplicity of the term 'MSC surface adherence' belies a rather complex biological process (Shotorbani et al., 2017). Multiple factors influence this process. These include biological, chemical, and physical characteristics such as hydrophilicity, material roughness, physical stress, and electrical charge (Dong et al., 2013). As for the known adherence molecules, these largely belong to the following broad categories: integrins, transmembrane glycoproteins, and occludins (Shotorbani et al., 2017).

The relevance of surface adherence by MSCs in VRM is that if it is possible to mimic the natural environment of MSCs, then this is likely to enhance their survival and longevity within the recipient tissue. In so doing, the potential for a more potent regenerative effect of the MSCs seems likely, as does a longer duration of effect. An active branch of RM concerns itself with implantable biomaterials whose function is to enhance the effects of transplanted cells, such as MSCs, by providing a favourable locale for adherence and biological thriving. A detailed discussion of biomaterials is beyond the scope of this present publication.

Spindle-shaped morphology

Under light microscopy, MSCs have a spindle-shaped morphology and resemble fibroblasts. In culture, they often form a monolayer as each cell tends to adhere to the surface. The density of the cell population on the plastic surface is referred to as 'confluency'. This is expressed as a percentage of the area occupied by the cells compared to the available area. Confluency is important for deciding when to subculture a cell colony.

Gene expression profile

A detailed discussion of the methodology by which gene expression profiles are determined is beyond the scope of this book. It is worth noting that MSCs have transcriptomic profiles that can be determined by RNA sequencing. Such assays can be useful as gene expression may be influenced by manipulation of the *in vitro* conditions (such as when MSCs are 'preconditioned' by hypoxia to enhance their function before transplantation (Zielniok et al., 2021)).

Multiple *in vitro* passages of MSCs result in morphological, immunophenotypic, and genetic changes (Yang et al., 2018). This drift away from the desirable MSC characteristics with successive passages and extended laboratory culture is a challenge in VRM.

Paracrine effects

The primary modus operandi of MSCs is using short-range, cell-to-cell communication, referred to as paracrine signalling. This is illustrated and compared with other categories (autocrine and endocrine) in Figure 4.3 in Chapter 4.

Table 7.1 lists many of the effects of MSCs along with the secreted factors that have been elucidated as mediating these processes. The upper part of the table lists some of the known factors that have been isolated and the specific activities they exhibit. The lower part of the table cites papers where the effects of MSC-derived extra-cellular vesicles (EVs) have been demonstrated to have the various biological effects described. In the latter case, the EVs contain multiple factors.

Figure 7.2 (adapted from Mancuso et al., 2019) summarises the proposed mechanism by which endogenous MSCs, derived from pericytes,

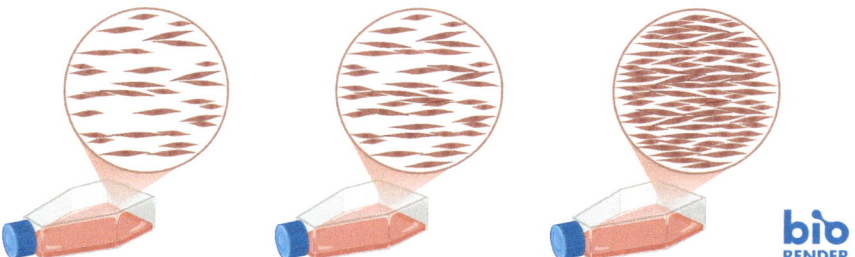

Fig. 7.1 Diagrammatic representation of MSCs in culture. From left to right: low confluency, medium confluency and high confluency.

Table 7.1 MSC secretome: selected known MSC's actions in OA and bioactive molecular factors involved. Redrawn from Mancuso et al. 2019. STC-1 stanniocalcin-1; bFGF basic fibroblast growth factor; AMD adrenomedullin; HGF hepatocyte growth factor; TIMP-1 tissue inhibitor of metalloproteinases-1; TIMP-2 tissue inhibitor of metalloproteinases-2; PGE2 prostaglandin E2; TSG-6 thromosponin-6 EVs extra-cellular vesicles.

Activity	Factor	References
Anti-apoptosis	STC-1	Rehman et al., 2004; Block et al., 2009
Anti-fibrosis	bFGF, AMD, HGF	Li et al., 2009; Suga et al., 2009; Maumus et al., 2013
Tissue metabolism	TIMP-1, TIMP-2	Lozito & Tuan, 2011
Chondrogenesis	TSP-2	Jeong et al., 2013; Jeong et al., 2015
Immunosuppression	PGE2	Aggarwal & Pittenger, 2005; Sotiropoulou et al., 2008; Martinet et al., 2009
Immunosuppression	TSG-6	Mindrescu et al., 2000; Bàrdos et al., 2001; Lee et al., 2009
Anti-apoptosis	EVs	Liu et al., 2018[a]; Liu et al., 2018[b]
Immunosuppression	EVs	Mokarizadeh et al., 2012; Budoni et al., 2013; Zhang et al., 2014
Chondrogenesis	EVs	Zhu et al., 2017
Chondroprotection/ anti-inflammatory	EVs	Cosenza et al., 2017

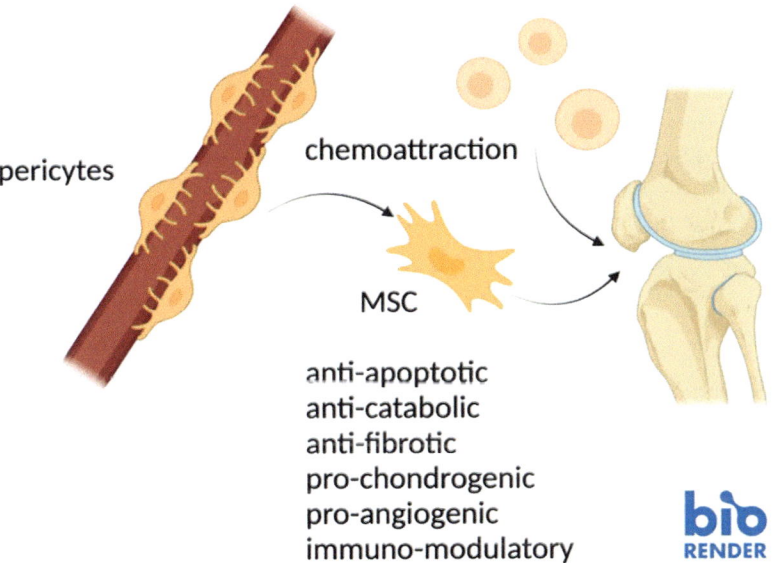

Fig. 7.2 Endogenous pericytes from tissue capillaries are the source of MSCs. The MSCs have multiple beneficial effects in the tissues. Redrawn from Mancuso et al. (2019).

effect joint tissue repair. The principal direct effects include anti-apoptotic, anti-catabolic, anti-fibrotic, pro-chondrogenic, pro-angiogenic, and immunomodulatory actions. Additionally, the chemoattraction of other endogenous cell types further enhances the healing process.

Immune evasion by mesenchymal stem cells (MSCs)

The administration of expanded populations of autologous MSCs appears logical, given the almost non-existent risk of immune rejection. This is because the auto-transplanted MSCs and the host tissues theoretically share an identical immunophenotype. However, this may not be entirely accurate, as *in vitro* culture and expansion of cells can be associated with genetic changes that may alter cell surface markers (Jeske et al., 2021). Nevertheless, a high degree of confidence in the immune compatibility between transplanted MSCs and the host can be expected with autologous MSC injections.

Turning to allogeneic MSCs, which are obviously 'foreign' to the recipient animal. In this case, 'immune privilege' has been a term ascribed to MSCs, due to their apparent very low immunogenicity when transplanted allogeneically or even xenogeneically. However, this convenient and popular term is somewhat inaccurate; MSCs may be better described as hypoimmunogenic when interacting with the recipient's immune system.

MSCs are certainly capable of largely evading the immune system. Their lack of MHC-II surface markers may substantially explain this observation. MHC-II plays a key role in the innate immune system's ability to recognise and respond to foreign cells. Thus, these MHC-II negative MSCs can evade detection to a higher degree than other MHC-II positive cell types.

The immune evasion capability of MSCs is a crucially important feature in VRM. Since allogeneic and even xenogeneic cell transplantation is often considered, being able to enter the host tissues relatively undetected by the immune system is of enormous importance. This contrasts with whole-organ, allogeneic transplant surgery in humans, which typically requires life-long, post-transplant immunosuppressive therapy. In the case of MSC transplantation, no such follow-up medication is necessary.

'Licensing' of mesenchymal stem cells (MSCs)

The interactions of transplanted MSCs with the immune system are complex. It is accepted that resident MSCs in tissue can have either pro-inflammatory or anti-inflammatory effects. In this context, the slightly confusing term of 'licensing' of MSCs refers not to the acquisition of regulatory permission for a commercial product but instead to the process of maturation that the cells undergo after transplantation (Krampera, 2011). Depending on the environment in which the injected MSCs find themselves, especially with regard to the degree and stage of inflammation (acute versus chronic), the MSC phenotype can be polarised differently. Thus, the MSC 'licensing' process can lead to the acquisition of immunomodulatory instead of immune-stimulatory functions.

Immunomodulatory properties of mesenchymal stem cells (MSCs)

When MSCs are transplanted into the host environment, such as an osteoarthritic joint, multiple interactions are possible with the resident cells and the immune system. Of the known effects on macrophages, a well-established effect is the ability of MSCs to favour the polarisation of the phenotype from the M1 (inflammatory) macrophage to the M2 (anti-inflammatory) version. Figure 2.5 in Chapter 2 summarises this phenomenon and, in addition, illustrates the effects of MSCs on other immune cells, including T-cells, T-reg cells, natural killer cells, dendritic cells, and B-cells.

Mesenchymal stem cell (MSC) secretome

The secretome of a cell or tissue refers to the total collection of all the bioactive molecules and factors released into the extra-cellular space (Merlo & Iacono, 2023). These may be soluble or contained within membrane-bound EVs. The secretome includes proteins, lipids, and free nucleic acids such as microRNAs, which are important non-protein-coding RNA molecules that regulate the translation of mRNA in the endoplasmic reticulum of the cell.

Extra-cellular vesicles (EVs) of mesenchymal stem cells (MSCs)

As already alluded, cells, including MSCs, secrete small, phospholipid membrane-surrounded structures termed 'extra-cellular vesicles' (EVs) (Thornton, 2023). The EV cargo comprises various molecules, including growth factors, cytokines, lipids, mRNAs, and microRNAs (Toh et al., 2017). A significant portion of the paracrine cell-to-cell communication is now understood to be mediated by these EV-contained molecules (Merlo & Iacono, 2023). It has been suggested, this being the case, that MSC-derived EVs may be effective as an orthobiologic instead of requiring the whole of the parent MSC. Using EVs instead of MSCs would have several advantages, including that they can be produced in large quantities, the costs of manufacture may be reduced, and the risk of adverse immunologic effects is even lower than with MSCs *per se* (Li et al., 2019; Merlo & Iacono, 2023).

Mitochondrial transfer by mesenchymal stem cells (MSCs)

The donation, by MSCs, of viable mitochondria to various recipient cells is well established (Velarde et al., 2022). Different modes of mitochondrial transfer may occur, such as by apoptotic bodies, EVs, microvesicles, fusion of cells, across gap junctions, and by the formation of intracellular nanotubes. Such provision of mitochondria to cells in the target tissue may be another mechanism by which beneficial regenerative effects could be produced by MSC transplantation.

Necrobiology of mesenchymal stem cells (MSCs)

MSCs are generally considered to be a 'living medicine'. This is logical since it is live cells that are typically injected or implanted into the target tissue. Transplanted MSCs can influence host tissue via dead or dying cells or their released subcellular particles (Weiss & Dahlke, 2019). The processes associated with MSC death, autophagy, and apoptosis may be a requirement for therapeutic efficacy. Indeed, it may be the host response to these processes that affects the downstream positive consequences seen. Apoptosis is a controlled process distinct from the much less desirable uncontrolled and pro-inflammatory cell necrosis (Fig. 7.3).

Efferocytosis

The removal of apoptotic cells by phagocytes may be performed without an immunological response. This is termed 'efferocytosis', and leads to a tissue repair response (Yin et al., 2021).

Mesenchymal stem cell (MSC) autophagy

Autophagy is a process by which cells can recycle their constituents, including organelles, in a controlled manner. MSCs, when transplanted into the host environment, such as the inflammatory milieu of an osteoarthritic joint, are likely to activate their 'autophagy program'. In so doing, structures such as membrane-bound vesicles and even mitochondria become available for donation from the MSCs to the resident

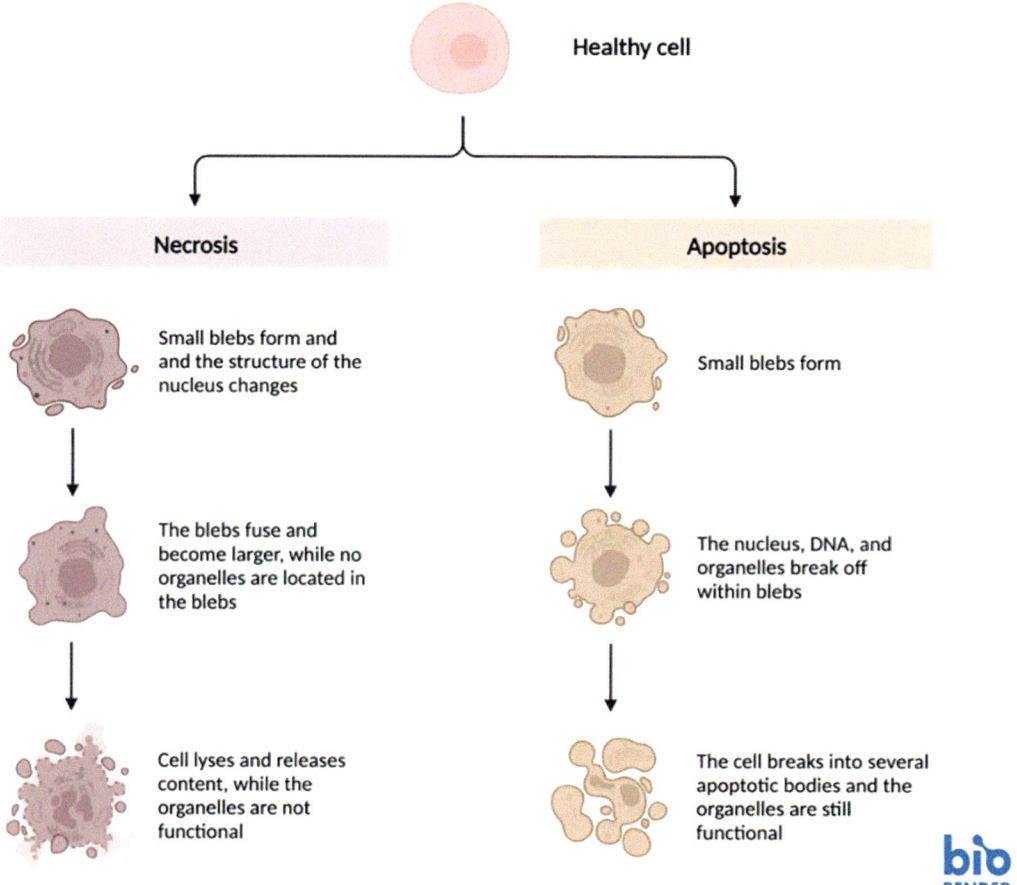

Fig. 7.3 Graphical representation of the differences between cell death by necrosis and by apoptosis (modified after Gaia Lugano – BioRender).

cells. By undergoing this autophagic process, the demise of the MSCs actually promotes the beneficial effects such as the immunomodulation characteristic of MSC therapy.

Homing of mesenchymal stem cells (MSCs)

MSCs can migrate towards the site of tissue damage (Ullah et al., 2019). While this is a useful trait in VRM, it is rather inefficient for systemic administration of MSCs, such as by intravenous (IV) injection. Only a low percentage of IV-injected MSCs typically reach their target, as the majority become 'trapped' in the pulmonary capillary bed. Various methods have been investigated to improve MSC homing. Readers are referred to the review by Ullah et al. (2019). Due to the significant challenges associated with systemic administration of MSCs, targeted administration by injecting the cells directly into the damaged tissue remains the primary means of applying this therapy.

It is hoped that this chapter has imparted a flavour of the complexities of MSC biology. It would be easy to become overwhelmed by the sheer amount of scientific information that is known about these remarkable cells. The author has attempted to navigate through the relevant material in a way that explains the principles of MSC function as they pertain to clinical veterinary practice. To round up the section, a concise précis is offered. The multitude of potential actions of transplanted MSCs in the recipient tissues was neatly summarised by Arnold Caplan (1991) – he succinctly described MSCs as 'site-regulated multi-drug dispensaries'.

> ## Chapter 7 key points
>
> - Stem cells may be classified by their pluri-, multi-, or oligo-potency.
> - There are conventional characteristics that define MSCs.
> - Self-replication of stem cells occurs by symmetrical division.
> - Stem cell senescence is associated with repeated divisions.
> - There is a specific immunophenotype of MSCs.
> - Adherence to plastic surfaces is a feature of MSCs.
> - MSCs have a spindle-shaped morphology *in vitro*.
> - MSCs have a recognised gene expression profile.
> - The actions of MSCs occur via their paracrine effects.
> - Immune evasion by MSCs accounts for their lack of immunogenicity.
> - Immunomodulatory properties of MSCs allow them to interact with the host immune system.
> - The necrobiology of MSCs is integral to their function.
> - Efferocytosis is a process whereby apoptotic cells may be removed without inflammation.
> - MSC autophagy facilitates the recycling of organelles such as mitochondria.
> - Homing of MSCs may occur, allowing them to move to the site of tissue damage.

Chapter 7 references

Aggarwal, S., & Pittenger, M. F. (2005). Human mesenchymal stem cells modulate allogeneic immune cell responses. *Blood*, *105*(4), 1815–1822. https://doi.org/10.1182/blood-2004-04-1559

Bárdos, T., Kamath, R. V., Mikecz, K., & Glant, T. T. (2001). Anti-inflammatory and chondroprotective effect of TSG-6 (tumor necrosis factor-α-stimulated gene-6) in murine models of experimental arthritis. *The American Journal of Pathology*, *159*(5), 1711–1721. https://doi.org/10.1016/s0002-9440(10)63018-0

Block, G. J., Ohkouchi, S., Fung, F., Frenkel, J., Gregory, C., Pochampally, R., DiMattia, G., Sullivan, D. E., & Prockop, D. J. (2009). Multipotent stromal cells are activated to reduce apoptosis in part by upregulation and secretion of stanniocalcin-1. *Stem Cells*, *27*(3), 670–681. https://doi.org/10.1002/stem.20080742

Budoni, M., Fierabracci, A., Luciano, R., Petrini, S., Di Ciommo, V., & Muraca, M. (2013). The immunosuppressive effect of mesenchymal stromal cells on B lymphocytes is mediated by membrane vesicles. *Cell Transplantation*, *22*(2), 369–379. https://doi.org/10.3727/096368911X582769

Caplan, A. I. (1991). Mesenchymal stem cells. *Journal of Orthopaedic Research*, *9*(5), 641–650. https://doi.org/10.1002/jor.1100090504

Cosenza, S., Ruiz, M., Toupet, K., Jorgensen, C., & Noël, D. (2017). Mesenchymal stem cells derived exosomes and microparticles protect cartilage and bone from degradation in osteoarthritis. *Scientific Reports*, *7*(1), 16214. https://doi.org/10.1038/s41598-017-15376-8

Dominici, M. L. B. K., Le Blanc, K., Mueller, I., Slaper-Cortenbach, I., Marini, F. C., Krause, D. S., Deans, R., Keating, A., Prockop, Dj., & Horwitz, E. M. (2006). Minimal criteria for defining multipotent mesenchymal stromal cells. The International Society for Cellular Therapy position statement. *Cytotherapy*, *8*(4), 315–317. https://doi.org/10.1080/14653240600855905

Dong, S., Guo, H., Zhang, Y., Li, Z., Kang, F., Yang, B., Kang, X., Wen, C., Yan, Y., Jiang, B., & Fan, Y. (2013). rFN/Cad-11-modified collagen type II biomimetic interface promotes the adhesion and chondrogenic differentiation of mesenchymal stem cells.

Tissue Engineering. Part A, *19*(21–22), 2464–2477. https://doi.org/10.1089/ten.tea.2012.0447

Guest, D. J., Dudhia, J., Smith, R. K. W., Roberts, S. J., Conzemius, M., Innes, J. F., Fortier, L. A., & Meeson, R. L. (2022). Position statement: Minimal criteria for reporting veterinary and animal medicine research for mesenchymal stromal/stem cells in orthopaedic applications. *Frontiers in Veterinary Science*, *9*, 817041. https://doi.org/10.3389/fvets.2022.817041

Hayflick, L., & Moorhead, P. S. (1961). The serial cultivation of human diploid cell strains. *Experimental Cell Research*, *25*(3), 585–621. https://doi.org/10.1016/0014-4827(61)90192-6

Jeong, S. Y., Ha, J., Lee, M., Jin, H. J., Kim, D. H., Choi, S. J., Oh, W., Yang, Y. S., Kim, J.-S., Kim, B.-G., Chang, J. H., Cho, D.-H., & Jeon, H. B. (2015). Autocrine action of thrombospondin-2 determines the chondrogenic differentiation potential and suppresses hypertrophic maturation of human umbilical cord blood-derived mesenchymal stem cells. *Stem Cells*, *33*(11), 3291–3303. https://doi.org/10.1002/stem.2120

Jeong, S. Y., Kim, D. H., Ha, J., Jin, H. J., Kwon, S.-J., Chang, J. W., Choi, S. J., Oh, W., Yang, Y. S., Kim, G., Kim, J. S., Yoon, J.-R., Cho, D. H., & Jeon, H. B. (2013). Thrombospondin-2 secreted by human umbilical cord blood-derived mesenchymal stem cells promotes chondrogenic differentiation. *Stem Cells*, *31*(10), 2136–2148. https://doi.org/10.1002/stem.1471

Jeske, R., Yuan, X., Fu, Q., Bunnell, B. A., Logan, T. M., & Li, Y. (2021). In vitro culture expansion shifts the immune phenotype of human adipose-derived mesenchymal stem cells. *Frontiers in Immunology*, *12*, 621744. https://doi.org/10.3389/fimmu.2021.621744

Krampera, M. (2011). Mesenchymal stromal cell "licensing": A multistep process. *Leukemia*, *25*(9), 1408–1414. https://doi.org/10.1038/leu.2011.108

Lee, R. H., Pulin, A. A., Seo, M. J., Kota, D. J., Ylostalo, J., Larson, B. L., Semprun-Prieto, L., Delafontaine, P., & Prockop, D. J. (2009). Intravenous hMSCs improve myocardial infarction in mice because cells embolized in lung are activated to secrete the anti-inflammatory protein TSG-6. *Cell Stem Cell*, *5*(1), 54–63. https://doi.org/10.1016/j.stem.2009.05.003

Li, J. J., Hosseini-Beheshti, E., Grau, G. E., Zreiqat, H., & Little, C. B. (2019). Stem cell-derived extracellular vesicles for treating joint injury and osteoarthritis. *Nanomaterials*, *9*(2), 261. https://doi.org/10.3390/nano9020261

Li, L., Zhang, S., Zhang, Y., Yu, B., Xu, Y., & Guan, Z. (2009). Paracrine action mediates the antifibrotic effect of transplanted mesenchymal stem cells in a rat model of global heart failure. *Molecular Biology Reports*, *36*(4), 725–731. https://doi.org/10.1007/s11033-008-9235-2

Liu, J., Ding, Y., Liu, Z., & Liang, X. (2020). Senescence in mesenchymal stem cells: Functional alterations, molecular mechanisms, and rejuvenation strategies. *Frontiers in Cell and Developmental Biology*, *8*, 258. https://doi.org/10.3389/fcell.2020.00258

Liu, Y., Lin, L., Zou, R., Wen, C., Wang, Z., & Lin, F. (2018[a]). MSC-derived exosomes promote proliferation and inhibit apoptosis of chondrocytes via lncRNA-KLF3-AS1/miR-206/GIT1 axis in osteoarthritis. *Cell Cycle*, *17*(21–22), 2411–2422. https://doi.org/10.1080/15384101.2018.1526603

Liu, Y., Zou, R., Wang, Z., Wen, C., Zhang, F., & Lin, F. (2018[b]). Exosomal KLF3-AS1 from hMSCs promoted cartilage repair and chondrocyte proliferation in osteoarthritis. *The Biochemical Journal*, *475*(22), 3629–3638. https://doi.org/10.1042/BCJ20180675

Lozito, T. P., & Tuan, R. S. (2011). Mesenchymal stem cells inhibit both endogenous and exogenous MMPs via secreted TIMPs. *Journal of Cellular Physiology*, *226*(2), 385–396. https://doi.org/10.1002/jcp.22344

Mancuso, P., Raman, S., Glynn, A., Barry, F., & Murphy, J. M. (2019). Mesenchymal stem cell therapy for osteoarthritis: The critical role of the cell secretome. *Frontiers in Bioengineering and Biotechnology*, *7*, 9. https://doi.org/10.3389/fbioe.2019.00009

Martinet, L., Fleury-Cappellesso, S., Gadelorge, M., Dietrich, G., Bourin, P., Fournié, J.-J., & Poupot, R. (2009). A regulatory cross-talk between Vγ9Vδ2 T lymphocytes and mesenchymal stem cells. *European Journal of Immunology*, *39*(3), 752–762. https://doi.org/10.1002/eji.200838812

Maumus, M., Manferdini, C., Toupet, K., Peyrafitte, J.-A., Ferreira, R., Facchini, A., Gabusi, E., Bourin, P., Jorgensen, C., Lisignoli, G., & Noël, D. (2013). Adipose mesenchymal stem cells protect chondrocytes from degeneration associated with osteoarthritis.

Stem Cell Research, *11*(2), 834–844. https://doi.org/10.1016/j.scr.2013.05.008

Merlo, B., & Iacono, E. (2023, November 19). Beyond canine adipose tissue-derived mesenchymal stem/stromal cells transplantation: An update on their secretome characterization and applications. *Animals (Basel)*, *13*(22), 3571. https://doi.org/10.3390/ani13223571

Mindrescu, C., Thorbecke, G. J., Klein, M. J., Vilček, J., & Wisniewski, H. G. (2000). Amelioration of collagen-induced arthritis in DBA/1J mice by recombinant TSG-6, a tumor necrosis factor/interleukin–1–inducible protein. *Arthritis and Rheumatism*, *43*(12), 2668–2677. https://doi.org/10.1002/1529-0131(200012)43:12<2668::AID-ANR6>3.0.CO;2-E

Mokarizadeh, A., Delirezh, N., Morshedi, A., Mosayebi, G., Farshid, A.-A., & Mardani, K. (2012). Microvesicles derived from mesenchymal stem cells: Potent organelles for induction of tolerogenic signaling. *Immunology Letters*, *147*(1–2), 47–54. https://doi.org/10.1016/j.imlet.2012.06.001

Rehman, J., Traktuev, D., Li, J., Merfeld-Clauss, S., Temm-Grove, C. J., Bovenkerk, J. E., Pell, C. L., Johnstone, B. H., Considine, R. V., & March, K. L. (2004). Secretion of angiogenic and antiapoptotic factors by human adipose stromal cells. *Circulation*, *109*(10), 1292–1298. https://doi.org/10.1161/01.CIR.0000121425.42966.F1

Shotorbani, B. B., Alizadeh, E., Salehi, R., & Barzegar, A. (2017). Adhesion of mesenchymal stem cells to biomimetic polymers: A review. *Materials Science and Engineering. C, Materials for Biological Applications*, *71*, 1192 1200. https://doi.org/10.1016/j.msec.2016.10.013

Sotiropoulou, P. A., Perez, S. A., Gritzapis, A. D., Baxevanis, C. N., & Papamichail, M. (2006). Interactions between human mesenchymal stem cells and natural killer cells. *Stem Cells*, *24*(1), 74–85. https://doi.org/10.1634/stemcells.2004-0359

Suga, H., Eto, H., Shigeura, T., Inoue, K., Aoi, N., Kato, H., Nishimura, S., Manabe, I., Gonda, K., & Yoshimura, K. (2009). IFATS collection: Fibroblast growth factor-2-induced hepatocyte growth factor secretion by adipose-derived stromal cells inhibits postinjury fibrogenesis through a c-Jun N-terminal kinase-dependent mechanism. *Stem Cells*, *27*(1), 238–249. https://doi.org/10.1634/stemcells.2008-0261

Thornton, O. R., & Li, W. (2023). Revolutionizing arthritis treatment: The synergy of iPSCs and extracellular vesicles-based acellular therapies for joint tissue repair. *Revolutionizing arthritis treatment: The synergy of iPSCs and extracellular vesicles-based acellular therapies for joint tissue repair*, *8*, *4*, 33–38.

Toh, W. S., Lai, R. C., Hui, J. H. P., & Lim, S. K. (2017, July). MSC exosome as a cell-free MSC therapy for cartilage regeneration: Implications for osteoarthritis treatment. In *Seminars in Cell and Developmental Biology*. Academic Press, *67*. https://doi.org/10.1016/j.semcdb.2016.11.008

Ullah, M., Liu, D. D., & Thakor, A. S. (2019). Mesenchymal stromal cell homing: Mechanisms and strategies for improvement. *iScience*, *15*, 421–438. https://doi.org/10.1016/j.isci.2019.05.004

Velarde, F., Ezquerra, S., Delbruyere, X., Caicedo, A., Hidalgo, Y., & Khoury, M. (2022). Mesenchymal stem cell-mediated transfer of mitochondria: Mechanisms and functional impact. *Cellular and Molecular Life Sciences*, *79*(3), 177. https://doi.org/10.1007/s00018-022-04207-3

Weiss, A. R. R., & Dahlke, M. H. (2019). Immunomodulation by mesenchymal stem cells (MSCs): Mechanisms of action of living, apoptotic, and dead MSCs. *Frontiers in Immunology*, *10*, 1191. https://doi.org/10.3389/fimmu.2019.01191

Yang, Y. K., Ogando, C. R., Wang See, C., Chang, T.-Y., & Barabino, G. A. (2018). Changes in phenotype and differentiation potential of human mesenchymal stem cells aging in vitro. *Stem Cell Research and Therapy*, *9*(1), 131. https://doi.org/10.1186/s13287-018-0876-3

Yin, C., & Heit, B. (2021). Cellular responses to the efferocytosis of apoptotic cells. *Frontiers in Immunology*, *12*, 631714. https://doi.org/10.3389/fimmu.2021.631714

Zhang, B., Yin, Y., Lai, R. C., Tan, S. S., Choo, A. B. H., & Lim, S. K. (2014). Mesenchymal stem cells secrete immunologically active exosomes. *Stem Cells and Development*, *23*(11), 1233–1244. https://doi.org/10.1089/scd.2013.0479

Zhu, Y., Wang, Y., Zhao, B., Niu, X., Hu, B., Li, Q., Zhang, J., Ding, J., Chen, Y., & Wang, Y. (2017). Comparison of exosomes secreted by induced pluripotent stem cell-derived mesenchymal stem cells and synovial membrane-derived mesenchymal stem cells for the treatment of osteoarthritis. *Stem Cell Research and*

Therapy, *8*(1), 64. https://doi.org/10.1186/s13287-017-0510-9

Zielniok, K., Burdzinska, A., Murcia Pienkowski, V., Koppolu, A., Rydzanicz, M., Zagozdzon, R., & Paczek, L. (2021, July 29). Gene expression profile of human mesenchymal stromal cells exposed to hypoxic and pseudohypoxic preconditioning-an analysis by RNA sequencing. *International Journal of Molecular Sciences*, *22*(15), 8160. https://doi.org/10.3390/ijms22158160

Chapter 7 further reading

Takahashi, K., & Yamanaka, S. (2006). Induction of pluripotent stem cells from mouse embryonic and adult fibroblast cultures by defined factors. *Cell*, *126*(4), 663–676. https://doi.org/10.1016/j.cell.2006.07.024

Chapter 8

Sources of mesenchymal stem cells (MSCs)

In VRM, the most common tissue sites for MSC harvesting are the BM, adipose tissue, and umbilical cord (Fig. 8.1).

Classification of mesenchymal stem cells (MSCs) by source

MSCs are classified, in addition to their tissue origin, by the donor animal from which they are harvested (Fig. 8.2).

Tissue sources of mesenchymal stem cells (MSCs)

Tissues derived from the mesenchymal (mesodermal) embryonic cell layer contain a reservoir of MSCs. The MSCs typically occupy certain MSC niches where there is a conducive physical as well as biological environment. The tissue sources of MSCs for transplantation may include, among others:

- Bone marrow (BM)
- Adipose tissue
- Umbilical cord
- Peripheral blood
- Dental pulp

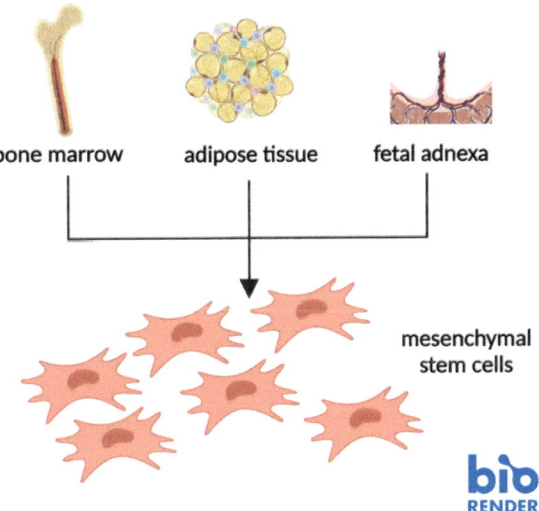

Fig. 8.1 Common tissue sites for harvesting MSCs in VRM.

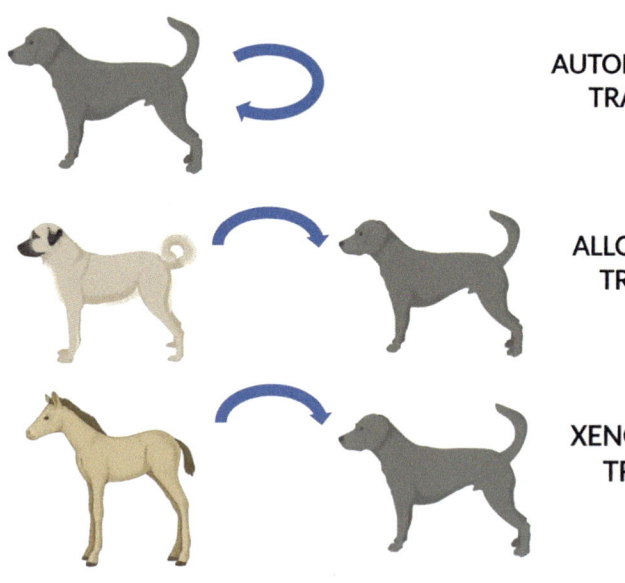

AUTOLOGOUS MSC
TRANSPLANT

examples available in UK
Adishot™, Biobest™, Orthostem™

ALLOGENEIC MSC
TRANSPLANT

examples available in UK
none yet

XENOGENEIC MSC
TRANSPLANT

examples available in UK
DogStem™

Fig. 8.2 Animal donor sources of MSCs in VRM.

Autologous MSCs

In the case of autologous MSC transplantation, the donor and the recipient (the patient) are the same animal. This is a common practice in veterinary orthobiologic medicine for MSCs and PRPs. One major advantage, at least theoretically, is the lack of immune rejection since the transplanted cells and recipient tissues have the same immunophenotype (at least before the laboratory processing). A potential disadvantage is that the older the patient, the older and less potent the MSCs, as MSC potency declines with age, (Maged et al., 2024). Additionally, autotransplanting these cells may be less effective than using cells from a younger donor. Another disadvantage is that when MSC therapy is required, a surgical procedure is necessary to harvest tissue for MSC extraction, culture, and expansion. There is also a delay of several weeks before the injectable MSC product is available.

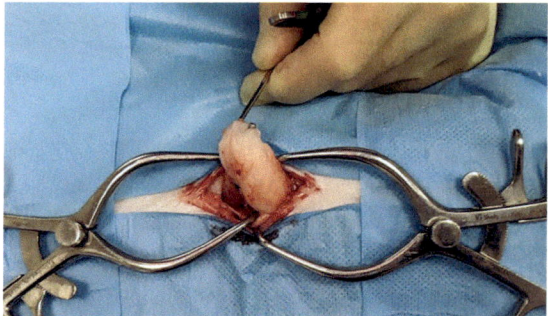

Fig. 8.3 Aseptic surgical collection of feline falciform fat for the harvesting of MSCs for autologous use. Minimal handling of the tissue is practised, maximising cell viability and minimising contamination risk.

Allogeneic MSCs

Using a donor cell source of another animal from the same species is referred to as an 'allogeneic cell transplant'. The theoretical disadvantage of adverse immune reaction and immune rejection is greater than with its autologous counterpart, though this may not be an important concern in practice. MSCs have been described as immune privileged due to their low immunogenicity when transplanted. A major reason for this is a feature of MSCs, namely that they do not express the major histocompatibility factor complex II (MHC-II). This cell surface protein acts as an identifying marker, indicating that the cell is foreign and triggering allorecognition. The presence of MHC-II would trigger the adaptive immune system and, particularly the T-cells, initiating a cascade of processes leading to the rejection of transplanted cells.

Donors can be selected for their health status and will preferably be relatively young. In this regard, cells from the fetal adnexa, such as the umbilical cord, are a relevant source of allogeneic MSCs.

Xenogeneic MSCs

The use of donor MSCs from a mammalian species different from the patient is a reality. To date, even the xenogeneic cells that are currently available appear to not elicit any noteworthy graft-versus-host disease associated with immune responses (Punzón et al., 2023). The reported advantages of, for example, equine umbilical cord (EUC) MSCs include the ready availability of large numbers of younger, potent cells.

Mesenchymal stem cell (MSC) niches

Native MSCs exist in specific locations referred to as niches. The niche provides for both the physical and physiological requirements of the MSCs. The three-dimensional structural characteristics of the extra-cellular components and the neighbouring cells permit adherence of the MSCs, which is essential for their survival and function.

The BM is a rich source of stem cells. The majority of these, however, are HSCs, which are responsible for producing, by multiple stages of differentiation, every kind of circulating blood cell and platelets. In an overwhelming numerical minority is another kind of stem cell, the BM-derived MSC, which have been used extensively in human, equine, and canine RM.

Adipose tissue is a rich source of MSCs. Some controversy still exists as to the lineage of these MSCs. A common cell type associated with the extraluminal surface of capillaries is the **pericyte**. Pericytes share many of the phenotypic cell-surface markers with MSCs. The exact relationship between these cells is uncertain, though it is probable that pericytes and MSCs may be one and the same cell (Crisan et al., 2008).

The umbilical cord is also a rich source of adult MSCs. One advantage of these umbilical cord MSCs is their youth, as younger stem cells are relatively more potent than their older, more mature counterparts.

Properties of mesenchymal stem cells (MSCs) and their fate after transplantation

After the transplantation of MSCs, the following effects may be observed in the recipient tissues.

Immunomodulation

MSCs can influence various immune cells through the secretion of bioactive molecules, helping to reduce cellular and tissue damage. Their effects extend to natural killer cells, B-lymphocytes, macrophages, T-reg cells, dendritic cells, and T-lymphocytes.

Effects on inflammation and oxidative stress

Oxidative stress significantly influences the OA disease process (Koike et al., 2018). The superoxide dismutase (SOD) enzymes are involved in removing harmful superoxide species.

In humans, ageing is the main risk factor for the downregulation of SOD activity, which likely explains the increased risk of OA with age. However, even accounting for age, OA-affected joints still show reduced SOD levels. In mice, endogenous synovial MSCs have been found to not only increase in number in the synovial fluid but also their gene expression profiles show upregulated SOD expression in response to OA (Furuoka et al., 2023). Logically, exogenously derived therapeutic MSCs could have similar beneficial effects regarding reduced oxidative stress in an OA-affected joint.

MSC apoptosis after injection

The vast majority of injected MSCs undergo rapid death (Zhu et al., 2023). At first, this may seem counter-intuitive if MSC transplantation aims to be 'regenerative'. So how can these injected MSCs benefit the target tissues when they almost immediately die? The answer lies in how they die and what materials result from their death. The MSCs predominantly undergo a process called apoptosis. This is a form of programmed cell death and is the organism's way of removing cells, which is constantly necessary in the body. Apoptotic processes are not associated with cell necrosis and therefore do not result in inflammation. This 'clean' form of cell death allows the recycling of the cell constituents (Fig. 7.3). In the case of post-apoptotic MSCs, a large collection of 'apoptotic bodies' are produced. In essence, it is these various apoptotic bodies that interact with the resident cells in a paracrine fashion, influencing the latter and resulting in the observed MSC effects.

Chapter 8 key points

- There is a variety of tissue sources for MSCs.
- MSC transplants may be autologous, allogeneic, or xenogeneic.
- The native MSCs reside in specialised niches.
- The main advantages to the donor tissue following MSC transplantation are anti-inflammatory, immunomodulatory, and trophic.
- MSCs are considered to rapidly perish after transplantation, mainly by apoptosis.
- The apoptotic products are essential for the MSC effects.
- Only a small number of MSCs survive after a few hours post-injection.

Chapter 8 references

Crisan, M., Yap, S., Casteilla, L., Chen, C.-W., Corselli, M., Park, T. S., Andriolo, G., Sun, B., Zheng, B., Zhang, L., Norotte, C., Teng, P.-N., Traas, J., Schugar, R., Deasy, B. M., Badylak, S., Buhring, H.-J., Giacobino, J.-P., Lazzari, L., . . . & Péault, B. (2008). A perivascular origin for mesenchymal stem cells in multiple human organs. *Cell Stem Cell*, *3*(3), 301–313. https://doi.org/10.1016/j.stem.2008.07.003

Furuoka, H., Endo, K., & Sekiya, I. (2023). Mesenchymal stem cells in synovial fluid increase in number in response to synovitis and display more tissue-re-parative phenotypes in osteoarthritis. *Stem Cell Research and Therapy*, *14*(1), 244. https://doi.org/10.1186/s13287-023-03487-1

Koike, M., Nojiri, H., Kanazawa, H., Yamaguchi, H., Miyagawa, K., Nagura, N., Banno, S., Iwase, Y.,

Kurosawa, H., & Kaneko, K. (2018). Superoxide dismutase activity is significantly lower in end-stage osteoarthritic cartilage than non-osteoarthritic cartilage. *PLOS ONE*, *13*(9), e0203944. https://doi.org/10.1371/journal.pone.0203944

Maged, G., Abdelsamed, M. A., Wang, H., & Lotfy, A. (2024). The potency of mesenchymal stem/stromal cells: Does donor sex matter? *Stem Cell Research and Therapy*, *15*(1), 112. https://doi.org/10.1186/s13287-024-03722-3

Punzón, E., García-Castillo, M., Rico, M. A., Padilla, L., & Pradera, A. (2023, May 17). Local, systemic, and immunologic safety comparison between xenogeneic equine umbilical cord mesenchymal stem cells, allogeneic canine adipose mesenchymal stem cells and placebo: A randomized controlled trial. *Frontiers in Veterinary Science*, *10*, 1098029. https://doi.org/10.3389/fvets.2023.1098029, PubMed: 37266387, PubMed Central: PMC10229832

Zhu, Y., Chen, X., & Liao, Y. (2023). Mesenchymal stem cells-derived apoptotic extracellular vesicles (ApoEVs): Mechanism and application in tissue regeneration. *Stem Cells*, 41(9), 837–849. https://doi.org/10.1093/stmcls/sxad046

Chapter 9

Laboratory manufacture of mesenchymal stem cells (MSCs)

Overview of mesenchymal stem cell (MSC) manufacture

Adherence to Good Manufacturing Practice (GMP) is mandatory in MSC manufacture (Ivanovska et al., 2022). The detailed series of necessary laboratory procedures involved in the manufacture of MSCs is beyond the scope of this book. It is, however, useful to have some rudimentary understanding of the steps involved and the principles associated with these. These steps are outlined in Figure 9.1.

The MSC product is only as good as the process that was used to manufacture it (Pittenger et al., 2019; Ivanovska et al., 2022). Thus, meticulous adherence to established laboratory protocols is imperative. Since MSC-containing orthobiologics are a 'living medicine', they cannot be sterilised at any stage of the process. It is therefore essential that the tissues are collected with excellent aseptic technique and that bacterial contaminants are excluded at every stage of processing.

The process typically proceeds along the following pattern:

- Donor screening
- Tissue collection
- Tissue processing
- Cell isolation
- Cell culture
- Cell expansion
- Cell passage
- Further cell expansion
- Cryo-storage in a master cell bank
- Release tests

Donor screening

Stem cell products, once produced, cannot be filtered or sterilised as they are composed of living cells. It is therefore incumbent upon the clinician and the laboratory team to ensure that donor animals used for harvesting allogeneic or xenogeneic cells are screened for infectious diseases. Any infective micro-organisms that enter the manufacturing process are likely to remain and be present in the final product (Ivanovska et al., 2022).

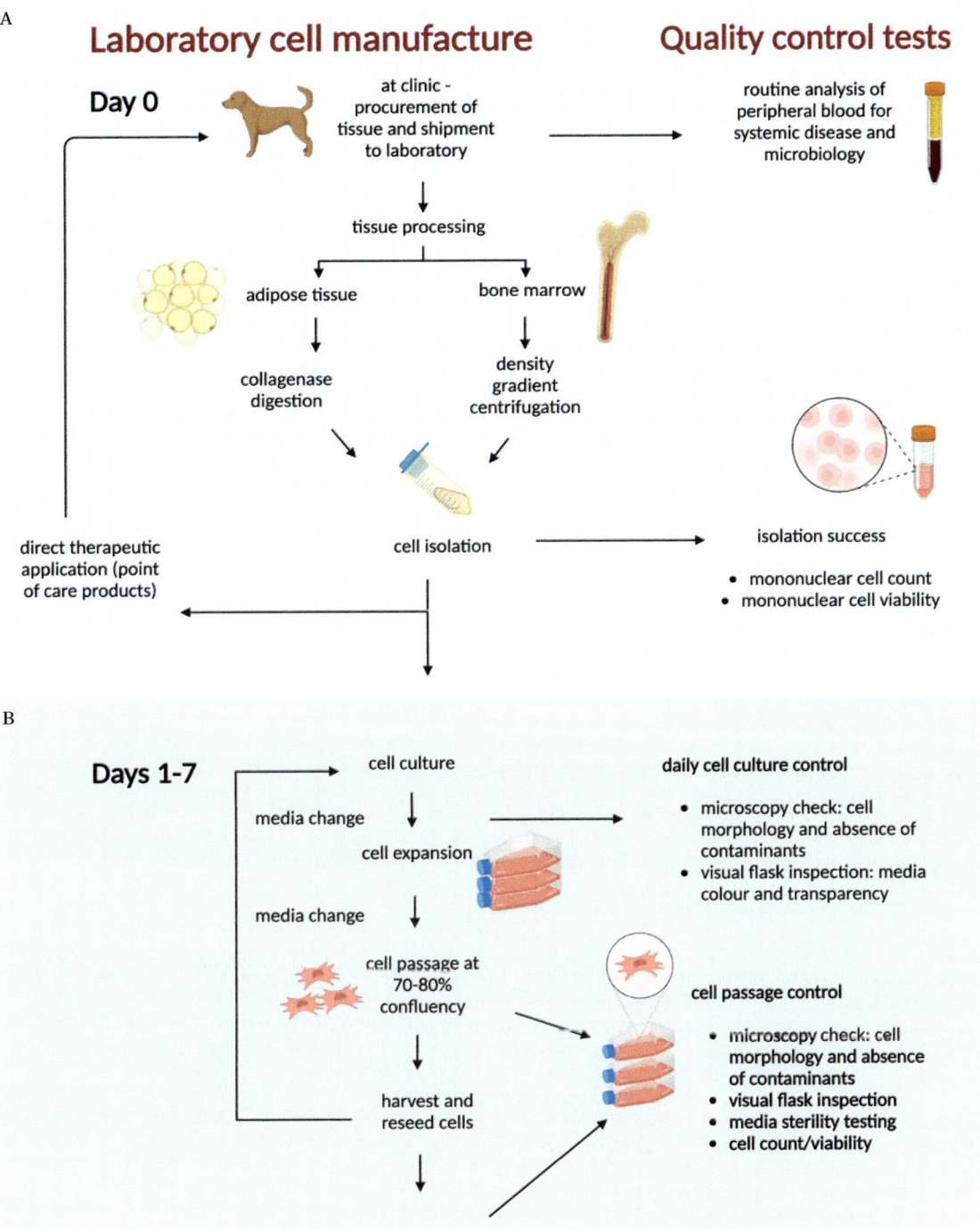

Fig. 9.1 Autologous MSC cell manufacturing flow diagram. Redrawn and adapted from Ivanovska et al. (2022). Initially the sample is collected at the clinic. Quality control and sterility testing are essential at every step. If at any step there is failure, the sample is discarded, and the process is recommenced with a fresh sample.

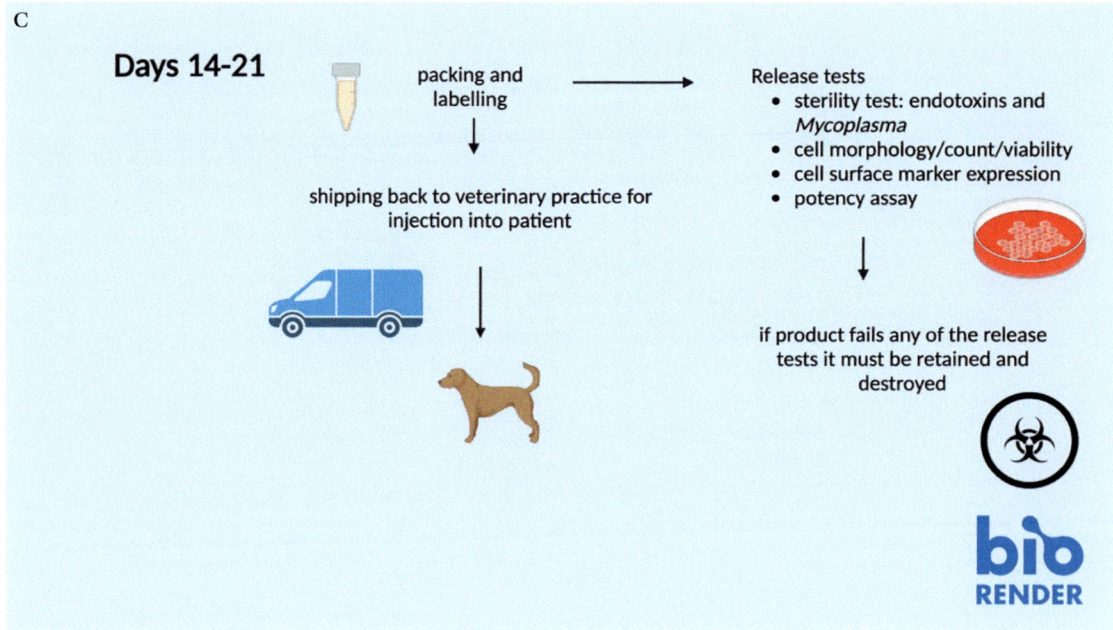

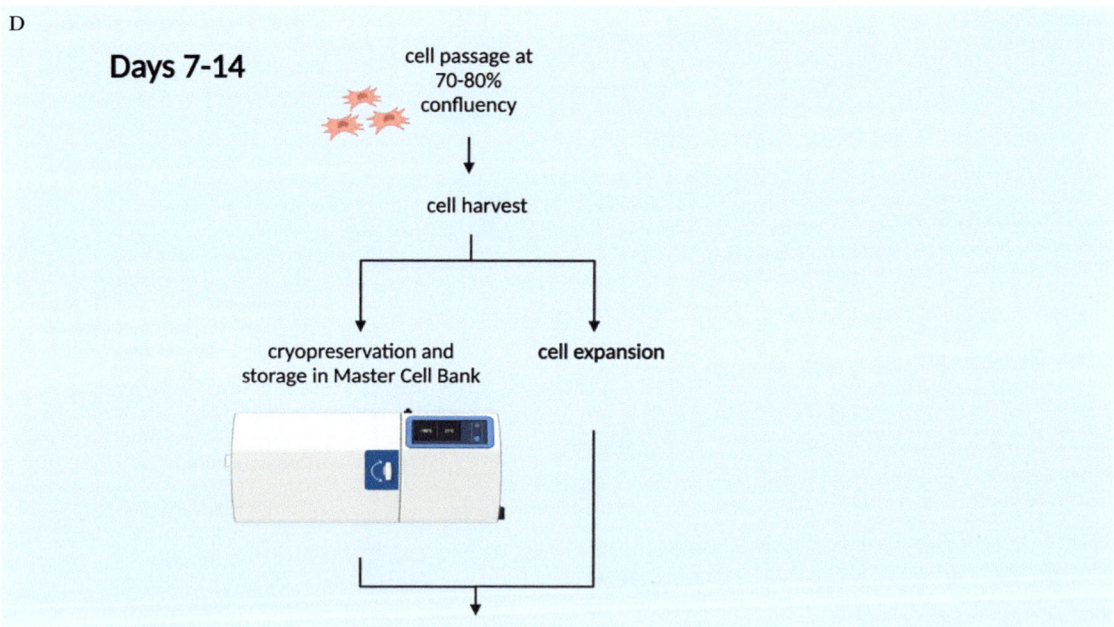

Fig. 9.1 (continued).

The Committee for Veterinary Medicinal Products (CVMP) of the European Medicines Agency (EMA) publishes guidelines for canine and equine donor screening (Tables 9.1 & 9.2).

The donor animal's geographical location and medical history may be relevant in the choice of pathogens added to the screening panel (Ivanovska et al., 2022) and should be scrutinised on a case-by-case basis.

Even with demonstrably healthy donors, from the pathogen-screening viewpoint, this does not eliminate the pathogen risk. Environmental micro-organisms that may be airborne, surface-borne, or from the animal's skin can enter the sample. Minimising this risk by strict attention to operating theatre asepsis is essential.

Tissue collection for mesenchymal stem cells (MSC)

MSCs are found in a wide range of tissues. These include, among many others:

Table 9.1 Guidelines for canine donor screening for RM. CVMP of the EMA.

Viruses	Bacteria	Rickettsia	Protozoa	Helminths
Canid herpesvirus Canine adenovirus Canine coronavirus Canine distemper virus Canine oral papilloma virus Canine parainfluenza 2 virus Canine parvovirus Rabies virus Swine herpesvirus 1 Canine influenza viruses	*Brucella canis* *Leptospira* spp. *Borrelia* spp. *Ehrlichia* spp. *Bartonella vinsonii*	*Anaplasma* spp. *Neorickettsia* spp. other *Rickettsia* spp.	*Babesia* spp. *Leishmania* spp. *Trypanosoma cruzi* *Neospora caninum*	*Dirofilaria immitis*

Table 9.2 Guidelines for equine donor screening for RM. CVMP of the EMA.

Viruses	Bacteria and rickettsia
African horse sickness virus Borna disease virus Endogenous retrovirus (replication competent) Equine adenovirus Equine arteritis virus Equine encephalomyelitis alphavirus Equine encephalosis virus Equine herpesvirus (EHV-1, EHV-4) Equine infectious anaemia virus Equine influenza virus Equine rotavirus Hendra virus Japanese encephalitis virus Rabies virus Vesicular stomatitis virus West Nile virus Hepaciviruses Pegiviruses	*Burkholderia mallei* *Burkholderia pseudomallei* *Neorickettsia risticii* *Borrelia* spp. *Anaplasma phagocytophilum*

- Bone marrow (BM)
- Peripheral blood
- Adipose tissue
- Dental pulp
- Fetal adnexa

The classical tissue source for HSC collection is the BM. BM also contains MSCs. The use of BM for MSC collection has several disadvantages when compared to HSC collection.

Firstly, the HSC population in BM vastly outnumbers the MSCs, with only approximately 1 MSC per 100 to 1,000 HSCs (Pittenger et al., 1999). This, at least theoretically, makes for more of a challenge in the laboratory extraction of sufficient numbers of MSCs to be practically useful. When BM aspiration is undertaken, this generally yields high numbers of nucleated cells. The downside is that relatively few of these are verifiably MSCs. Sullivan et al. (2016) investigated the canine MSC yield in BM aspirates from various bones (humerus, ilium, and tibia) and adipose tissue harvests for SVF extraction from several locations (inguinal, subcutaneous tissue over the caudal scapular area, and falciform ligament). The aim was to determine which site was the easiest for MSC collection and which would yield the most MSCs. The authors concluded that the BM aspirates resulted in the largest absolute numbers of MSCs collected, while the falciform fat harvest yielded the highest percentage of MSCs relative to other nucleated cells. This led them to recommend falciform fat as the optimal option for MSC collection, as more consistent results could be expected. Even when canine SVF is produced, 92.3% of the cells injected are undefined (Sullivan et al., 2016).

Furthermore, BM aspiration is a relatively painful procedure (Pittenger et al., 2019). This technique mandates a robust pre-emptive multimodal analgesic regimen, and this is usually combined with general anaesthesia. Its execution requires a certain level of skill: this may be somewhat daunting for veterinarians in primary care practice.

The laboratory culture and expansion of MSCs is described (by the EMA) as major manipulation. Alternatively, minimally manipulated MSC-containing products may be produced at point-of-care.

Point-of-care mesenchymal stem cell (MSC) products

The collection of autologous cells for point-of-care orthobiologic application is possible. The product yields a heterogeneous mixture of cells of various kinds, including some percentage of MSCs. Examples of donor tissues for harvesting include BM and adipose tissue.

BM concentrate

Autologous BM may be aspirated, and its cellular portion concentrated patient-side. The cell populations so produced are a varied mixture of various nucleated cells. Some of these will be MSCs, but the percentage is unknowable unless every sample undergoes analysis, which is not the case in patient-side, point-of-care orthobiologics. The BM concentrate may then be injected into the target area, such as a joint. The sterility of the BM concentrate when used as a point-of-care therapy is reliant on the aseptic technique, as this cannot be verified by laboratory testing before application.

Stromal vascular fraction (SVF)

Another point-of-care product containing autologous cells, a proportion presumed to be MSCs, is to use the SVF of adipose tissue. An example of this is the Lipogems® process, which is described in more detail in Chapter 11.

Culture-expanded autologous adipose-derived mesenchymal stem cells (AD-MSCs)

An example of a United Kingdom-based laboratory active in manufacturing autologous MSCs is Cell Therapy Sciences (CTS) in Coventry. The 'product' (in inverted commas since each cell production is unique) from CTS has the trade name AdiShot®. While parts of the process are proprietary (that is, intellectual property belonging to the company), it broadly follows the well-worn path of MSC manufacture (see Fig. 9.1). The starting cell source is adipose tissue from one of the subcutaneous areas (inguinal, lateral thorax) or the intra-abdominal falciform ligament.

Adipose tissue harvesting

The most common tissue currently harvested from pet animals for MSC manufacture is adipose tissue. Adipose tissue is metabolically active and is accordingly supplied with a rich capillary network. The perivascular niche is where the MSCs are located. There is a good deal of overlap in the characteristics of MSCs and the cells resident on the adventitial surface of the capillary, namely the pericytes. It is not clear whether pericytes and MSCs are the same or whether one is a progenitor of the other. Nonetheless, adipose tissue harvesting allows the extraction of genuine MSCs in the laboratory.

Reported locations for adipose tissue harvesting are:

- inguinal subcutaneous fat
- falciform fat
- lateral thoracic subcutaneous fat.

All the above locations are accessible by relatively simple surgery.

Inguinal fat harvesting

The photographs in Figures 9.2 to 9.8 depict the aseptic harvesting of inguinal fat from a dog for MSC culture, and the process is summarised in Figure 9.12. Other locations for surgical harvest of adipose tissue are possible, including the subcutaneous tissue caudal to the scapula and the falciform ligament. Current opinion tends to favour the latter as the optimal site for tissue collection (Sullivan et al., 2016; Armitage et al., 2023). In the author's experience, falciform fat collection, anecdotally, appears to be less prone to surgical site complications such as seroma formation and patient interference than collection from the inguinal area.

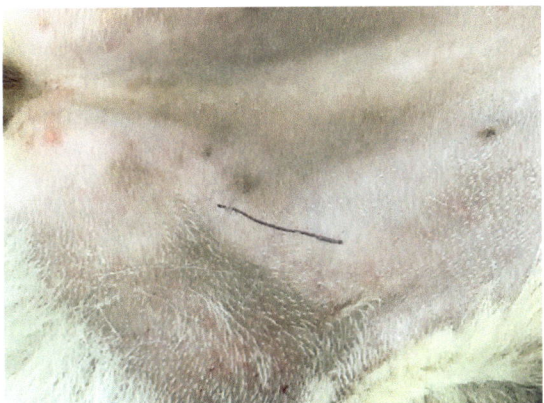

Fig. 9.2 Surgical site clipped, aseptically prepared, and proposed incision site marked with surgical marker.

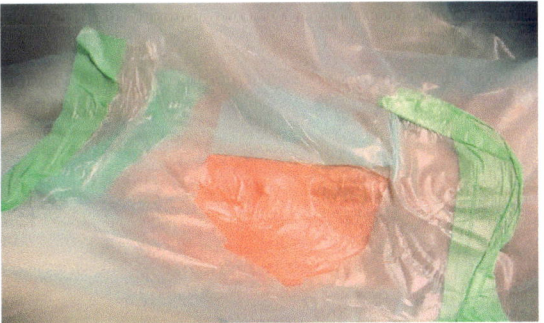

Fig. 9.3 Standard surgical draping with two layers of Opsite® (Smith & Nephew) and transparent surgical drapes.

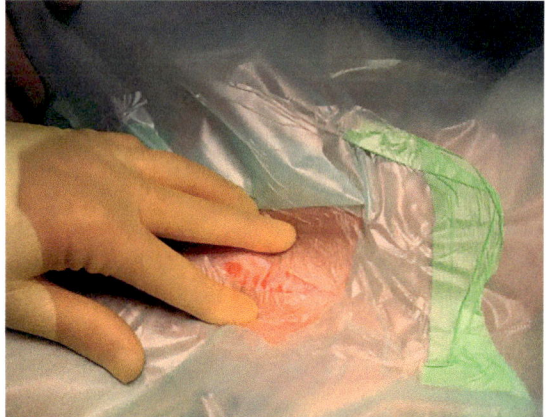

Fig. 9.4 Skin incised and wound gently spread, avoiding handling of the fat tissue.

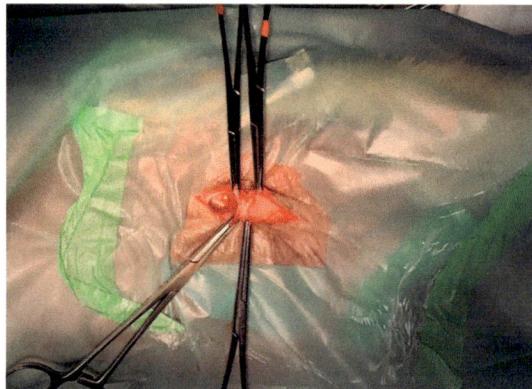

Fig. 9.5 Strict haemostasis applied using artery forceps.

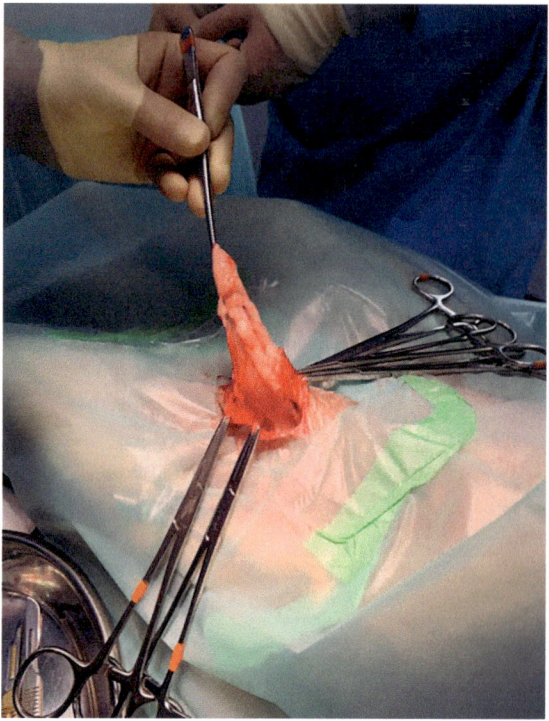

Fig. 9.6 Gentle elevation of fat tissue with minimal handling.

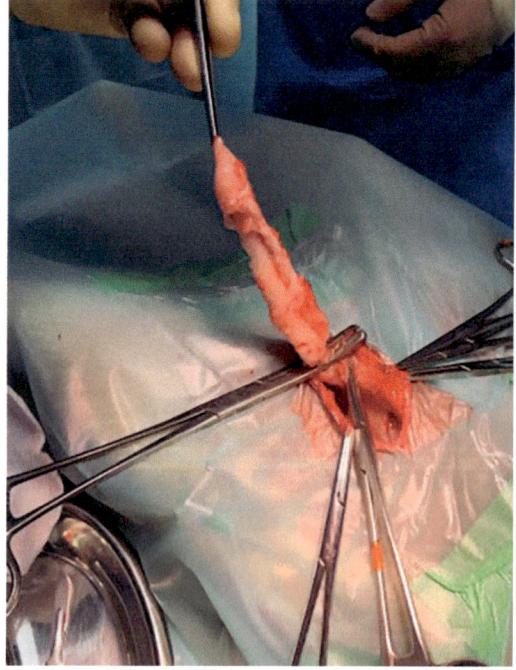

Fig. 9.7 Clamping of fat before sharply separating sample.

Donor screening

For allogeneic and xenogeneic transplantation of MSCs, donor screening tests are required (Tables 9.1 & 9.2.).

Tissue processing

Adipose tissue is first subjected to collagenase digestion, while BM undergoes density gradient centrifugation. The clinician does not ordinarily require detailed knowledge of these laboratory processes.

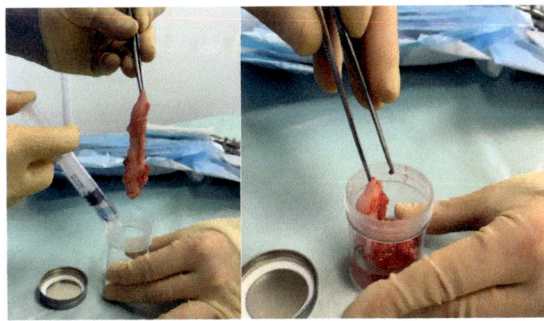

Fig. 9.8 Immediate transfer of sample into sterile transport vessel with 10ml of sterile saline.

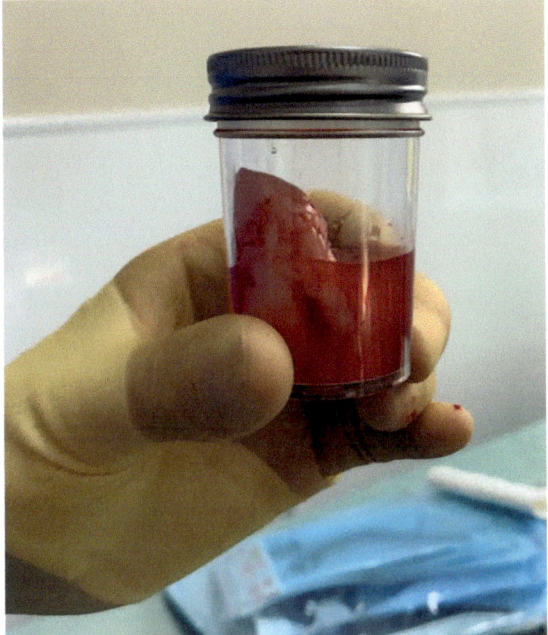

Fig. 9.9 Sample sealed for shipping. An autologous jugular blood sample is also collected (not depicted) and submitted along with the fat tissue sample.

Cell isolation

Enrichment of the extracted cell population to retain MSCs and discard other cell types can be performed using one of the following methods:

- Magnetic cell separation systems such as autoMACS® and CliniMACS® (Miltenyi Biotech, Germany),

- CD271 MicroBead® Kits (Miltenyi Biotech, Germany),
- or adherence to the surface of a plastic flask, which allows other non-MSCs to be washed away, leaving a very enriched sample of MSCs.

Cell culture

The culture of cells in a laboratory has been possible for many decades. Optimal media have been established and are commercially available. It is common to use fetal bovine serum as one of the components, which is xenogeneic (to all but bovine cells). Alternatives include various xeno-free media. The isolated (MSC) cell culture contains a heterogeneous population of microscopically spindle-shaped cells with several processes that adhere to the plastic flask. They have large nuclei and prominent nucleoli.

If allowed to become fully confluent (that is, the cells have fully carpeted the dish surface without space in between them), growth arrests and the viability and potency of the cells decline.

Cell passage

At around 70–80% confluency, it is appropriate to subculture some MSCs into a new flask with fresh medium. This is referred to as 'passaging'. This promotes the expansion of cell numbers by repeated mitotic divisions. Too many cycles of passage result in reduced cell viability, genetic and phenotypic drift, and reduced cell potency. An optimal number of passages that permit expansions of a 'healthy' population of MSCs while minimising the above risks is likely to be around four. With excessive numbers of passages, cell senescence can be expected.

Cell expansion

In order to have therapeutically meaningful numbers of MSCs for injection (consensus is lacking on the optimal 'dose' of MSCs, though it is usual to inject several million at a time in the

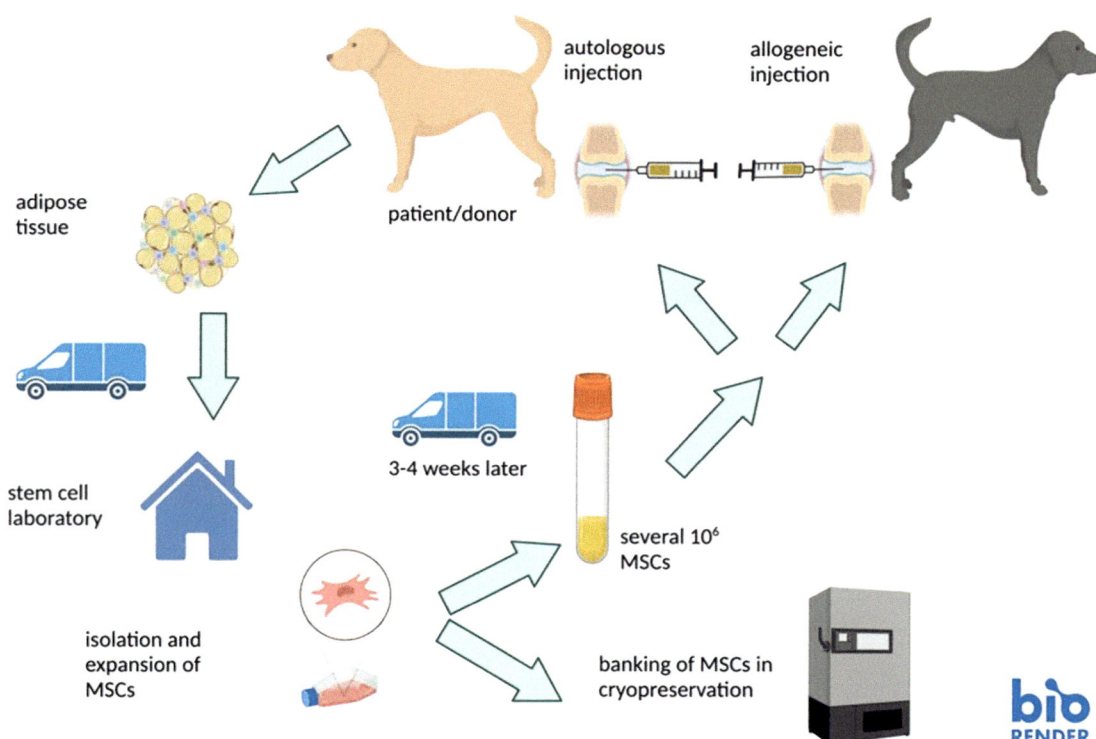

Fig. 9.10 Summary of workflow to administer IA culture-expanded canine autologous or xenogeneic MSCs from the clinician's viewpoint. Where allogeneic donors are used, appropriate screening is imperative. (A more detailed graphical depiction of the laboratory side of the process is shown in Fig. 9.1).

final orthobiologic product), MSCs once isolated require expansion of their numbers. Conditions are provided for the MSCs to divide, and in so doing, population doubling (PD) occurs. There is a limit on the optimal number of PDs, as *in vitro* the successive generations of cells tend to be affected by ageing and senescence (Yang et al., 2018). This manifests as morphologic, genetic, and phenotypic changes and affects the cells' differentiation capability.

Cryo-storage in a master cell bank

MSCs may be cryopreserved and stored for subsequent use (Cooper & Viswanathan, 2011). At GMP-compliant facilities, liquid nitrogen preservation is used to maintain the cells at -80 to −196°C. This method allows for the retrieval

of MSC orthobiologic 'doses' when needed. A cryoprotectant chemical is required, and several have been described. The agent of choice is dimethyl sulphoxide. However, this chemical has drawbacks, as *in vitro* studies have shown it can affect gene expression and DNA methylation, which leads to dysregulation of cellular processes. Despite these effects, dimethyl sulphoxide remains widely used in both research and clinical settings (Erol et al., 2021).

Release tests

The MSC product needs to have its sterility maintained at every stage of the process. This commences with the aseptic collection of the donor tissue and follows on throughout the laboratory processing. This is part of what constitutes GMP.

Investment in the necessary laboratory facilities and skilled personnel is essential, as is the stringent adherence to protocols. Before release from the laboratory, a variety of microbiological tests are undertaken to verify that the orthobiologic is free from contamination by bacteria and other pathogens.

Keeping MSC products sterile

Sterility of the final MSC product for injection is essential. Otherwise, IA injections would be fraught with the risk of iatrogenic infection from micro-organism contaminants. This is facilitated by strict attention to sterility at every step of the harvest and cell manufacturing process.

The tissue sample, such as adipose tissue or BM, must be aseptically harvested and shipped in a sterile container. At the laboratory, the sample needs to be handled in a laboratory hood at every stage to prevent contamination with bacteria.

At certain stages of the processing, antibiotics are added to the media. This is permitted early in the process but avoided in the later stages lest the final MSC product could contain traces of these substances (Ivanovska et al., 2022).

Rationale for release tests

As previously mentioned, MSCs are considered a 'living medicine' and cannot be terminally sterilised before release, as this would kill the very cells being produced. This makes stem cell manufacturing akin to a hybrid of aseptic surgery and sterile laboratory practice. Existing at this intersection mandates that the sample remains uncontaminated by micro-organisms, especially known pathogens. While the laboratory assumes, as a matter of good practice, that surgery is performed aseptically, it would be unwise to dismiss the possibility of mishaps occurring in the operating room. Therefore, the laboratory process must include built-in safeguards to confirm and verify that the final product is uncontaminated.

Bacterial testing

Testing for the absence of bacteria is mandatory. When allogeneic or xenogeneic MSCs are used, a standardised master cell bank is employed. This bank has been previously tested by conventional bacterial culturing methods (Punzón et al., 2022), so the MSCs are guaranteed sterile.

Verifying the absence of bacteria can be more challenging when autologous MSCs are used since the manufacture and release of the MSCs for injection is time-critical due to the short shelf life after manufacture. The recommendation is that a period of 48–72 hours of bacterial culture is performed before the sample can be certified as negative for bacterial presence. More rapid tests for the detection of bacteria are available, including, for example, BACT/ALERT® (BioMérieux), Milliflex® Rapid System (Merck Millipore), and BD BACTEC™ (Becton Dickinson) (Ivanovska et al., 2022). Even when using these assays, testing may take up to 72 hours, meaning even these may not meet the required time frame. In practice, the use of such rapid microbiological tests in combination with Gram staining may be a reasonable compromise. Even with this approach, the release and potentially the injection of an autologous MSC product could occur before the final receipt of the microbiology report, which is clearly unacceptable.

Overcoming the delay of test results for bacteriology

A preferable solution to the 72-hour window for cell use post-thawing is to ship the MSCs while they are still frozen (this must be below -60C). The microbiological tests can be undertaken well ahead of injecting the product, which is thawed patient-side immediately before being injected.

Viability testing

A test to prove that the MSCs are viable when dispatched is essential. The trypan blue test is a commonly used method for this purpose. Trypan blue is a dye that cannot penetrate living cells but readily enters and stains the degenerate membranes of dead cells. These dead cells are stained blue and can be counted. This allows the release certificate to accurately report that the cell product contains, for example, 99% viable cells.

Ethical considerations for mesenchymal stem cell (MSC) donors

Autologous MSC donors

Since autologous MSCs originate from the patient, it is easy to forget that they have not 'volunteered' for the procedure. Instead, they have been vicariously put forward for tissue harvest and MSC administration by their owners. Affording these patient donors/recipients the appropriate care in recognition of this fact is fundamentally appropriate. Suitable analgesia and anaesthetic management need to be undertaken, along with meticulous attention to detail in all aspects of the process. Informed owner consent relies on a full explanation of all the implications of MSC therapy.

Allogeneic MSC donors

At the time of writing, no allogeneic small animal MSC product was available in the United Kingdom. In the equine sector, several such products have thus far come to market (such as HorStem®, Arti-Cell® Forte, and RenuTend™). Regarding available and licensed MSC products, it is accurate to state that the equine RM sector leads both the companion animal and the human RM discipline. A detailed discussion of the ethics of equine allogeneic MSC transplantation is beyond the scope of this book. However, where canine or feline allogeneic donors are used, it is essential to ensure that all their welfare requirements are adequately addressed.

Xenogeneic MSC donors

Several observations can be made regarding the xenogeneic product available in the United Kingdom and European Union, namely DogStem® (Dômes Pharma). The disadvantage of using allogeneic canine umbilical cord MSCs for transplantation is that the fetal adnexa, post-whelping, are typically consumed by the post-partum bitch. To circumvent this natural series of events, when caesarean surgery is undertaken, the umbilical cord materials may be retained for MSC harvesting. Thus, only fetal adnexa from caesareans will be reliably available for this purpose. However, the ethics of elective caesarean surgery would not allow such practice, solely for the purpose of MSC procurement (Punzón et al., 2022). This is the rationale that is cited for the use of EUC-MSCs. The EUC is long and rich in MSCs. It is typically regarded as waste tissue and discarded after foaling, yet, instead of being thrown away, this tissue can be collected by laboratory personnel and processed in a sterile manner. From an ethical viewpoint, this practice is appealing because it repurposes a 'waste product' into a valuable source of MSCs (Punzón et al., 2022).

In summary, where autologous MSCs are used, the same considerations apply to any potentially painful surgical procedure, including pre-emptive and post-surgery analgesic medication. For xenogeneic MSCs, the logic of taking a waste tissue and using this as a source of MSCs seems to make ethical sense.

Chapter 9 key points

- Donor screening is mandatory for allogeneic and xenogeneic MSC products.
- All MSC products, including autologous MSCs, require bacteriological testing before administration.
- The possible sites of cell and tissue collection should be known so that a considered decision on which to select can be made in each situation.
- A rudimentary understanding of the tissue processing for MSC manufacture is useful.
- Meticulous attention to asepsis and minimally traumatic surgical technique is essential.
- Cryo-storage of culture-expanded MSCs in a master cell bank can provide for multiple future administrations of MSCs.
- Release tests must be performed and certified as negative for micro-organisms and especially pathogens before the MSCs are used.

Chapter 9 references

Armitage, A. J., Miller, J. M., Sparks, T. H., Georgiou, A. E., & Reid, J. (2023). Efficacy of autologous mesenchymal stromal cell treatment for chronic degenerative musculoskeletal conditions in dogs: A retrospective study. Frontiers in Veterinary Science, 9, 1014687. https://doi.org/10.3389/fvets.2022.1014687.

Committee for Veterinary Medicinal Products (CVMP) of the European Medicines Agency (EMA) (87). (accessed 22.4.23)

Cooper, K., & Viswanathan, C. (2011). Establishment of a mesenchymal stem cell bank. *Stem Cells International*, *2011*, 905621. https://doi.org/10.4061/2011/905621

Erol, O. D., Pervin, B., Seker, M. E., & Aerts-Kaya, F. (2021). Effects of storage media, supplements, and cryopreservation methods on quality of stem cells. *World Journal of Stem Cells*, *13*(9), 1197–1214. https://doi.org/10.4252/wjsc.v13.i9.1197, https://www.ema.europa.eu/en/documents/scientific-guideline/reflection-paper-stem-cell-based-medicinal-products_en.pdf

Ivanovska, A., Wang, M., Arshaghi, T. E., Shaw, G., Alves, J., Byrne, A., Butterworth, S., Chandler, R., Cuddy, L., Dunne, J., Guerin, S., Harry, R., McAlindan, A., Mullins, R. A., & Barry, F. (2022). Manufacturing mesenchymal stromal cells for the treatment of osteoarthritis in canine patients: Challenges and recommendations. *Frontiers in Veterinary Science*, *9*, 897150. https://doi.org/10.3389/fvets.2022.897150

Pittenger, M. F., Discher, D. E., Péault, B. M., Phinney, D. G., Hare, J. M., & Caplan, A. I. (2019). Mesenchymal stem cell perspective: Cell biology to clinical progress. *npj Regenerative Medicine*, *4*(1), 22. https://doi.org/10.1038/s41536-019-0083-6

Pittenger, M. F., Mackay, A. M., Beck, S. C., Jaiswal, R. K., Douglas, R., Mosca, J. D., Moorman, M. A., Simonetti, D. W., Craig, S., & Marshak, D. R. (1999). Multilineage potential of adult human mesenchymal stem cells. *Science*, *284*(5411), 143–147. https://doi.org/10.1126/science.284.5411.143

Punzón, E., Salgüero, R., Totusaus, X., Mesa-Sánchez, C., Badiella, L., García-Castillo, M., & Pradera, A. (2022). Equine umbilical cord mesenchymal stem cells demonstrate safety and efficacy in the treatment of canine osteoarthritis: A randomized placebo-controlled trial. *Journal of the American Veterinary Medical Association*, *260*(15), 1947–1955. https://doi.org/10.2460/javma.22.06.0237

Sullivan, M. O., Gordon-Evans, W. J., Fredericks, L. P., Kiefer, K., Conzemius, M. G., & Griffon, D. J. (2016). Comparison of mesenchymal stem cell surface markers from bone marrow aspirates and adipose stromal vascular fraction sites. *Frontiers in Veterinary Science*, *2*, 82. https://doi.org/10.3389/fvets.2015.00082

Yang, Y. K., Ogando, C. R., Wang See, C., Chang, T.-Y., & Barabino, G. A. (2018). Changes in phenotype and differentiation potential of human mesenchymal stem cells aging *in vitro*. *Stem Cell Research and Therapy*, *9*(1), 131. https://doi.org/10.1186/s13287-018-0876-3

Chapter 10

Clinical applications of mesenchymal stem cells (MSCs) in musculoskeletal (MSK) conditions

Cellular mechanisms of tissue damage and repair

Our understanding of the biological mechanisms occurring during tissue damage and repair has developed into a rich bank of knowledge and information. At the biochemical level, the identification of novel molecular interactions has broadened and deepened our appreciation of how tissues are both damaged and repaired. Furthermore, where a receptor-ligand interaction or biochemical pathway is identified, then a novel 'druggable target' may be revealed. Such processes may be amenable to the modifying effects of the molecules released by VRMs.

OA is a complex set of disease phenotypes. Despite this, many of the pathological biochemical dysregulations are well established. It is therefore possible to envisage some of the mechanisms by which VRMs may be beneficial. The diarthrodial joint is a complex organ containing multiple cell types and tissues. While cartilage damage is clearly involved in the pathophysiology of the disease, focusing too narrowly on this tissue in isolation does not describe the whole of the disorder. It is more realistic to consider the whole joint, including all the associated tissues and structures, as well as the downstream effects joint pathology has on local and distant areas of the body.

Osteoarthritis (OA) at the cellular and subcellular level

In essence, small animal OA results from overloading of the joint in some way, which is often the result of conformational variations and/or joint congruence abnormalities. Typical originating conditions include dysplasias and/or instabilities. These result in excessive localised joint stresses (in this context, 'stress' refers to the force per unit area) that lead to activation of the B synoviocytes. The increased synovial fluid secretion (also known as synovial effusion) that follows is rich in inflammatory cytokines, including IL-1, IL-6, and

TNF-alpha. The downstream effects of these events include the polarisation of the invading macrophages into the M1 phenotype, which is pro-inflammatory *per se*. Further effects are the upregulation of metalloproteinases such as MMP-13 and MMP-9, which mediate cartilage destruction and bone remodelling. In summary, there is inflammation of the synovial membrane and a self-perpetuating cycle of cartilage destruction.

An ideal orthobiologic would combat the pathological events described here. While the anatomical and functional abnormalities may not be corrected or reversed, the biochemical and cellular molecular pathways are often amenable to amelioration. For example, MSCs can counteract the pro-inflammatory combination of molecules that fuels the OA cascade. The tendency for the macrophages to adopt

an M1 phenotype is reduced. A different set of interleukins may predominate, including IL-10, IL-4, and IL-5, along with TGF-beta. The irritation of the B synoviocytes is thus suppressed, and the metalloproteinases are downregulated. This gives the articular cartilage some respite and possibly the opportunity to self-repair.

Over recent years, the importance of canine OA has been increasingly recognised. The current paradigm for canine OA management is multimodal (Fox, 2017) (Fig. 10.1). A significant component of this approach involves the use of pharmaceuticals. These are highly effective for controlling pain, but they are, as a rule, symptom-modifying therapies. The quest for a genuinely disease-modifying therapy has been relatively unfruitful to date. The advent of RM represents a potentially *bona fide* disease-modifying OA therapy.

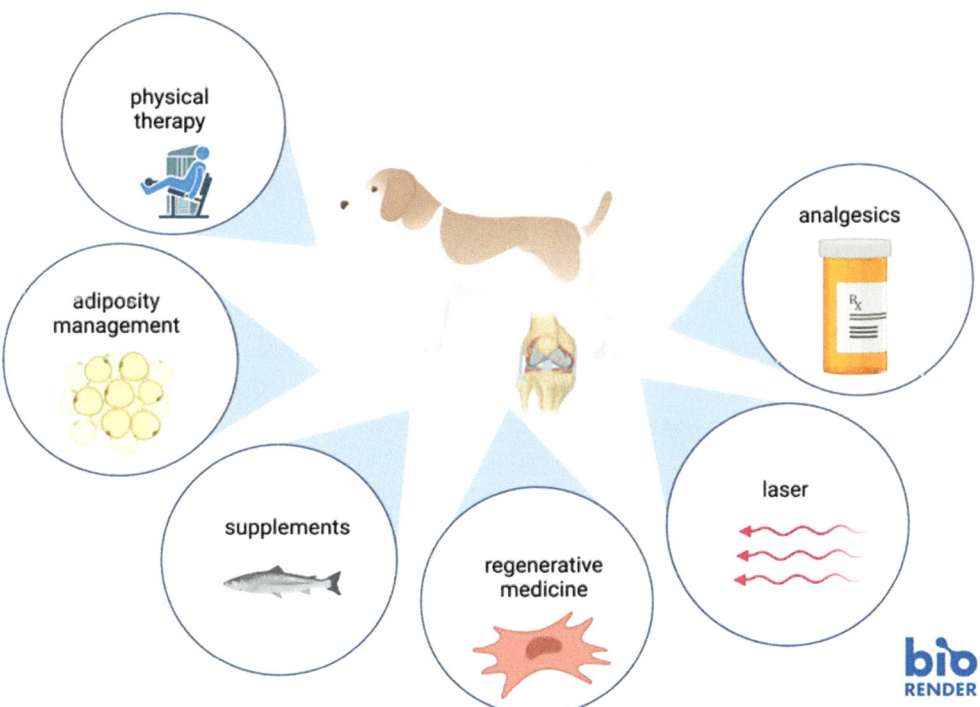

Fig. 10.1 Some of the different 'modes' of management that may be typically combined for osteoarthritis in dogs (adapted from Fox, 2017). Laser refers to therapeutic photobiomodulation. Dietary supplementation often includes omega-3 fatty acids from fish or crustaceans.

When and where does regenerative medicine (RM) fit in the management of canine osteoarthritis (OA)?

RM can be expected to have its best effect when used relatively early in the OA disease process. Intuitively, waiting until there is end-stage degeneration and remodelling of the joint with extreme cartilage loss and bone-on-bone contact would be much less likely to yield favourable results. To this end, the earlier the RM is applied in the course of the OA disease, the higher the likelihood of improvement in joint comfort and function.

The 'age' of the MSCs transplanted is also relevant. Younger cells are relatively more biologically active and have greater potential for proliferation and differentiation. Conversely, probably associated with the well-accepted Hayflick limit that cells have a natural limit to how many cell divisions they can undergo, older cells have diminished function. The reason for the Hayflick limit appears to be the age-related shortening of chromosomal telomeres. The practical implication of this is that the younger the MSCs that are harvested and used for RM cell transplantation, the better. Many aged canine OA patients may be considered for MSC therapy. Theoretically at least, a more effective paracrine effect within the injected joint may be predicted if younger cells (either allogeneic or xenogeneic) are applied. The youngest 'adult' MSCs currently available are derived from perinatal tissues such as the umbilical cord. From the age of implanted cells point of view, at least, umbilical cord MSCs represent an attractive source for cellular transplantation.

It seems logical that RM should be considered early in the course of OA and the younger the transplanted cells the better. Furthermore, the environment into which the cells are injected is also relevant. The recipient's joint is a hostile environment for transplanted MSCs, particularly in the cases of chronic or advanced OA. The effects of the MSCs are paracrine, meaning their effects depend on the by-proxy activities of the resident population cells within the recipient joint.

The transplanted cells interact with the innate immune system (macrophages, dendritic cells, natural killer cells, and natural killer T-cells) and the adaptive immune system (T-cells and B-cells) (Hu & Li, 2019). This occurs by cell-to-cell interactions, requiring proximity between cells, and by paracrine mechanisms, where soluble secreted cytokines and other molecules are required.

Some of the cellular mechanisms involved in OA pathogenesis, along with some of the known beneficial influences of transplanted MSCs, are summarised in Figure 10.2.

The importance of an accurate diagnosis

As clinicians responsible for managing MSK conditions in small animals, it is incumbent on us to determine the cause of the MSK problem as accurately as is practically possible. All manner of obstacles to this may be involved, such as financial constraints or unwillingness of the owner to consent to sedation or anaesthesia of their animal. Nonetheless, veterinarians – the only members of the multidisciplinary team who are legally able to diagnose a medical problem – should endeavour to establish as accurate a diagnosis, for example, of the cause of lameness, as possible. The diagnostic process has been discussed earlier; however, in essence, the sequence includes the patient's history and signalment, the owner's description of the problem, observation of the patient lying, rising, walking, and moving at faster gaits, hands-on palpation, and manipulation of the limbs, especially the joints, range of motion assessments, muscle bulk determinations, and so forth. Usually, a tentative primary diagnosis can be proposed, along with several differential diagnoses from which it should be distinguished.

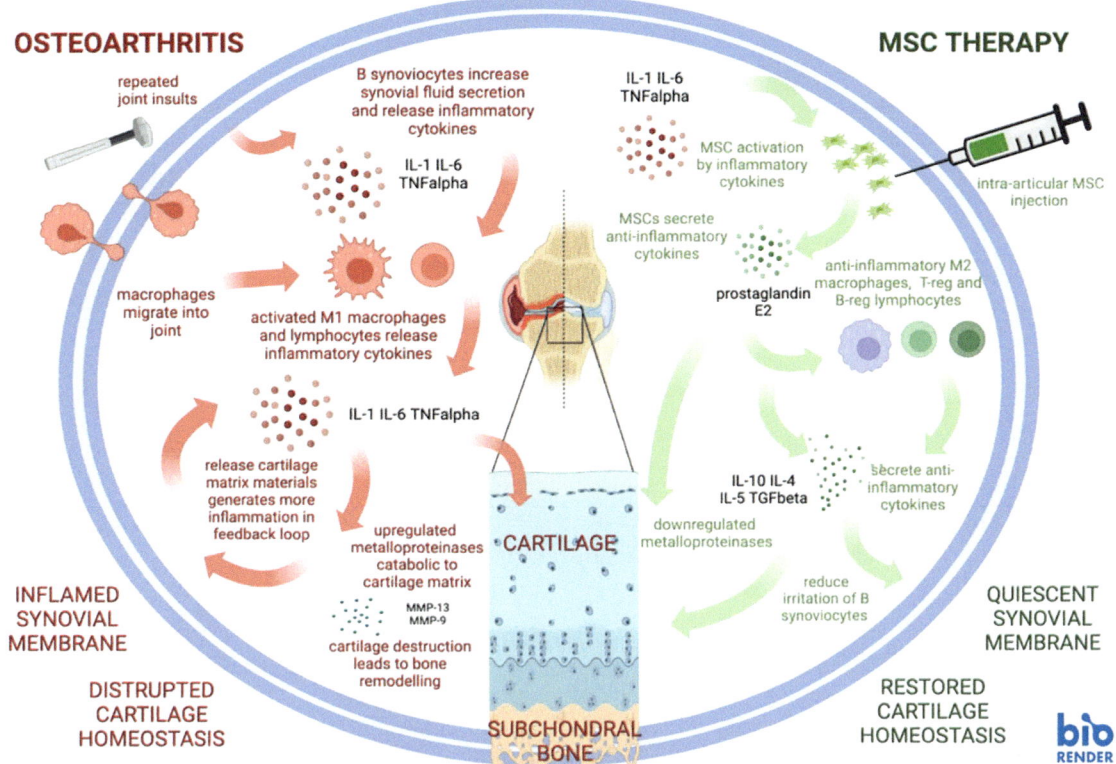

Fig. 10.2 Some of the cellular mechanisms involved in OA pathogenesis and their remediation by MSC therapy. The image is inspired by, modified from, and redrawn with permission following an image presented by Almudena Pradera in 2023 (created by Equicord®). IL-1 = interleukin-1; IL-4 = interleukin-4; IL-5 = interleukin-5; IL-6 = interleukin-6; IL-10 = interleukin-10; TNFalpha = tumour necrosis factor-alpha; TGFbeta = transforming growth factor-beta.

Contra-indications for regenerative medicine (RM)

When not to use MSCs for OA:

- Absence of a definitive diagnosis.
- Presence of severe systemic disease that contra-indicates sedation or anaesthesia.
- Active joint infection.
- Skin infection at or near the intended injection site.
- Current cancer diagnosis.
- Haemostatic disorders that increase bleeding risk.
- Use of anticoagulant medication.
- Possibly polyarthritis.

Diagnostic tests are chosen on a case-by-case basis to confirm or refute the tentative diagnosis and, where possible, to rule in or out the differentials. Diagnostic imaging is commonly practised, and radiography is the foremost of these. Where more detailed imaging of the osseous elements of the joint is required, such as in cases of elbow dysplasia, then computed tomography (CT) is useful. Soft tissue pathology may be investigated by MSK ultrasound.

Arthrocentesis and synovial fluid analysis may help distinguish inflammatory arthropathies from their degenerative counterparts. A cytology picture in which neutrophils predominate is consistent with inflammatory joint disease. This category includes immune-mediated conditions such as polyarthritis, where multiple joints are affected. If only a single joint is involved, then bacterial infective arthritis is more likely. A degenerative cytology picture in which mononuclear cells (synoviocytes and macrophages) are the dominant type is seen in conditions such as OA and where there is instability or incongruence of the joint. The latter includes, for example, CCL degeneration, elbow dysplasia, and patellar luxation.

Joint infection

Joint infections are most likely to have a bacterial aetiology. The diagnosis is confirmed by a positive culture of synovial fluid. In these cases, an appropriate antibiotic can be selected for systemic use. Saline lavage of the joint can also help reduce the bacterial load. Many cases do not yield growth of bacterial isolates in the laboratory. Instead, the diagnosis is implied by the history, clinical findings, and a neutrophilic synovial infiltrate.

During the phase of the joint disease in which there is an infection present, RM is generally considered to be contra-indicated. There are circumstances, however, in which MSCs may be effective against septic arthritis. This is exemplified by Johnson et al. (2017), who showed that TLR-activated (TLR = Toll-like receptor) MSCs may be useful in combination with antibiotics in managing chronic bacterial infections associated with biofilms.

Skin infection

To minimise the risk of iatrogenic bacterial arthritis, the injection of joints in the presence of macroscopically apparent skin infection is best avoided. Topical and systemic dermatological therapies may be required to eliminate skin infections before joint injections are contemplated.

Cancer

While MSCs may, in the future, have a role in cancer therapy, for example, as a vehicle for gene therapy delivery, in the current veterinary context, it is not recommended that MSCs are injected into MSK tissues or joints where cancer has been diagnosed.

Haemostatic disorders

PRP relies on the concentration of the circulating platelets. In cases where there is thrombocytopenia, there is clearly a reduced number of these. Drawing blood may be hazardous from the risk of haemorrhage point of view. Similarly, hemarthrosis is a likely complication of joint injection in a thrombocytopenic patient. Furthermore, establishing a platelet product with sufficient concentration is less likely if standard procedures, which assume a normal starting platelet concentration, are followed.

Anticoagulants

Animals receiving anticoagulants may be at higher risk of haemorrhage from venepuncture. Bleeding could also occur as a result of IA injection; if this happens inside the joint, then hemarthrosis may result.

Polyarthritis

In human rheumatoid arthritis, MSCs combined with disease-modifying antirheumatic drugs (DMARDs) represent a promising therapeutic approach (Wang et al., 2019). In the veterinary situation, MSCs are ordinarily used to target an affected joint or joints using their predominantly locally acting paracrine effects. In cases of polyarthritis, a systemic disease potentially affecting all the joints in the body, such an approach is not especially practical. The systemic use of VRMs in future could apply to autoimmune conditions such as polyarthritis.

In the human field, MSCs have been administered to patients with refractory polyarthritides of various kinds (Wong et al., 2021). The authors emphasise that this paper did not involve a controlled study; instead, it reports on three cases where MSC treatments appeared to produce profoundly positive outcomes, albeit anecdotally. Additionally, the authors highlight that the treatments were carried out as the families' choice, without the recommendation of the conventional rheumatology clinicians. It has been suggested that the autologous MSCs derived from patients who already suffer from an autoimmune disease may themselves have impaired immunomodulatory and regenerative function (Zaripova et al., 2023). Therefore, allogeneic MSCs, such as those from the fetal adnexa, are likely to show better efficacy.

Administration of regenerative medicine (RM)

Synovial joint injections

To achieve the maximum effectiveness of the injected orthobiologic, accurate positioning of the needle is essential. As already discussed, we cannot rely on the limited capabilities of the MSCs to 'home' to the affected area.

Most of the main canine and feline synovial joints are amenable to 'blind injection', meaning that appropriate locations for joint penetration can be determined by the palpation of anatomical landmarks.

Strict adherence to the principles of aseptic technique for joint injection is mandatory. Concurrent bacterial or yeast infection of the skin over the joint is a contra-indication for an intra-synovial injection. Injecting through infected skin intuitively increases the risk of iatrogenic joint infection, which is likely to damage the joint, even if effectively treated subsequently.

The hair coat should be widely and carefully clipped over the planned joint injection site. It is worth avoiding the creation of dermal inflammation by excessive or rough handling of the skin. Standard surgical skin preparation is employed before injection. The operating surgeon dons sterile surgical gloves and ensures that the aseptic process is unbroken during the procedure. Sterile draping that does not obscure the target location or bony landmarks is recommended.

Post-injection complications are, in the author's experience, rare. When these do occur, they are mild and short-lived. The most common adverse events are joint pain and swelling.

Post-injection care includes analgesic medication, activity restriction, and careful observation at home. Follow-up veterinary examinations are scheduled to monitor progress, and CMIs are used, preferably at every visit.

Ultrasound-guided injections

Musculotendinous conditions for which orthobiologics are being administered require a targeted application of the product. Ultrasound guidance is the standard of care in human sports medicine (Czyrny, 2017). Even for large joints, such as the human knee, ultrasound guidance outperforms 'blind' injection for accuracy of administration (Fang et al., 2021). In the small animal veterinary context, however, the use of ultrasound guidance is less common due to limited access to equipment and expertise at the time of writing. This situation is likely to improve as specific MSK ultrasonography training becomes more available and widespread. Veterinary clinicians involved in VRM are encouraged to acquire the skills of MSK ultrasonography not only for targeting orthobiologic administration but also for the diagnosis and monitoring of MSK cases.

Chapter 10 key points

- VRM has the potential to be a disease-modifying OA therapy.
- VRM is part of the multimodal management of canine OA.
- An accurate diagnosis is essential if VRM is to be applied.
- There are contra-indications for VRM which need to be considered.

Chapter 10 references

Czyrny, Z. (2017, September). Standards for musculoskeletal ultrasound. *Journal of Ultrasonography*, *17*(70), 182–187. https://doi.org/10.15557/JoU.2017.0027

Fang, W. H., Chen, X. T., Vangsness, C. T., Jr., & Knee, U.-G. (2021, June 26). Ultrasound-Guided Knee Injections are more accurate than blind injections: A systematic review of randomized controlled trials. *Arthroscopy, Sports Medicine, and Rehabilitation*, *3*(4), e1177–e1187. https://doi.org/10.1016/j.asmr.2021.01.028

Fox, S. M. (2017). *Multimodal management of canine osteoarthritis*. CRC Press. ISBN 978184076.

Hu, C., & Li, L. (2019). The immunoregulation of mesenchymal stem cells plays a critical role in improving the prognosis of liver transplantation. *Journal of Translational Medicine, 17*(1), 412. https://doi.org/10.1186/s12967-019-02167-0

Johnson, V., Webb, T., Norman, A., Coy, J., Kurihara, J., Regan, D., & Dow, S. (2017). Activated mesenchymal stem cells interact with antibiotics and host innate immune responses to control chronic bacterial infections. *Scientific Reports*, *7*(1), 9575. https://doi.org/10.1038/s41598-017-08311-4

Wang, L., Huang, S., Li, S., Li, M., Shi, J., Bai, W., Wang, Q., Zheng, L., & Liu, Y. (2019). Efficacy and safety of umbilical cord mesenchymal stem cell therapy for rheumatoid arthritis patients: A prospective phase I/II study. *Drug Design, Development and Therapy*, 13, 4331–4340. https://doi.org/10.2147/DDDT.S225613

Wong, S. C., Medrano, L. C., Hoftman, A. D., Jones, O. Y., & McCurdy, D. K. (2021). Uncharted waters: Mesenchymal stem cell treatment for pediatric refractory rheumatic diseases; a single center case series. *Pediatric Rheumatology Online Journal*, *19*(1), 87. https://doi.org/10.1186/s12969-021-00575-5

Zaripova, L. N., Midgley, A., Christmas, S. E., Beresford, M. W., Pain, C., Baildam, E. M., & Oldershaw, R. A. (2023). Mesenchymal stem cells in the pathogenesis and therapy of autoimmune and autoinflammatory diseases. *International Journal of Molecular Sciences*, *24*(22), 16040. https://doi.org/10.3390/ijms242216040

Section IV

Chapter 11

Other veterinary regenerative medicines (VRMs) in musculoskeletal (MSK) conditions

This book focuses on the most commonly used VRMs in small animal practice, namely PRP and MSCs. While alternative VRMs are available and may be appropriate in certain circumstances, only a few examples are discussed here. As science and technology in the field of VRM advances, the range of options is likely to expand.

Micro-fragmented adipose tissue and stromal vascular fraction (SVF)

A technique of preparing autologous, minimally manipulated, micro-fragmented adipose tissue has been developed as a point-of-care procedure (Lipogems®, Lipocast, UK). This therapy is available for use in human, canine, and equine patients (Zeira et al., 2018). The rationale is that the MSC niche in adipose tissue is the perivascular zone and that pericytes are the putative MSC precursors in this juxta-capillary location.

Since adipose tissue is typically amply available in subcutaneous tissues, and because it is richly supplied with capillaries, then the harvesting of this adipose tissue will contain numerous pericytes/MSCs.

A mini-liposuction technique is used to collect adipose tissue. A specifically designed device is employed to physically break down the fat tissue into a micro-fragmented suspension containing the desired pericytes/MSCs, known as 'Lipogems®'. This suspension can be immediately injected into the target tissue, such as a joint, where the intended beneficial stem cell effects can be produced. The presence of fragmented adipose cells and extra-cellular matrix may enhance the beneficial effects of the pericytes/MSCs by providing a three-dimensional extra-cellular substrate for attachment.

Zeira et al. (2018) reported on a large retrospective series involving 130 dogs with naturally occurring OA treated with a single IA dose of micro-fragmented adipose tissue using the Lipogems® device. These were consecutive cases treated by the authors in real-world, multicentred, private veterinary practice across seven veterinary hospitals in four countries. The primary outcome measures were veterinary clinical metrology and owner questionnaires. No controls were included in the study. Despite this obvious limitation, the results were very positive for both safety and efficacy, and the effects were reasonably long-lasting, persisting for six months, and in some cases up to 24 months.

The micro-fragmented adipose tissue system described here is worthy of consideration in situations where a one-step VRM treatment is required. The harvesting of tissue (mini-liposuction), minimal physical processing, and injection into the target location can all be done under one general anaesthetic. This eliminates the requirement for a stem cell laboratory, and the delays associated with stem cell manufacture. This technique may find a niche in areas of the world where such stem cell laboratories are not readily accessible.

An alternative means of producing an adipose-derived SVF for transplant relies not on the physical means of preparation of the product but on enzymatic digestion (Sharun et al., 2022). This method is more time-consuming than the physical method described above, although a higher concentration of cells may be yielded. After collection, the adipose tissue is minced and incubated with collagenase. Centrifugation separates a 'pellet' containing a mixture of MSCs, pericytes, haemopoietic cells, pre-adipocytes, and endothelial progenitor cells. Resuspension of the cells in PRP, phosphate-buffered saline, or saline produces a ready-to-use orthobiologic product for injection.

Bone marrow (BM) aspirate concentrate

BM aspirate concentrate can be used as an alternative method of VRM. It has distinct advantages in terms of its lower cost compared to, for example, cultured and expanded MSCs. In addition, since it can be prepared patient-side, there is minimal delay between collection and administration, and since it is an autologous product, adverse immune incompatibility issues are circumvented. Finally, BM aspirate concentrate may be combined with PRP (Canapp et al., 2016; Canapp, 2018).

BM aspirate concentrate has been shown to be safe and efficacious in several species, such as humans, horses, and dogs (Fortier et al., 2010; Canapp et al., 2016; Holton et al., 2016). A recent study by Pintore et al. (2023) found no difference in results measuring the positive effects on human knee OA between lipoaspirate, SVF, and AD-MSCs. How BM aspirate concentrate exerts its effects on the damaged tissues is a subject of conjecture. While MSCs are present in niches within the BM, they are hugely outnumbered by other cell types, including HSCs. The concentration of MSCs in BM aspirate is a paltry 0.001% to 0.01% (Pittenger et al., 1999). Rather than injecting native BM aspirate into the target tissue, the BM aspirate concentrate processing uses centrifugation to concentrate the product.

The concentrated cell profile of the BM aspirate concentrate has been investigated. In studies of human BM aspirate concentrate, the rank order of cellular composition is broadly polymorph neutrophils, erythroblasts, lymphocytes, eosinophils, and basophils. A variable number of platelets are found, though the platelet concentration is similar to PRP (Cassano et al., 2018). Interestingly, the same authors report that compared to peripheral blood, the leukocyte count is increased by 11.8 times, and when neutrophils are considered, these are concentrated by 19.4 times. The question therefore arises: if it is the cellular components of the BM aspirate concentrate that are responsible for its beneficial effects in, for example, OA, what are the mechanisms by which such a concentrated source of leukocytes may act? To the author's knowledge, this remains unknown. However, one could postulate that the platelets could have similar benefits to those of PRP by using their alpha-granule cargo, which is rich in growth factors.

Turning to the non-cellular components of BM aspirate concentrate, the following has been reported in the human context (Holton et al., 2016). Various beneficial growth factors and cytokines are concentrated in the concentrate, including VEGF (by 172.5x), IL-8 (by 78x), IL-1-beta (by 4.6x), TGF-beta (by 3.4x), and PDGF

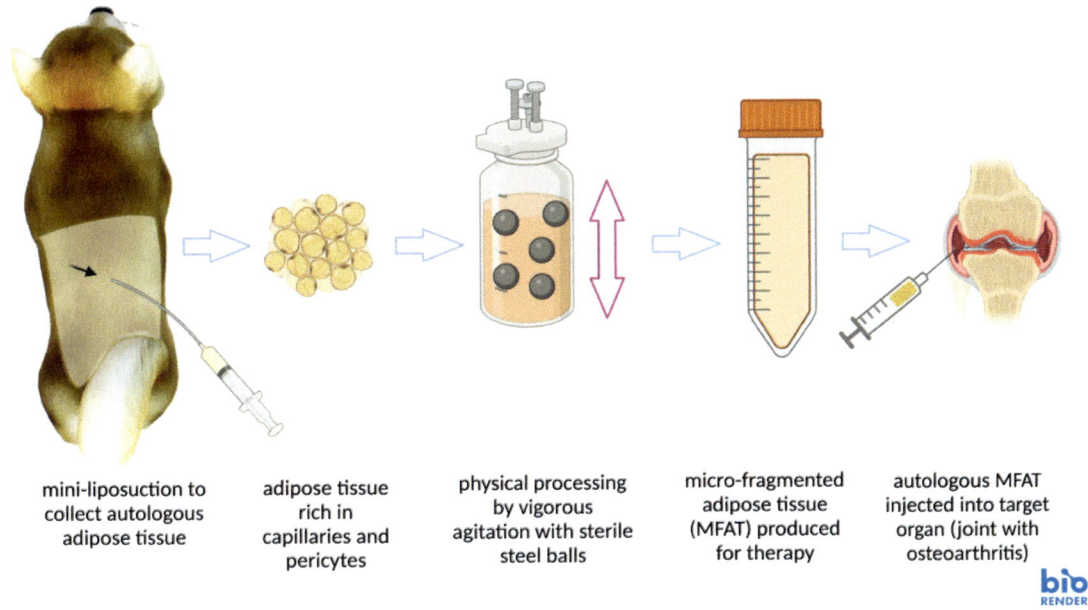

mini-liposuction to collect autologous adipose tissue | adipose tissue rich in capillaries and pericytes | physical processing by vigorous agitation with sterile steel balls | micro-fragmented adipose tissue (MFAT) produced for therapy | autologous MFAT injected into target organ (joint with osteoarthritis)

Fig. 11.1 Micro-fragmented adipose tissue flow diagram. Aseptic harvesting of subcutaneous adipose tissue from the dog's dorsum and flanks is undertaken first. The adipose tissue is vigorously bombarded by sterile steel balls to fragment the tissue. The resultant micro-fragmented adipose tissue is immediately injected into the target tissues (Zeira et al., 2018).

(by 1.3x). It is likely that these molecular components of the concentrate, which are richly contained within the platelet alpha-granules in addition, are the instrumental factors in its efficacy as a VRM.

BM aspirate concentrate in combination with PRP has been demonstrated to be effective in the management of partial CCL rupture (meaning that less than 50% of the ligament is ruptured) (Canapp et al., 2016). Typically, the concentrate involves the injection of a heterogeneous combination of 30,000 BM cells. The relative importance of these cells and the PRP platelets in the regeneration of the damaged CCL is unknown.

Autologous conditioned serum

A major inflammatory mediator in OA is interleukin-1β (IL-1β). A natural antagonist for IL-1β exists, namely interleukin-1 receptor antagonist (IL-1ra). An orthobiologic containing supraphysiological levels of IL-1ra may be produced by collecting autologous blood in a simple in-house process. The blood is harvested into an acid citrate dextrose (ACD) syringe (such as one that is available from Orthokine® Vet IRAP, Dechra) and incubated for 24 hours at 37°C. The following day, the blood is centrifuged at 2,100-g for ten minutes. The supernatant is the autologous conditioned serum (ACS), which contains high levels of IL-1ra and a high IL-1ra: IL-1β ratio (Sawyere et al., 2016). The product can be injected immediately or stored at -18°C for up to a year.

Plasma rich in growth factors (PRGFs)

PRGFs is a relatively recent development and a derivative of PRP. An example of this is the product PRGF-ENDORET® (BTI Biotechnology).

This method produces an orthobiologic containing platelets that are two to three times more concentrated than the starting blood. In addition, the plasma portion is highly concentrated in growth factors. Cuervo et al. (2020) determined that PRGFs has a beneficial effect on canine OA, which lasts around 90 days or 180 days if combined with physiotherapy.

Blood cell secretome

Yet another potentially useful orthobiologic may be autologous blood cell secretome. Efficacy for IA blood cell secretome in canine OA has been demonstrated (Alves et al., 2022a; Alves et al., 2022b), the effect being enhanced by co-injection with triamcinolone. The preparation method involves extended coagulation by incubation at 37°C for 4.5 hours followed by centrifugation at 1,500-g for three minutes. The serum is filtered, and a sterile blood cell secretome sample is available for IA injection, freezing of the remainder at -18°C provides aliquots for future use.

> ### Chapter 11 key points
>
> - Several VRMs other than PRP and MSCs are currently available.
> - These may be considered when PRP equipment or stem cell laboratory access is unavailable.
> - Some alternatives, such as BM aspirate concentrate, can be used in combination with PRP.
> - It is foreseeable that future variations on the existing VRMs will be innovated and introduced to the market.

Chapter 11 references

Alves, J. C., Santos, A., Jorge, P., & Carreira, L. M. (2022a). A first report on the efficacy of a single intra-articular administration of blood cell secretome, triamcinolone acetonide, and the combination of both in dogs with osteoarthritis. *BMC Veterinary Research*, *18*(1), 1–10.

Alves, J. C., Santos, A., Jorge, P., & Carreira, L. M. (2022b). A Comparison of Intra-Articular Blood Cell Secretome and Blood Cell Secretome with Triamcinolone Acetonide in Dogs with Osteoarthritis: A Crossover Study. *Animals*, *12*(23), 3358.

Barfod, K. W., & Blønd, L. (2019). Treatment of osteoarthritis with autologous and microfragmented adipose tissue. *Danish Medical Journal*, *66*(10), A5565.

BTI Biotechnology. https://bti-biotechnologyinstitute.com/

Canapp, Jr., S. O., Leasure, C. S., Cox, C., Ibrahim, V., & Carr, B. J. (2016). Partial cranial cruciate ligament tears treated with stem cell and platelet-rich plasma combination therapy in 36 dogs: A retrospective study. *Frontiers in Veterinary Science*, *3*, 112. https://doi.org/10.3389/fvets.2016.00112

Canapp, S. O. (2018). Conservative treatment options for partial and complete CCL tears in dogs. *Veterinary practice news*.

Cassano, J. M., Kennedy, J. G., Ross, K. A., Fraser, E. J., Goodale, M. B., & Fortier, L. A. (2018). Bone marrow concentrate and platelet-rich plasma differ in cell distribution and interleukin 1 receptor antagonist protein concentration. *Knee Surgery, Sports Traumatology, Arthroscopy*, *26*(1), 333–342. https://doi.org/10.1007/s00167-016-3981-9

Cuervo, B., Rubio, M., Chicharro, D., Damiá, E., Santana, A., Carrillo, J. M., Romero, A. D., Vilar, J. M., Cerón, J. J., & Sopena, J. J. (2020). Objective comparison between platelet-rich plasma alone and in combination with physical therapy in dogs with osteoarthritis caused by hip dysplasia. *Animals: An Open Access Journal from MDPI*, *10*(2), 175. https://doi.org/10.3390/ani10020175

Fortier, L. A., Potter, H. G., Rickey, E. J., Schnabel, L. V., Foo, L. F., Chong, L. R., Stokol, T., Cheetham, J., & Nixon, A. J. (2010). Concentrated bone marrow aspirate improves full-thickness cartilage repair compared with microfracture in the equine model. *The Journal of Bone and Joint Surgery. American Volume*, *92*(10), 1927–1937. https://doi.org/10.2106/JBJS.I.01284

Holton, J., Imam, M., Ward, J., & Snow, M. (2016). The basic science of bone marrow aspirate concentrate in chondral injuries. *Orthopedic Reviews*, *8*(3), 6659. https://doi.org/10.4081/or.2016.6659

Pintore, A., Notarfrancesco, D., Zara, A., Oliviero, A., Migliorini, F., Oliva, F., & Maffulli, N. (2023, May). Intra-articular injection of bone marrow aspirate concentrate (BMAC) or adipose-derived stem cells (ADSCs) for knee osteoarthritis: A prospective comparative clinical trial. *Journal of Orthopaedic Surgery and Research*, *18*(1), 350. https://doi.org/10.1186/s13018-023-03841-2

Pittenger, M. F., Mackay, A. M., Beck, S. C., Jaiswal, R. K., Douglas, R., Mosca, J. D., Moorman, M. A., Simonetti, D. W., Craig, S., & Marshak, D. R. (1999). Multilineage potential of adult human mesenchymal stem cells. *Science*, *284*(5411), 143–147. https://doi.org/10.1126/science.284.5411.143

Sawyere, D. M., Lanz, O. I., Dahlgren, L. A., Barry, S. L., Nichols, A. C., & Werre, S. R. (2016). Cytokine and growth factor concentrations in canine autologous conditioned serum. *Veterinary Surgery*, *45*(5), 582–586. https://doi.org/10.1111/vsu.12506

Sharun, K., Jambagi, K., Kumar, R., Gugjoo, M. B., Pawde, A. M., Tuli, H. S., Dhama, K., & Amarpal. (2022). Clinical applications of adipose-derived stromal vascular fraction in veterinary practice. *The Veterinary Quarterly*, *42*(1), 151–166. https://doi.org/10.1080/01652176.2022.2102688

Zeira, O., Scaccia, S., Pettinari, L., Ghezzi, E., Asiag, N., Martinelli, L., Zahirpour, D., Dumas, M. P., Konar, M., Lupi, D. M., Fiette, L., Pascucci, L., Leonardi, L., Cliff, A., Alessandri, G., Pessina, A., Spaziante, D., & Aralla, M. (2018). Intra-articular administration of autologous micro-fragmented adipose tissue in dogs with spontaneous osteoarthritis: Safety, feasibility, and clinical outcomes. *Stem Cells Translational Medicine*, *7*(11), 819–828. https://doi.org/10.1002/sctm.18-0020

Chapter 11 further reading

Sembronio, S., Tel, A., Tremolada, C., Lazzarotto, A., Isola, M., & Robiony, M. (2021). Temporomandibular joint arthrocentesis and microfragmented adipose tissue injection for the treatment of internal derangement and osteoarthritis: A randomized clinical trial. *Journal of Oral and Maxillofacial Surgery*, *79*(7), 1447–1456. https://doi.org/10.1016/j.joms.2021.01.038

Tremolada, C., Colombo, V., & Ventura, C. (2016). Adipose tissue and mesenchymal stem cells: State of the art and Lipogems® technology development. *Current Stem Cell Reports*, *2*(3), 304–312. https://doi.org/10.1007/s40778-016-0053-5

Tremolada, C. (2022). Microfractured adipose tissue graft (Lipogems®) and regenerative surgery. *J. Orthop. Re. s Ther*, *7*, 1210.

Chapter 12

Evidence for the usefulness of veterinary regenerative medicine (VRM)

Background

VRM is an attractive, even exciting concept for clinicians managing MSK conditions. The idea of being able to administer a genuine disease-modifying OA therapy appears, *prima facie*, to fill an obvious unmet clinical need. This begs the question: in its current iteration, how efficacious is VRM in small animal patients in practice? To answer this in as balanced and unbiased a way as possible, it is necessary to examine the evidence objectively.

The placebo effect in veterinary therapeutics

In human medicine, the placebo effect is a well-known phenomenon. While its mechanisms may be obscure, the consequences are powerful and significant. The apparent positive outcomes that result from 'dummy pills', or sham treatments, need to be considered when testing the effects of a pharmaceutical, surgical intervention, or other form of therapy. The conventional way of correcting the placebo effect is through careful experimental design. The most robust form of clinical trial is one that is randomised, double-blinded, and has suitable controls. The controls are a cohort of non-test subjects, as closely matched to the test subjects as possible. While the test subjects receive the test treatment, the controls, by contrast receive an inactive substitute referred to as a placebo. Theoretically, any placebo effect, that is, improvement in the condition unrelated to the treatment, should be equal in both the test and the placebo group. Double-blinding removes bias since neither the test subjects nor the researchers or clinicians are aware of which subjects received the treatments and which received the placebo.

Similarly, a kind of placebo effect influences the evaluation of the efficacy in veterinary therapeutics. When a novel veterinary treatment is applied to an animal in a real-world situation, such as in clinical veterinary practice, this is always confounded by the caregiver placebo effect. Thus, the owner-caregiver placebo effect and the veterinary-caregiver placebo effect will both markedly interfere with the perceived efficacy of treatment unless strict and robust experimental methodology is applied when testing VRMs.

The legal description of autologous therapies for injection (auto-transplant), that is autologous PRP and autologous MSCs, is different from the injection (transplant) of allogeneic or xenogeneic MSCs. Autologous therapies are not usually categorised as a 'medicine' by licensing authorities in many jurisdictions since the biological materials come from the patient themselves, although the degree of laboratory 'manipulation' is also considered. Accordingly, while GMP is needed, a medicine licence for autologous transplants may not be essential. In the case of allogeneic MSCs and xenogeneic MSCs, since these originate from a different animal (and species in the case of xenogeneic MSCs), a product licence needs to be sought.

Where autologous orthobiologics are studied, the inherent heterogeneity of the product represents a significant obstacle to the performance of RCTs. This is because every subject in the test group will inevitably be receiving a different formulation of cells and/or platelets.

Evidence pyramid

Not all scientific, medical, and veterinary 'evidence' is equal in terms of its 'weight' (Phillips, 2014; Brennan et al., 2020). When considering any veterinary intervention, the highest level of evidence is derived from systematic reviews, preferably with meta-analyses (Fig. 12.1). These rely on having a series of RCTs on which to base the review and to undertake the statistical analysis required for the meta-analysis. In VRM, this is where the situation becomes challenging. For studies to be compared and for their findings to be combined or amalgamated, there needs to be a high degree of similarity between them. Since no 'standard experimental protocol' currently exists in VRM studies, the literature contains a 'mixed bag' of reports, all of which vary in the details of, for example, the product administered and the outcome measures selected, among many other aspects.

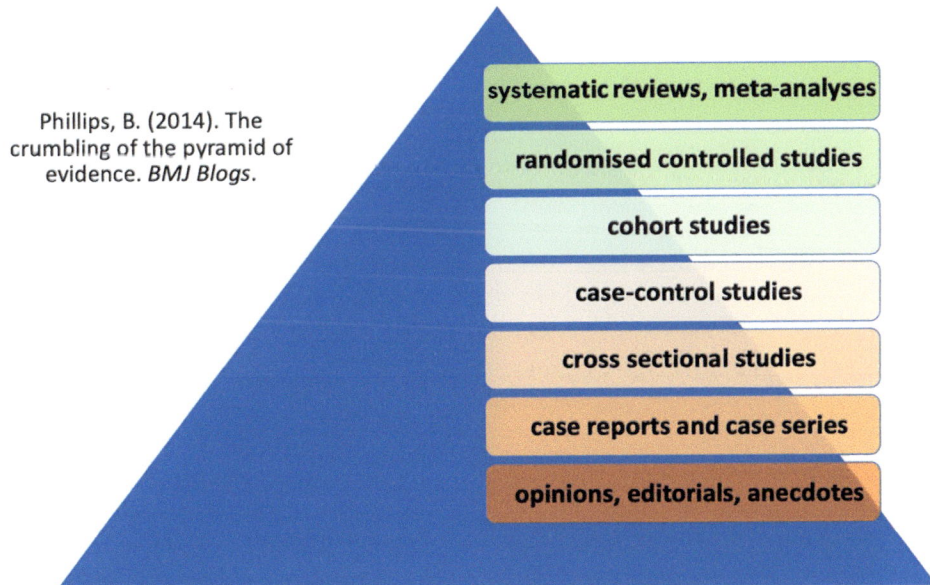

Phillips, B. (2014). The crumbling of the pyramid of evidence. *BMJ Blogs.*

systematic reviews, meta-analyses

randomised controlled studies

cohort studies

case-control studies

cross sectional studies

case reports and case series

opinions, editorials, anecdotes

Fig. 12.1 Evidence categories in veterinary orthopaedics. Redrawn after Phillips (2014).

Suitable controls are an important part of high-level studies and essential in RCTs. The ethics of taking animals with a painful disease such as OA and selecting some of them as controls so that they receive a placebo only is debatable. This problem may be circumvented by undertaking a comparison study in which a treatment of established efficacy is tested head-to-head with the orthobiologic in question.

In an unpublished literature search conducted by the author in 2022, only seven controlled studies were identified that examined the use of MSCs administered via IA injection in dogs with OA, without the concurrent use of other IA orthobiologics or viscosupplements. Even this collection of studies defied meta-analysis due to their heterogeneity.

In veterinary clinical practice, we should strive, wherever and whenever possible, to apply the principles of evidence-based veterinary medicine. In so doing, we ensure that our chosen therapies meet safety standards, to the degree that any intervention can be. It also promotes their efficacy. We should be able to point to published literature to support our decision-making and underpin our clinical reasoning for our choices. The application of VRM, a relatively novel area of clinical practice, must be similarly underpinned by robust evidence.

When considering the use of a VRM, two fundamental considerations are important:

- Is the proposed treatment safe for the patient?
- Does the proposed treatment work effectively?

Published studies typically report adverse events and any other untoward outcomes. VRMs are generally considered safe (Armitage et al., 2023).

The question of the efficacy of VRM is crucially important to answer as comprehensively as possible. An enormous amount of literature has grown on the science of stem cells. Matters relating to PRP and MSCs in humans and veterinary species have been extensively reported. When clinicians make evidence-based decisions, the range of publications can be overwhelming. It is therefore useful to filter the available research using one of the accepted conventions of evidence appraisal. The evidence pyramid is a familiar means by which research can be 'weighted' (Table 12.1). The highest level of evidence from a clinical trial is gained from an RCT. If several of these are available, then a meta-analysis of these may provide further robust evidence. Unfortunately, in VRM, as with many other veterinary disciplines, sound RCTs are relatively few in number. This may require

Table 12.1 Level of evidence proposed by Aragon and Budsberg for evaluation of orthopaedic surgery (modified from Aragon & Budsberg (2005)).

Evidence class	Study design	Examples
I	Multiple, randomised, blinded, placebo-controlled trials in target species	Systematic reviews with meta-analysis
II	High-quality clinical trials with historical controls	RCTs on animals with naturally occurring disease, in the laboratory
III	Uncontrolled case series	Non-randomised, prospective case comparison studies; prospective comparison studies that are not randomised with limited subjective influence; prospective case series that include subjective clinical impressions to objective gait analysis
IV	Expert opinion, or extrapolated from physiological studies	Retrospective comparison of cases, non-client owned studies

us to move further down the evidence pyramid to cohort studies, case-control studies, and so forth.

The critically appraised topic format for answering a clinical question may be readily applied in VRM as in other domains of veterinary clinical practice.

Levels of clinical evidence

The strength of evidence for the efficacy of a particular clinical intervention in veterinary orthopaedic research can also be categorised according to the hierarchy proposed by Aragon and Budsberg (2005).

Uncontrolled studies

A considerable number of uncontrolled studies on VRM exist. These represent a large majority of the reports. While these obviously fall short of the 'gold standard' ascribed to RCTs, they still have considerable value to offer when considering the safety and applicability of VRM and, to a lesser extent, efficacy. Such uncontrolled studies include the evidence pyramid layers that are below RCTs, namely cohort, case-controlled, and cross-sectional studies.

Controlled studies

Removing bias, as far as is practical, by having credible blinding and placebo controls is the ideal means to produce robust evidence. When designing an experiment for a VRM, the EMA has specific guidelines. Below is a description of the components of a theoretically excellent clinical study of MSC therapy for canine OA that follows the EMA guidelines:

- Use a prospective study format.
- Include pet dogs of various breeds and sexes with naturally occurring limb joint OA.
- Ensure sufficient subject numbers to provide adequate statistical power.

- Apply appropriate diagnostic criteria to confirm the presence of OA and preferably defining the severity of the joint pathology.
- Preferably include cases with unilateral OA and ensure uniform joint types (e.g., all elbows or all hips).
- Implement double blinding for both clinicians and owners.
- Use randomisation or pairing methods.
- Establish specific inclusion and exclusion criteria for subjects.
- Incorporate appropriate control groups to compare results.
- Conduct the study across multiple centres to enhance reliability and generalisability.
- Use objective measurements for primary end points to assess efficacy.
- Ensure the study duration is sufficient.
- Ensure the study design allows for reproducibility of results.
- Verify compliance with GMP standards.
- Clearly define the cell type and the number of cells used.
- Screens for pathogens and toxins to ensure safety.
- Obtain ethical approval for the study where required.
- Publish findings in a peer-reviewed journal to contribute to the body of evidence.

By way of example, the excellent clinical study by Punzón et al. (2022) can be examined. It meets all the above criteria and therefore provides plausible evidence and reasonable conclusions relating to the efficacy of xenogeneic EUC-MSCs as therapy for canine OA. The study was randomised, placebo-controlled, and multicentred. Forty test subjects were used in both the test and the control group, which is sufficient in number. The test group received one IA dose of MSCs, while the IA injection administered to the controls contained a cell transport vehicle without MSCs. The cell manufacture complied with GMP, and the MSCs were of known immunophenotype. Force plate data provided the primary outcome measure for the study, which is currently the gold standard objective measure for canine lameness. In addition, secondary outcome measures were veterinary orthopaedic examination and owner questionnaires assessing quality of life. A relatively long study duration was reported; it was blinded for one year, followed by six months unblinded.

Evidence for mesenchymal stem cell (MSC) therapy in small animal musculoskeletal (MSK) disorders

In 2022, the author conducted a literature review on MSC therapies in OA as part of an MSc dissertation at the University of Bristol (unpublished). The review aimed to critically analyze the reliability of evidence supporting the therapeutic use of MSCs in canine OA. The inclusion criteria were IA-injected MSCs without being combined with any other orthobiologic. Only controlled studies that were classed as evidence level II according to Aragon and Budsberg (2005) were considered. Seven papers were retrieved, all from the most recent decade or so (Cuervo et al., 2014; Vilar et al., 2014; Harman et al., 2016; Kim et al., 2019; Maki et al., 2020; Okamoto-Okubo et al., 2021; Punzón et al., 2022).

The most significant obstacle to comparing the papers was the heterogeneity of the studies. The review focused on three key criteria: safety, efficacy, and applicability in real-world veterinary practice.

- Safety: Injecting MSCs for OA in dogs proved to be safe in a total of 137 test subjects. Where adverse events occurred, these were invariably mild and transient. No lasting treatment-associated morbidities were reported.
- Efficacy: Six of the seven studies revealed significant improvements in the treatment groups compared to placebos.
- Applicability: The use of autologous, allogeneic, or xenogeneic MSCs are all achievable in everyday veterinary practice.

This review concluded that, on the current evidence, a cautious endorsement of the use of IA-MSCs for canine OA can be made. MSC therapy does not replace existing modes of OA management. Instead, it enhances the offering available for this intractable condition and provides a genuine disease-modifying OA therapy that can have positive and possibly long-lasting effects. Proceeding with care should be advised as more MSC products become available. Meticulous recording of the outcomes, including adverse events in real-world clinical cases, may also add much-needed evidence and weight of numbers to the sum of knowledge on MSCs for canine OA.

Evidence for platelet-rich plasma (PRP) therapy in small animal musculoskeletal (MSK) disorders

Experimental transection of the canine CCL has served as a model for OA research, commonly referred to as the Pond-Nuki model (1973). Its naturally occurring CCL rupture counterpart may also be relevant for experimental study. PRP has been injected into the stifles of dogs affected by chronic rupture of the CCL (Venator et al., 2020). In this uncontrolled study, significant improvements were observed in hind limb peak vertical force symmetry at four, eight, and twelve weeks following a single PRP injection.

Tibial plateau levelling osteotomy is a common surgical intervention in dogs for the management of CCL insufficiency. This is a significant surgery involving osteotomy and stabilisation of the tibia with orthopaedic implants. A recent study has been reported in which intra-operative leukocyte-poor PRP was applied to the osteotomy site and inside the joint. The control group had identical surgery without the PRP (Aryazand et al., 2023). The PRP-treated group showed faster bone healing of the osteotomy, less OA progression, and lower lameness scores compared to the controls.

In the human PRP research field, Johal et al. (2019) undertook a review and meta-analysis of studies including 5,308 patients. The papers analysed covered a wide range of MSK indications for PRP. Pain was reduced across all these indications; however, the only conditions that demonstrated clinically significant PRP efficacy were lateral epicondylitis and knee OA.

Khurana et al. (2021) reported that both PRP and autologous conditioned serum were equivalently efficacious in relieving pain for six months in human knee OA. Both outperformed the control groups that received either IA steroid or IA hyaluronic acid.

> ## Chapter 12 key points
>
> - Clinicians should bear in mind the caregiver placebo effect, as it influences the perception of both the animal owners and the attending clinicians. This is especially important when introducing a novel therapeutic modality such as VRM.
> - When weighing evidence on VRM, it is useful to understand what an ideal study resembles.
> - The higher the quality of the evidence, the more reliable it will be. A limited amount of level II evidence is available for the effectiveness of MSC therapy in dogs.
> - RCTs are relatively few, though these are the preferred type of reports.
> - Clinicians should critically evaluate the information presented on VRM.
> - Standardisation of study parameters, wherever possible, would enable more direct comparisons.

Chapter 12 references

Aragon, C. L., & Budsberg, S. C. (2005). Applications of evidence-based medicine: Cranial cruciate ligament injury repair in the dog. *Veterinary Surgery*, *34*(2), 93–98. https://doi.org/10.1111/j.1532-950X.2005.00016.x

Armitage, A. J., Miller, J. M., Sparks, T. H., Georgiou, A. E., & Reid, J. (2023). Efficacy of autologous mesenchymal stromal cell treatment for chronic degenerative musculoskeletal conditions in dogs: A retrospective study. Frontiers in Veterinary Science, 9, 1014687. https://doi.org/10.3389/fvets.2022.1014687.

Aryazand, Y., Buote, N. J., Hsieh, Y., Hayashi, K., & Rosselli, D. (2023). Multifactorial assessment of leukocyte reduced platelet-rich plasma injection in dogs undergoing tibial plateau leveling osteotomy: A retrospective study. *PLOS ONE*, *18*(6), e0287922. https://doi.org/10.1371/journal.pone.0287922

Brennan, M. L., Arlt, S. P., Belshaw, Z., Buckley, L., Corah, L., Doit, H., Fajt, V. R., Grindlay, D. J. C., Moberly, H. K., Morrow, L. D., Stavisky, J., & White, C. (2020). Critically appraised topics (CATs) in veterinary medicine: Applying evidence in clinical practice. *Frontiers in Veterinary Science*, *7*, 314. https://doi.org/10.3389/fvets.2020.00314

Conzemius, M. G., & Evans, R. B. (2012). Caregiver placebo effect for dogs with lameness from osteoarthritis. *Journal of the American Veterinary Medical Association*, *241*(10), 1314–1319. https://doi.org/10.2460/javma.241.10.1314

Cuervo, B., Rubio, M., Sopena, J., Dominguez, J. M., Vilar, J., Morales, M., Cugat, R., & Carrillo, J. M. (2014). Hip osteoarthritis in dogs: A randomized study using mesenchymal stem cells from adipose tissue and plasma rich in growth factors. *International Journal of Molecular Sciences*, *15*(8), 13437–13460. https://doi.org/10.3390/ijms150813437

European Medicines Agency Reflection on stem cell-based medicinal products. (January 2011). https://www.ema.europa.eu/en/documents/scientific-guideline/reflection-paper-stem-cell-based-medicinal-products_en.pdf

Harman, R., Carlson, K., Gaynor, J., Gustafson, S., Dhupa, S., Clement, K., Hoelzler, M., McCarthy, T., Schwartz, P., & Adams, C. (2016). A prospective, randomized, masked, and placebo-controlled efficacy study of intraarticular allogeneic adipose stem cells for the treatment of osteoarthritis in dogs. *Frontiers in Veterinary Science*, *3*, 81. https://doi.org/10.3389/fvets.2016.00081

Johal, H., Khan, M., Yung, S. P., Dhillon, M. S., Fu, F. H., Bedi, A., & Bhandari, M. (2019). Impact of platelet-rich plasma use on pain in orthopaedic surgery: A systematic review and meta-analysis. *Sports Health*, *11*(4), 355–366. https://doi.org/10.1177/1941738119834972

Khurana, A., Goyal, A., Kirubakaran, P., Akhand, G., Gupta, R., & Goel, N. (2021). Efficacy of autologous conditioned serum (ACS), platelet-rich plasma (PRP), hyaluronic acid (HA) and steroid for early osteoarthritis knee: A comparative analysis. *Indian Journal of Orthopaedics*, *55* Suppl. 1, 217–227. https://doi.org/10.1007/s43465-020-00274-5

Kim, S. E., Pozzi, A., Yeh, J.-C., Lopez-Velazquez, M., Au Yong, J. A., Townsend, S., Dunlap, A. E., Christopher, S. A., Lewis, D. D., Johnson, M. D., & Petrucci, K. (2019). Intra-articular umbilical cord derived mesenchymal stem cell therapy for chronic elbow osteoarthritis in dogs: A double-blinded, placebo-controlled clinical trial. *Frontiers in Veterinary Science*, *6*, Art. no. 474. https://doi.org/10.3389/fvets.2019.00474

Maki, C. B., Beck, A., Wallis, C. C. C., Choo, J., Ramos, T., Tong, R., Borjesson, D. L., & Izadyar, F. (2020). Intra-articular administration of allogeneic adipose-derived MSCs reduces pain and lameness in dogs with hip osteoarthritis: A double blinded, randomized, placebo controlled pilot study. *Frontiers in Veterinary Science*, *7*, Art. no. 570. https://doi.org/10.3389/fvets.2020.00570

Okamoto-Okubo, C. E., Cassu, R. N., Joaquim, J. G. F., dos Reis Mesquita, L. D., Rahal, S. C., Oliveira, H. S. S., Takahira, R., Arruda, I., Maia, L., Cruz Landim, F. D., & Luna, S. P. L. (2021). Chronic pain and gait analysis in dogs with degenerative hip joint disease treated with repeated intra-articular injections of platelet-rich plasma or allogeneic adipose-derived stem cells. *The Journal of Veterinary Medical Science*, *83*(5), 881–888. https://doi.org/10.1292/jvms.20-0730

Phillips, B. (2014). The crumbling of the pyramid of evidence. *BMJ blogs*.

Pond, M. J., & Nuki, G. (1973). Experimentally induced osteoarthritis in the dog. *Annals of the Rheumatic Diseases*, *32*(4), 387–388. https://doi.org/10.1136/ard.32.4.387

Punzón, E., Salgüero, R., Totusaus, X., Mesa-Sánchez, C., Badiella, L., García-Castillo, M., & Pradera, A. (2022, October 4). Equine umbilical cord mesenchymal stem cells demonstrate safety and efficacy in the treatment of canine osteoarthritis: A randomized placebo-controlled trial. *Journal of the American Veterinary Medical Association*, *260*(15), 1947–1955. https://doi.org/10.2460/javma.22.06.0237

Venator, K. P., Frye, C. W., Gamble, L.-J., & Wakshlag, J. J. (2020). Assessment of a single intra-articular stifle injection of pure platelet-rich plasma on symmetry indices in dogs with unilateral or bilateral stifle osteoarthritis from long-term medically managed cranial cruciate ligament disease. *Veterinary Medicine*, 11, 31–38. https://doi.org/10.2147/VMRR.S238598

Vilar, J. M., Batista, M., Morales, M., Santana, A., Cuervo, B., Rubio, M., Cugat, R., Sopena, J., & Carrillo, J. M. (2014). Assessment of the effect of intraarticular injection of autologous adipose-derived mesenchymal stem cells in osteoarthritic dogs using a double blinded force platform analysis. *BMC Veterinary Research*, *10*(1), Art. no. 143. https://doi.org/10.1186/1746-6148-10-143

Chapter 12 further reading

Bosch, G., van Schie, H. T. M., de Groot, M. W., Cadby, J. A., van de Lest, C. H. A., Barneveld, A., & van Weeren, P. R. (2010). Effects of platelet-rich plasma on the quality of repair of mechanically induced core lesions in equine superficial digital flexor tendons: A placebo-controlled experimental study. *Journal of Orthopaedic Research*, *28*(2), 211–217. https://doi.org/10.1002/jor.20980

Gupta, S., Paliczak, A., & Delgado, D. (2021). Evidence-based indications of platelet-rich plasma therapy. *Expert Review of Hematology*, *14*(1), 97–108. https://doi.org/10.1080/17474086.2021.1860002

Sharun, K., Jambagi, K., Dhama, K., Kumar, R., Pawde, A. M., & Amarpal. (2021). Therapeutic potential of platelet-rich plasma in canine medicine. *Archives of Razi Institute*, *76*(4), 721–730. https://doi.org/10.22092/ari.2021.355953.1749

Section V

Chapter 13

Legal and regulatory aspects of veterinary regenerative medicine (VRM)

It is incumbent on the veterinary clinician to ensure the legality of all therapeutic interventions undertaken. VRM is no exception in this respect. The following is a brief and general commentary on the regulation of VRM. This is not intended as a definitive guide, and the field of VRM is progressing apace, so clinicians must make their own enquiries to verify the current rules that apply in their jurisdiction.

Good manufacturing practice (GMP)

A minimum standard for medicine manufacture and production has been established. This ensures the product is consistently of high quality, appropriate for the indication for which it is intended, and meets the criteria of the product specification.

The World Health Organization (WHO) has established guidelines for GMP in the production of medicinal products. Equivalent GMP guidelines for pharmaceutical products have been adopted by numerous countries and regions worldwide, including the United Kingdom (under the EMA), and the United States (under the Food and Drug Administration) (Bogers, 2018).

Veterinary stem cell laboratories should adhere to GMP. This gives the animal owners and attending clinicians the confidence to use stem cell preparation. A further level of compliance may be afforded by licensing of the laboratory by government-associated bodies.

Licensing of stem cell laboratories

Legislation pertaining to stem cells varies from country to country. The relevant regulations in the territory where the stem cell therapy is being performed need to be complied with. In the United Kingdom, the Veterinary Medicines Directorate has responsibility for issuing licences for the manufacture of stem cells for use in equine therapy. However, a licence is not mandatory to manufacture canine stem cells. Despite this, laboratories may voluntarily apply for such a licence as a means of verifying that the laboratory processes meet rigorous quality and safety standards. As another example, the Australian Veterinary Stem Cell Pty Ltd (Magellan Stem Cells) complies with the regulations set out by the Australian Pesticides and Veterinary Medicine Authority, a division of the Australian government.

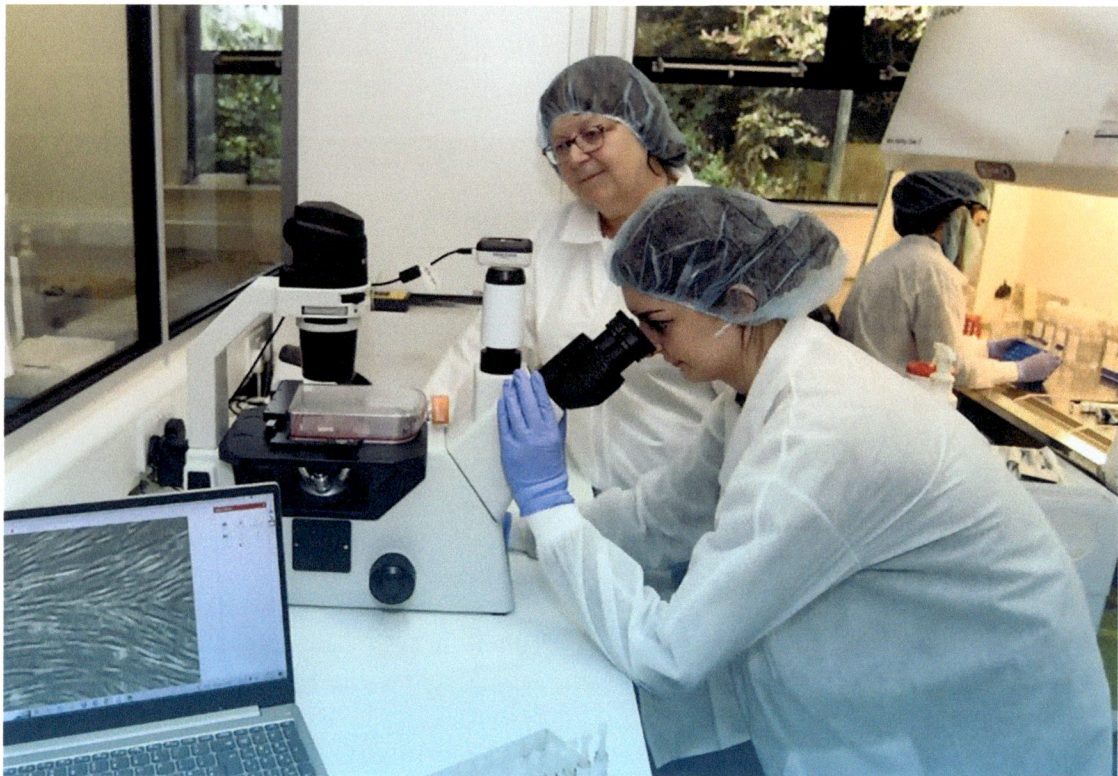

Fig. 13.1 A Veterinary Stem Cell Laboratory (photograph courtesy of Cell Therapy Sciences, Coventry, UK).

Legal categories for medicines

The administration of autologous products, including PRP and MSCs, since the biological products originate from the patient, could be considered a clinical procedure, rather than a medication administration. This is especially the case where patient-side preparation of the orthobiologic is performed. The Food and Drug Administration in the United States considers MSCs to be a drug therapy and therefore to fall under this agency's jurisdiction.

Allogeneic and xenogeneic products, such as the EUC-MSC product currently available in the United Kingdom and the EU (DogStem® Dômes Pharma), require appropriate medicine licensing. In this case, in the United Kingdom, the category is POM-V (Prescription Only Medicine-Veterinary).

Intellectual property and overseas affiliation

The processes involved in the laboratory manufacture of stem cells can be the subject of intellectual property that may be owned by private companies. Various aspects of these processes may be patented. An example of such a company is VetStem Biopharma Inc., Poway, California, which has multiple global patents. By collaborating with affiliate companies such as Chemaphor in Canada, Central Veterinary Research Laboratory in Dubai (giving access to fourteen countries in the Middle East), and Australian Veterinary Stem Cell (with markets in Australia, New Zealand, and Singapore), VetStem has an international reach for their stem cell products.

Chapter 13 key points

- The administration of autologous PRP and MSCs is more akin to a procedure rather than a 'pharmaceutical'.
- Allogeneic PRP and xenogeneic MSCs are prescription only medicines.
- Legislation and regulation of veterinary orthobiologics is likely to change so clinicians must seek the most current requirements in the relevant jurisdiction.
- Intellectual property pertaining to MSC processing may be privately owned and protected by patents.

Chapter 13 references

Australian Veterinary Stem Cell Pty. Ltd. *(Magellan Stem Cells)*. https://www.veterinarystemcells.com.au/

Bogers, S. H. (2018). Cell-based therapies for joint disease in veterinary medicine: What we have learned and what we need to know. *Frontiers in Veterinary Science*, *5*, 70. https://doi.org/10.3389/fvets.2018.00070

European Medicines Agency stem cell-based medicinal products – Scientific guideline https://www.ema.europa.eu/en/stem-cell-based-medicinal-products-scientific-guideline. https://www.ema.europa.eu/en/documents/scientific-guideline/reflection-paper-stem-cell-based-medicinal-products_en.pdf, https://www.gov.uk/guidance/good-manufacturing-practice-and-good-distribution-practice

European Medicines Agency. (January 14, 2011). *EMA/CAT/571134/2009 Committee for Advanced Therapies (CAT) Reflection paper on stem cell-based medicinal products.*

Food and Drug Administration (USA). *Regenerative medicine advanced therapy (RMAT) designation https://www.fda.gov/vaccines-blood-biologics/cellular-gene-therapy-products/regenerative-medicine-advanced-therapy-designation*

Royal Veterinary College website Retrieved 11/11/2023. https://www.rvc.ac.uk/small-animal-vet/specialist-referrals/advanced-techniques/stem-cell-clinic/information-for-dog-owners#:~:text=The%20Veterinary%20Medicines%

UK government Guidance Good manufacturing practice and good distribution practice.

Veterinary practice news November 2010. World Health Organization. https://www.veterinarypracticenews.com/vet-stem-inks-license-deal-with-aussie-affiliate/. https://www.who.int/

Chapter 14

Recommendations for the clinical use of veterinary regenerative medicine (VRM)

Management of expectations

RM in humans and animals has been the subject of a great deal of hype. This is not necessarily helpful to clinicians, as it could garner unrealistic owner expectations. One of the obligations of the clinician is to communicate, as clearly and accurately as possible, the current state of knowledge of the subject to colleagues, owners, and others. The nuances of VRM may be easily misunderstood by a lay audience, so providing printed and digital educational materials can be helpful. The appendices in this book contain some examples of pet owner information materials.

Preparations before establishing a veterinary regenerative medicine (VRM) service

As with all novel services that are to be integrated into everyday veterinary care, planning and preparation are advisable. Embarking upon a VRM enterprise without attention to these considerations is likely to yield less than optimal results and may even adversely affect patient outcomes or the reputation of the clinician, the veterinary practice, the veterinary profession, or VRM *per se*.

Training in veterinary regenerative medicine (VRM)

Veterinarians motivated to use RM need to equip themselves with the fundamental knowledge of the subject that will allow them to proceed with optimal effectiveness. Understanding the main VRM approaches available, namely PRP and MSCs, is mandatory. This will require some study of relevant materials, such as this book, and contact with experienced clinicians within the VRM field can be useful on a practical level. Proficiency in IA injections is mandatory where VRM is applied to joint diseases such as OA. Numerous published sources are available for directing the clinician's preliminary research, while practical courses are available to allow finessing of the technique. Where extra-articular soft tissue MSK lesions are to be treated with orthobiologics, ultrasound guidance is an indispensable tool for injection accuracy.

Diagnosis and application of evidenced-based veterinary medicine in veterinary regenerative medicine (VRM)

Veterinary clinicians are well versed in diagnosing and managing the wide-ranging conditions affecting their small animal patients. Furthermore, they are familiar with the principles of evidence-based veterinary medicine. From these aspects, VRM does not differ from any other sphere of veterinary medicine or surgery. Underpinning its application must be an accurate diagnosis. Only then can the optimal choices of evidence-based veterinary medicine be made.

Diagnosis in clinical musculoskeletal (MSK) cases

Regardless of the anticipated combination of therapeutic modalities, all MSK cases, including

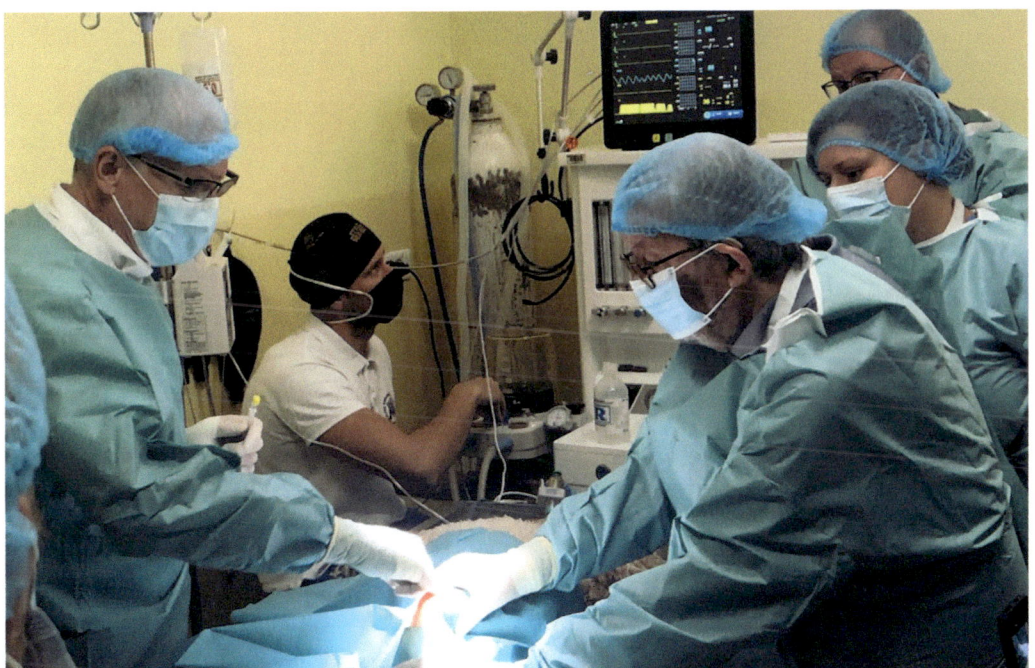

Fig. 14.1 Veterinarians demonstrating IA injection of PRP into a canine stifle to delegates on a training course. Photograph courtesy of Ksenjia Ilieska.

those where VRM is a possibility, merit the same precision in diagnostic work-up. However, clinicians may face constraints, such as financial limitations, which may restrict the extent to which a case is investigated. Under such circumstances, VRM may not be a feasible option anyway.

Sufficient time needs to be allocated for the full diagnostic work-up of an MSK case. If too little of this precious resource is made available, a reliable diagnosis may not be possible. When practising VRM, the highest standards of clinical diagnosis should be applied. This does not necessarily imply the excessive use of expensive imaging techniques; rather, it suggests that a combination of attention to detail and clinical acumen is consistently applied.

A logical diagnostic approach should include:

- History and signalment
- Owner's description of the problem
- Observation
- Gait assessment
- General examination
- Physique, muscle condition score, and body condition score
- Orthopaedic examination
- Neurological examination
- Clinical metrology
- Diagnostic imaging
- Laboratory analysis

History and signalment

Before a consultation, it is often possible to become familiarised with the patient's details, including age, breed, sex, and so forth, as well as the previous medical history. This should save time as well as provide some diagnostic insight.

Owner's description of the problem

The art of listening to the owner's remarks on how they see the pet's problem is an essential skill. Clinicians who are pressed for time will not be able to gather all the information from the owner, let alone distil down from this what is relevant to the case. A more accurate and thorough history may be gleaned from a well-designed owner questionnaire. This also has the advantage of efficiency since it takes much less of the clinician's time, especially if it is completed ahead of the consultation.

Observation

Patient observation often reveals clues indicating the diagnosis. This may even precede the consultation if owner video footage of the pet during rising or ambulation is available. One downside is that the owner's video is frequently not optimally filmed from the veterinarian's point of view. Nonetheless, 'seeing' the animal in their own environment can allow detection of subtleties that may elude us in the clinical situation. Observing pets sitting, rising, and moving is useful to assess posture and preferences to bear weight or not on any particular limb.

Gait assessment

The traditional veterinary lameness examination requires standardised ambulation that is preferably filmed (at least on a smartphone) and is observed from the front, either side, and the rear. Walking pace is most useful in the author's experience. Trotting and running may be added as needed. The more complex manoeuvres of turning and so on are beyond the scope of this brief description.

Watching and playing back the video footage, in slow motion if needed, usually allows a lameness to be narrowed down to one or more limbs. The severity of the lameness can be visually scored.

Lameness scoring

It is a convention in veterinary medicine that lameness is ascribed a score according to its perceived severity. Unfortunately, there are

Table 14.1 Example of a canine lameness score chart. Redrawn from Carr & Dycus (2016).

Numerical rating scale for lameness by visual assessment	
Grade of lameness	Description
1	Walks soundly, weight shifting, mild lameness at trot
2	Mild weight-bearing lameness
3	Weight-bearing lameness with head bob
4	Significant weight-bearing lameness
5	Toe touching lameness
6	Non-weight-bearing lameness

many different schemes for this. One such framework is described by Carr and Dycus (2016) (Table 14.1).

If available, more accurate lameness measurements can be made using specifically designed gait laboratory apparatuses (Fig. 14.2). Most practices are not equipped with force plate equipment, though many now have pressure mats.

General examination

Considering an orthopaedic problem in the absence of a basic clinical examination can be a costly error. All patients require an elementary assessment of their general health, especially as it may impact the diagnosis or management of the presenting MSK condition.

Physique, muscle condition score, and body condition score

MSK patients frequently present with changes in muscle and adipose tissue. Muscle loss may be physiological through disuse atrophy or pathological through neurogenic atrophy. In the former case, addressing the underlying cause of the disuse, such as a painful joint affected by OA, may allow the atrophy to be reversed. In the latter case, unless the nervous system input recovers, the atrophy will be permanent. Muscle loss may also be generalised; this is termed sarcopenia. Quantification of muscle loss may be aided by

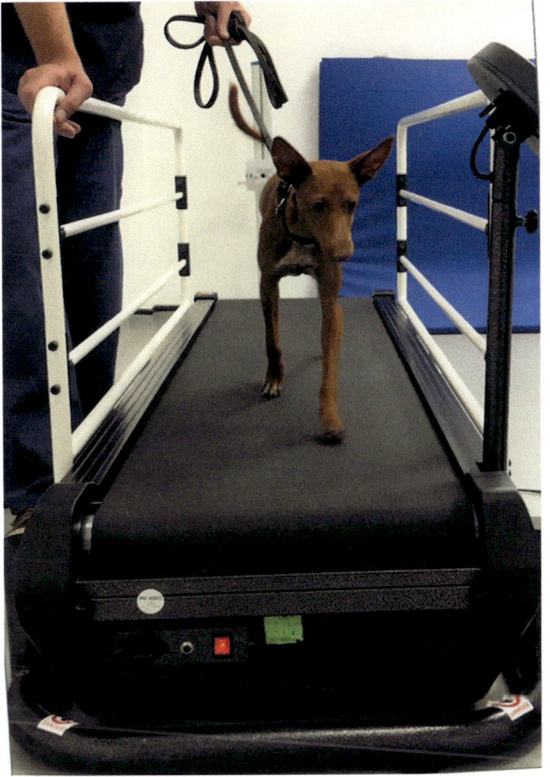

Fig. 14.2 Force plate analysis using a treadmill (CanidGait® Zebris Medical GmbH). Photograph courtesy of Nupsala MSK Clinic, Melton Mowbray, UK.

the WSAVA Muscle Condition Score Chart (see Fig. 14.3). Sarcopenia may be associated with systemic diseases such as renal insufficiency or hyperadrenocorticism. It is also strongly associated with ageing, especially during the final

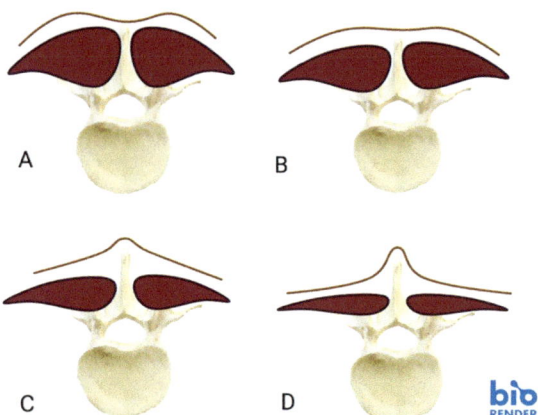

Fig. 14.3 Muscle Condition Score (Modified after World Small Animal Association Global Nutrition Committee Muscle Condition Score Chart. (www. wsava.org)). The muscle condition is assessed by visualisation of the skull, scapulae, spine, and pelvis. In addition, the caudal thoracic epaxial muscle mass is palpated and categorised according to the above diagrams. A. normal muscle mass; B. mild muscle loss; C. moderate muscle loss; D. severe muscle loss.

stage of life, potentially due in part to increased autophagy (Pagano et al., 2015).

Limb circumference measurements are commonly used to detect asymmetry caused by muscle atrophy. Measurement accuracy is confounded by multiple variables (Kim et al., 2022); nevertheless, serial measurements can be useful to monitor patient progress.

Excess adipose tissue has an enormous impact on pet health; therefore, assessing it is a critical part of the examination of an MSK patient. The WSAVA nine-point framework is widely used for this purpose (see Fig. 14.4). This framework allows for the identification of overweight or obese pets, and provides a numerical categorisation for the severity of the situation.

Adiposity management, whenever body condition scores exceed 5/9, is an essential part of OA management. The detrimental effects of excess adipose tissue are both physical and biological. Regarding the former, excess adiposity puts greater physical loads on the joints, which could be expected to increase the rate of joint tissue attrition. As for the latter, it is known that the plethora of adipokine molecules released from the adipose tissue has a pro-inflammatory effect on all parts of the body, including the joints. This upregulation of the inflammatory state in the joint tissues exacerbates pain and accelerates degeneration. Regardless of which other mode of OA management are combined in a patient, adiposity management is central to successful therapy.

Orthopaedic and neurological examination

The entire MSK system should be thoroughly examined, including the spine and all limbs. The aim is to detect 'all' issues affecting the locomotor system, as it is common for multiple conditions to coexist. For example, large-breed dogs may present with both bilateral hip OA and lumbosacral disease. Detecting only the hip OA may leave the lumbosacral disease untreated, leaving the dog in pain.

A basic neurological examination is advisable for the spine since spinal conditions need to be differentiated from other orthopaedic conditions. Foot placing tests are useful for assessing proprioception. Myotatic reflexes, such as the patellar reflex, can also have value. The entire spine can be palpated for signs of hyperaesthesia and muscle atrophy.

The most likely limb(s) affected by lameness-associated pathology is typically identified through observation of the animal's gait. It is worthwhile examining the sounder limbs first, since presumably this will be more comfortable and less likely to elicit a pain response and subsequent loss of patient cooperation. After assessing the sound limb(s), the affected limb(s) can then be examined.

The entire limb should be palpated, and the following should be noted:

- Lesions of the digits, footpads, or interdigital areas.

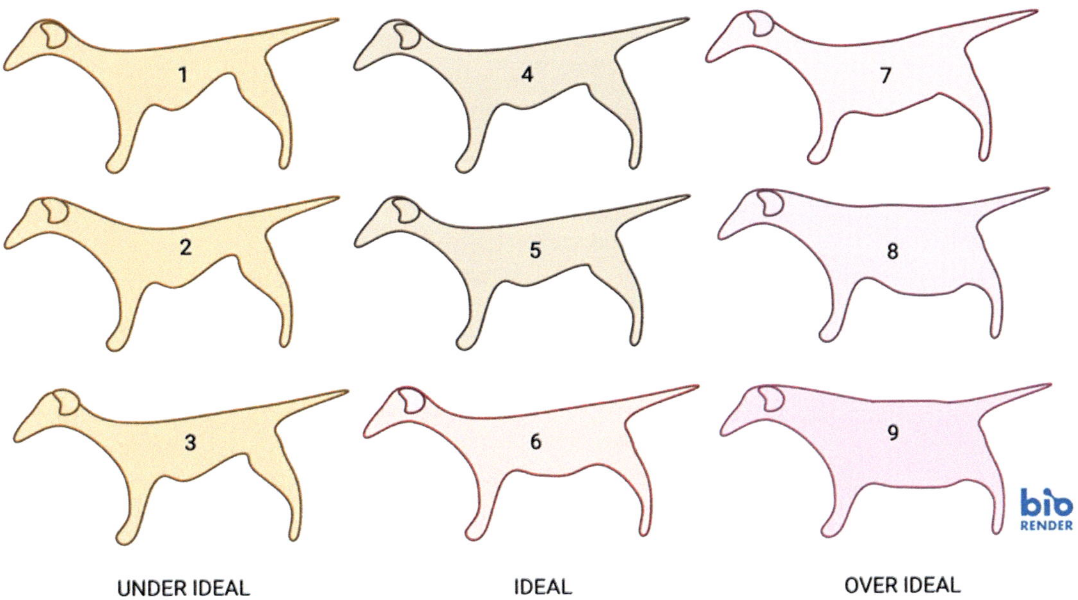

Fig. 14.4 Body Condition Score Chart (modified after World Small Animal Association Global Nutrition Committee Body Condition Score Chart (www.wsava.org)). 1. All bony prominences evident from afar, no noticeable body fat, clear muscle loss. 2. Ribs, lumbar vertebrae, and pelvic bones obviously visible, no palpable body fat, minor muscle loss. 3. Easily palpable ribs, lumbar spinous processes visible, pelvic bones prominent, clear waist and abdominal tuck. 4. Easily palpable ribs with minimal overlying body fat, waist seen from above, and abdominal tuck. 5. Ribs palpable, waist seen from above, abdominal tuck present. 6. Ribs palpable though obvious body fat covering, waist just discernible from above, abdominal tuck seen. 7. With difficulty due to heavy body fat covering ribs palpable, abdominal tuck may be seen. 8. Heavy body fat covering over ribs so ribs not palpable, fat over lumbar spine and tail base, no waist seen, no abdominal tuck, evidence of abdominal distension due to intra-abdominal fat. 9. Neck, chest, spine, tail base, and limbs all show body fat deposits. Enlarged abdomen due to intra-abdominal fat.

- Muscle bulk or degree of atrophy.
- Joint swelling.
- Joint ranges of motion.
- Pain anywhere associated with the soft tissues, joints or bones.

Joint range of motion

Joint range of motion is a useful parameter for measurement. This is done by goniometry, which is straightforward enough, though consistency is required for it to be useful. Normal limits of joint ranges of motion have been documented in the literature (Millis & Levine, 2013). Deviations from the reference range are useful to record. In OA, joint range of motion typically reduces as the articular pathology progresses;

therefore, the serial monitoring of this movement can serve as a measure of OA progression. Additionally, the application of VRM has been demonstrated to result in improved joint range of motion (Armitage, 2023).

Clinical metrology

Clinical metrology, in the form of owner and veterinarian questionnaires, is to be encouraged from the outset. This is best practice regardless of whether VRM is planned. If VRM is used, it can be an enormous benefit to the accumulation of knowledge on the effectiveness, or otherwise, of the therapy. An example of the excellent use of clinical metrology, among other outcome measures, can be found in a recent paper

Table 14.2 Examples of canine clinical metrology instruments (CMIs).

Canine clinical metrology instrument	Reference
LOAD Liverpool Osteoarthritis Assessment in Dogs	Walton et al. 2013
CBPI Canine Brief Pain Inventory	Brown et al. 2007
COI Canine Orthopaedic Index	Brown, 2014
HCPI Helsinki	Hielm-Björkman, 2009
Vetmetrica™	Armitage et al. 2023

by Armitage et al. (2023). Because the authors had been particularly diligent in recording the clinical metrology findings in all 245 cases in which VRM had been used, excellent data was accessible for review. Several different CMIs are available, and a selection of these are included in Table 14.2.

In addition to the CMIs listed above, it is also recommended that canine OA cases are 'staged' to allow for meaningful comparisons between similar cases. The current standard framework for staging is the four-point system provided by the Canine OsteoArthritis Staging Tool (COAST), which includes the evaluation of radiographs, or COASTeR, which excludes radiography (Cachon et al., 2018; Cachon et al., 2023).

Diagnostic imaging

The accurate diagnosis of MSK conditions usually requires the use of diagnostic imaging. The imaging modalities that may be commonly considered include:

- Radiography
- Ultrasonography
- Computed tomography (CT)
- Magnetic resonance imaging
- Arthroscopy

Of these, radiography is the most commonplace.

Radiographic diagnosis of osteoarthritis

Wessely et al. (2017) discovered 22 different OA radiographic scoring systems for canine and feline stifles alone. The authors recommended a relatively simple system (Mager, 2000; Matis et al., 2005). Simple and repeatable 1–4 or 0–3 scales can be used, mainly based on the presence and severity of osteophytes, to reduce interobserver variability. Whichever system is adopted, consistency is vital along the course of OA progression. It must always be borne in mind that radiographic severity for OA and the clinical compromise that the disease causes are relatively poorly correlated. In the human knee, a recent study found no correlation between WOMAC scores and radiological OA scores (Steenkamp et al., 2022).

Laboratory analysis

Before formulating a management plan for any MSK disease, relevant clinical pathology work-up may be indicated to identify MSK disease biomarkers, and/or to rule in or out concurrent systemic conditions.

Blood analysis
MSK biomarkers

- Inflammatory biomarker (C-reactive protein)
- Anti-nuclear antibody
- Rheumatoid Factor
- *Borrelia burgdorferi* antibodies
- Other serological assays (depending on your location in the world)

Systemic disease markers

- Blood biochemistry
- Haematology
- Endocrinological tests

Conditions associated with systemic inflammation, such as the various forms of polyarthritis, are often associated with raised circulating levels of C-reactive protein. Polyarthritis may be a feature of systemic lupus erythematosus (SLE). Anti-nuclear antibodies are typically elevated in this case. Rheumatoid arthritis, an erosive and highly destructive form of polyarthritis, is common in humans but relatively rare in canine patients. One criterion for a rheumatoid arthritis diagnosis is a raised circulating level of rheumatoid factor. Rheumatoid factor is measured using the Rose-Waaler test. Infectious diseases may manifest with MSK clinical signs. A classic example of this is Lyme disease, a tick-borne infection, and one of the clinical signs relates to inflammatory polyarthritis. Detection of seroconversion with *Borrelia* antibodies aids diagnosis.

Concurrent systemic conditions may influence the MSK disorder or may affect the choice of treatments. In dogs and cats affected by OA, it is worthwhile undertaking routine haematology and biochemistry to assess the patient for any coexisting pathologies, since this is a lifelong condition. Of particular importance may be renal or hepatic disease since one or both may contra-indicate NSAIDs. Common endocrinopathies could also be of significance, including hypothyroidism, hyperadrenocorticism, and diabetes mellitus. All of these require management alongside MSK therapy.

Synovial fluid analysis

- Physical characteristics such as colour, clarity, and viscosity.
- Cytology and cell counts.
- Bacterial culture and extended culture in blood culture medium.

Synovial fluid analysis is crucial to confirm the diagnosis of several articular conditions. In essence, synovial fluid cytology may broadly show degenerative or inflammatory changes. Light microscopy of fresh synovial fluid smears

Table 14.3 Potential biomarkers in synovial fluid (Huňáková et al., 2020).

Potential biomarkers in synovial fluid	
TIMP-1	Tissue inhibitor of metalloproteinases
MMP-3	Matrix metalloproteinase-3
FGF-1	Fibroblast growth factor-1
IGF-1	Insulin-like growth factor-1
PDGF	Platelet-derived growth factor
IL-2	Interleukin-2
IL-6	Interleukin-6
IL-8	Interleukin-8
IL-10	Interleukin-10
IL-12	Interleukin-12
TNF-α	Tumour necrosis factor-α
INF-γ	Interferon-γ

can be undertaken patient-side. The relevant cell types under microscopy are broadly mononuclear (macrophages and synoviocytes) and polymorph neutrophils. Mononuclear cells predominate in degenerative conditions such as OA, while inflammatory conditions such as polyarthritis or bacterial infection show a prevalence of neutrophils. Multiple molecular biomarkers of joint disease may be measured in experimental research on OA and regenerative therapies (Huňáková et al., 2020, Table 14.3).

To the author's knowledge, these proposed synovial fluid biomarkers are not generally used in individual clinical cases in practice currently, though this may change.

Pharmacovigilance

As VRM becomes increasingly common in veterinary practice, there is a significant opportunity to collect large amounts of real-world clinical data. It is important that, as more cell products become licensed, the clinicians administering the products are involved, to as great a degree as the constraints of clinical practice allow, in data recording. The information so gathered is useful in the early detection of adverse events, which could be detrimental to animal health. If such events go unnoticed or unreported, further patients may suffer the same effects. The suggested minimum data collection and follow-up for all cases receiving VRM is as follows:

- A thorough clinical and orthopaedic examination.
- Confirmation of the diagnosis with imaging and/or laboratory tests, as appropriate.
- Clinical metrology.
- Follow-up at, for example, one month, two months, three months, six months, nine months, and twelve months post-orthobiologic administration.
- Reporting of suspected adverse events.
- Pressure mat and force plate measurements are also desirable, if available.

How to develop a veterinary regenerative medicine (VRM) service in practice

Establishing a VRM service is relatively straightforward. However, it requires an investment in time to upskill and a relatively modest amount of capital. PRP is a reasonable place to start when considering VRM. Many different centrifuges can be purchased for different prices. There are several validated for veterinary use for the production of PRP. Some training in the use of your chosen centrifuge device is required to ensure consistent results. PRP has many advantages as an introductory VRM, which include that it is autologous, it can be prepared patient-side and immediately administered, and it can be combined with MSC products.

How to obtain information on VRM

This book aims to provide enough background information to facilitate any veterinarian's journey from no experience or familiarity with VRM to being able to reliably and safely administer either or both PRP and MSCs. The references sections at the end of each chapter provide multiple sources of further information for those wishing to explore the subject in greater depth. It is worth contacting veterinarians in your region who have already integrated VRM into their MSK treatment offering. Such colleagues may be able to offer practical demonstrations of the skills required for VRM. As the field of VRM continues to grow and mature, continuing professional development courses are becoming available in areas such as practical joint injection techniques. Attending these courses is highly recommended. Digital education platforms have similarly embraced VRM, and webinars and podcasts are becoming commonplace.

When to use VRM

The question of when to use VRM in small animal MSK cases is frequently asked. In essence, VRM can be used in almost any case where a disease-modifying therapy would be beneficial. Acute injuries may benefit from a prompt application of PRP alone. At the other end of the spectrum, end-stage OA cases that are unresponsive to conventional multimodal management may be beyond the point where VRM can be expected to be effective. However, Armitage et al. (2023) described 245 cases of MSK disease all of which were refractory to conventional management. So, it has been shown to be the case that even chronic, advanced cases with severe joint pathology, can still benefit from VRM.

In the author's opinion, the earlier in the course of the MSK disease the VRM is administered, the more likely it is to be associated with a favourable outcome. Each case needs to be judged on its merits. If a joint sprain or muscle strain settles down within a short time span using activity reduction and NSAIDs, then VRM is not justified. In cases with more severe injury and or limited response to initial treatments then VRM can legitimately be considered.

VRM does not replace conventional multimodal medical management in the case of OA, instead, the two are complementary. VRM is another 'mode' of management that can be added to the existing array of treatment categories.

Which VRM to use

The choice of VRM can be confusing. This may become more so as additional products enter the market. The orthobiologic selected will depend largely on what is hoped to be achieved from the VRM. Determining this will help to identify the most suitable product. For example, the main effects of PRP are stimulatory. The alpha-granule-derived collection of growth factors promotes angiogenesis, cell recruitment, and trophic effects. PRP may also be integral in the production of a fibrin 'scaffold', which may be relevant for providing for the attachment of cells. MSCs, as already described, release paracrine molecules that are profoundly anti-inflammatory and immunomodulatory. Accordingly, MSCs are an excellent choice in OA to downregulate the inflammation involved in the disease process and to influence macrophages to polarise from M1 to M2 phenotype.

Table 14.4 compares two MSC products that are available in the United Kingdom. Each has advantages and disadvantages. Using an autologous source of cells would intuitively be less likely to trigger an adverse immune reaction after injection. Furthermore, multiple recipient sites may be injected, and cryo-banking allows this to be done on multiple occasions. It does, however, require a surgical collection of tissue before the cells can be prepared. EUC-MSCs are convenient since they are supplied ready for administration. The concentration of cells within the preparation is relatively standardised at around 7.5 million MSCs per vial. The downsides are that the product licence only permits their injection into the canine elbow or hip, and repeat injections are not allowed.

Table 14.4 Comparison of two MSC products available in the UK. EUC-MSCs = equine umbilical cord mesenchymal stem cells; Auto AD-MSCs = autologous adipose-derived mesenchymal stem cells.

	EUC-MSCs	Auto AD-MSCs
Legally licensed	Yes	Not needed
Single dose only	Yes	No
Multiple joints	No	Yes
Repeat treatments	No	Yes
Off-the-shelf	Yes	No
Needs surgery to collect	No	Yes
Cryo-banked MSCs	No	Yes

How to monitor progress after VRM

As previously discussed, it is good practice to adhere to the principles of evidence-based veterinary medicine. Where good scientific evidence for a particular therapeutic approach exists in the literature, then the clinician is on firm ground. In VRM, most studies have limitations such as small number of subjects and typically lack controls. It therefore falls on the attending clinician to be as objective as possible, which is challenging considering the strength of the veterinarian caregiver placebo effect. The author recommends that clinicians make use of as many validated measures as possible when managing chronic MSK cases, such as those with OA. There are many CMIs available, and these are quick and easy to implement. The baseline data collection should be performed at the initial consultation and repeated at standard intervals whenever practical. This permits 'charting' of the individual's progress. Consistency is vital, so having the same owner complete the CMI each time is preferred. The more information collected on the effects of VRM, the higher the quality of information available, which significantly enhances the overall knowledge base on the subject. A notable example of how retrospective data can be reviewed and analysed is provided by Armitage et al. (2023).

Future possible veterinary regenerative medicine (VRM) approaches in small animal musculoskeletal (MSK) conditions

Induced pluripotent stem cells (iPSCs)

So far, we have discussed the current use of MSCs, which has included autologous, allogeneic, and xenogeneic cells. They are all adult cells that were collected from various tissues in different anatomical locations, with a common origin in the mesoderm. The understanding is that these MSCs were derived from various areas of the mesodermal embryonic layer. They are capable of symmetrical division to self-renew and divide asymmetrically to give rise to daughter cells that can differentiate into various cell lines. One of the hallmarks of MSCs is their multipotency, exemplified by the ability of their daughter cells to differentiate into different adult cells such as chondrocytes, osteoblasts, and adipocytes. This typical differentiation through generations of cells with a progressively greater differentiation along a cell-fate path was considered a 'one-way street', in other words, once cells were on the differentiation pathway, they would not be able to reverse this process to become less differentiated.

In 2006, Takahashi and Yamanaka demonstrated that this unidirectional process could be reversed. They developed a means where fully differentiated and functional adult cells could be induced to undergo reversal of the differentiation process and become artificially created pluripotent cells. These iPSCs have properties almost identical to embryonic stem cells. Both embryonic stem cells and iPSCs demonstrate pluripotency. That is to say that their descendant cells can potentially differentiate into any mature cell type of any of the three embryonic cell layers. The discovery that iPSC manufacture is possible was such a groundbreaking piece of scientific work that it resulted in the award of a Nobel Prize.

iPSCs have been studied extensively in mice and humans. Their uses to date include *in vitro* disease modelling, the testing of novel drugs, and potentially cell transplant therapy. In comparison, progress in the iPSC field for veterinary species has hitherto lagged behind that of humans. The multiple reasons for this have been reviewed by Barrachina et al. (2023).

Induced MSCs

One useful approach using iPSCs may, somewhat ironically, be that of generating MSCs, referred to as induced MSCs (Barrachina et al., 2023). The induced MSCs could be used therapeutically or further differentiated into specialised cells of mesenchymal lineage for laboratory use, such as chondrocytes or osteoblasts. The automation of the manufacturing process of iPSCs and induced MSCs has recently been described by Herbst et al. (2023). This promises to greatly enhance the efficient and timely delivery of these cell products.

Cell-free VRM products and EVs

Sharun et al. (2022) reviewed cell-free regenerative therapies for canine OA. The literature search conducted by these authors yielded two papers (Huňáková et al., 2020; Mocchi et al., 2021) in which a total of nine dogs were injected intra-articularly with allogeneic products of MSC-conditioned medium or MSC-secretome.

Huňáková et al. (2020) produced a conditioned medium from cultured allogeneic AD-MSCs. This was administered to twelve elbow joints in six dogs with naturally occurring OA. The researchers used synovial fluid biomarkers and kinematic range of motion measurements for the affected elbow joints. Despite the lack of controls, encouraging results were demonstrated as several biomarkers had favourable changes in synovial fluid concentrations (reduced MMP-3, increased TIMP-1, and reduced TNF-alpha). The range of motion in the elbow joints showed significant improvements.

Mocchi et al. (2021) provided a proof of concept for the feasibility of producing a lyosecretome-based injectable product. IA injection was devoid of major adverse events; however, no evidence for efficacy against canine OA could be determined.

Combination of veterinary regenerative medicine (VRM) with other modalities

Orthobiologics such as PRP and MSCs may be used individually or in combination, provided they are compatible and this does not contravene data sheet recommendations. An example of this is the licensed EUC-MSC product, DogStem® (Dômes Pharma). In this instance, the product licence is for IA administration without being mixed with another product. It may also be the case that an orthobiologic can be injected with a viscosupplement, such as hyaluronic acid; however, specific advice from manufacturers would be advisable before this is considered.

The use of IA-PRP with MSCs is widely practised, as exemplified by the cases reported by Armitage et al. (2023). One of the advantages of having PRP in the mixture is that the fibrin forms a mesh-like matrix soon after injection that may provide a physical structure for MSC attachment, perhaps akin to the naturally occurring MSC niches found in mesenchymal tissues. This could, at least theoretically, prolong the longevity of these transplanted cells and thereby enhance their activity. Even if this effect is minimal, as transplanted MSCs are known to have very low survival times after administration, at the minimum the fibrin network can provide a reservoir of growth factors and cytokines. In summary, it would appear to be reasonable to combine freshly prepared PRP

and culture-expanded, autologous MSCs immediately before injection. As stated previously, PRP will coagulate rapidly in the presence of an MSC culture medium, so delaying the injection is to be avoided.

The question may arise as to whether other therapeutic categories of the multimodal approach are indicated alongside VRM. It has been suggested that NSAID administration before, during, and after PRP administration may have a detrimental effect on platelet activation and growth factor release due to its anti-inflammatory activity, since the initial phase of healing involves inflammation (Frey et al., 2020; Magruder & Rodeo, 2021). However, this recommendation is not as definitive as it once was (Carr, 2022), and it is the author's current practice not to withhold this class of medication when VRM is used.

Viscosupplements such as hyaluronic acid may be used in combination with PRP. To this end, some of the commercially available PRP systems, such as Vet-PRP®-hyaluronic acid, provide hyaluronic acid-containing collection tubes to aid the production of this combination.

Photobiomodulation therapy, delivered by Class IV therapeutic laser, is commonly combined with either PRP, MSCs, or both (Armitage et al., 2023). In the author's hands, such combination therapy appears to be very effective, suggesting there may be synergistic effects.

MSK conditions, and especially OA, typically require a multimodal approach to their management. Physiotherapy is an important pillar of the multimodal therapeutic combination that is frequently indicated (Carr, 2023). The combination of physiotherapy with orthobiologics is generally to be encouraged as their effects on tissue regeneration are likely to be synergistic.

A downside of multimodal therapy is the challenge it presents in identifying which, if any, of the therapeutic interventions is having a positive effect. Since the goal in clinical practice is to aim for a super-additive effect, this may not be of practical importance for the individual patient. The challenge is assessing the effectiveness of each component within the combination from an evidence-based veterinary medicine perspective, and this may not always be possible in the strictest sense. A means of mitigating this may be to engage a stepwise approach to the addition of therapies. It is logical to use CMIs at every stage, starting before any intervention. As each therapeutic intervention is introduced, after sufficient time is allowed for the observation of any effect, the CMI measurement is repeated. In so doing, the progress may be charted, and the effect, if any, of each therapy can be somewhat objectively determined.

> ## Chapter 14 key points
>
> - Pet owner expectations should be managed.
> - Clinicians should gain baseline knowledge before establishing a VRM service.
> - Training courses in VRM, where available, should be attended.
> - Accurate MSK diagnosis is a requirement for VRM.
> - Evidence-based veterinary medicine should be applied whenever possible.
> - Clinicians performing VRM must keep abreast of the rapidly changing developments in the field to maintain up-to-date knowledge.
> - The combination of VRM with other modalities is generally advisable.

Chapter 14 references

Armitage, A. J., Miller, J. M., Sparks, T. H., Georgiou, A. E., & Reid, J. (2023). Efficacy of autologous mesenchymal stromal cell treatment for chronic degenerative musculoskeletal conditions in dogs: A retrospective study. Frontiers in Veterinary Science, 9, 1014687. https://doi.org/10.3389/fvets.2022.1014687

Barrachina, L., Arshaghi, T. E., O'Brien, A., Ivanovska, A., & Barry, F. (2023). Induced pluripotent stem cells in companion animals: How can we move the field forward? *Frontiers in Veterinary Science*, *10*, 1176772. https://doi.org/10.3389/fvets.2023.1176772

Brown, D. C. (2014). The canine orthopedic index. Step 1: Devising the items. *Veterinary Surgery*, *43*(3), 232–240. https://doi.org/10.1111/j.1532-950X.2014.12142.x

Brown, D. C., Boston, R. C., Coyne, J. C., & Farrar, J. T. (2007). Development and psychometric testing of an instrument designed to measure chronic pain in dogs with osteoarthritis. *American Journal of Veterinary Research*, *68*(6), 631–637. https://doi.org/10.2460/ajvr.68.6.631

Cachon, T., Frykman, O., Innes, J. F., Lascelles, B. D. X., Okumura, M., Sousa, P., Staffieri, F., Steagall, P. V., Van Ryssen, B., & COAST Development Group. (2018). Face validity of a proposed tool for staging canine osteoarthritis: Canine OsteoArthritis Staging Tool (COAST). *Veterinary Journal*, *235*, 1–8. https://doi.org/10.1016/j.tvjl.2018.02.017

Cachon, T., Frykman, O., Innes, J. F., Lascelles, B. D. X., Okumura, M., Sousa, P., Staffieri, F., Steagall, P. V., & Van Ryssen, B. (2023). COAST Development Group's international consensus guidelines for the treatment of canine osteoarthritis. *Frontiers in Veterinary Science*, *10*, 1137888. https://doi.org/10.3389/fvets.2023.1137888

Carr, B. J. (2022). Platelet-rich plasma as an orthobiologic: Clinically relevant considerations. *The Veterinary Clinics of North America. Small Animal Practice*, *52*(4), 977–995. https://doi.org/10.1016/j.cvsm.2022.02.005

Carr, B. J. (2023). Regenerative medicine and rehabilitation therapy in the canine. *The Veterinary Clinics of North America. Small Animal Practice*, *53*(4), 801–827. https://doi.org/10.1016/j.cvsm.2023.02.011

Carr, B. J., & Dycus, D. L. (2016). Canine gait analysis. *Recovery & Rehab*, *6*(2), 93–100.

Frey, C., Yeh, P. C., & Jayaram, P. (2020). Effects of antiplatelet and nonsteroidal anti-inflammatory medications on platelet-rich plasma: A systematic review. *Orthopaedic Journal of Sports Medicine*, *8*(4), 2325967120912841. https://doi.org/10.1177/2325967120912841

Herbst, L., Groten, F., Murphy, M., Shaw, G., Nießing, B., & Schmitt, R. H. (2023). Automated production at scale of induced pluripotent stem cell-derived mesenchymal stromal cells, chondrocytes and extracellular vehicles: Towards real-time release. *Processes*, *11*(10), 2938. https://doi.org/10.3390/pr11102938

Hielm-Björkman, A. K., Rita, H., & Tulamo, R.-M. (2009). Psychometric testing of the Helsinki chronic pain index by completion of a questionnaire in Finnish by owners of dogs with chronic signs of pain caused by osteoarthritis. *American Journal of Veterinary Research*, *70*(6), 727–734. https://wsava.org/wp-content/uploads/2020/01/Muscle-Condition-Score-Chart-for-Dogs.pdf. https://doi.org/10.2460/ajvr.70.6.727

Huňáková, K., Hluchý, M., Špaková, T., Matejová, J., Mudroňová, D., Kuricová, M., Rosocha, J., & Ledecký, V. (2020). Study of bilateral elbow joint osteoarthritis treatment using conditioned medium from allogeneic adipose tissue-derived MSCs in Labrador retrievers. *Research in Veterinary Science*, *132*, 513–520. https://doi.org/10.1016/j.rvsc.2020.08.004

Kim, A. Y., Elam, L. H., Lambrechts, N. E., Salman, M. D., & Duerr, F. M. (2022). Appendicular skeletal muscle mass assessment in dogs: A scoping literature review. *BMC Veterinary Research*, *18*(1), 280. https://doi.org/10.1186/s12917-022-03367-5

Mager, F. W. (2000). *Zur Kniegelenksarthrose des Hundes nach vorderer Kreuzbandruptur – Ein retrospektiver Vergleich dreier Operationsmethoden* [Unpublished dissertation]. Ludwig-Maximilians University.

Magruder, M., & Rodeo, S. A. (2021). Is antiplatelet therapy contraindicated after platelet-rich plasma treatment? A narrative review. *Orthopaedic Journal of Sports Medicine*, *9*(6), 23259671211010510. https://doi.org/10.1177/23259671211010510

Matis, U., Brahm-Jorda, T., Jorda, C. et al. (2005). Radiographic evaluation of the progression of osteoarthritis after tibial plateau levelling osteotomy in 93 dogs. *Veterinary and Comparative Orthopaedics and Traumatology*, *18*, A32.

Millis, D., & Levine, D. (2013). *Canine rehabilitation and physical therapy*. Elsevier Health Sciences.

Mocchi, M., Bari, E., Dotti, S., Villa, R., Berni, P., Conti, V., Del Bue, M., Squassino, G. P., Segale, L., Ramoni, R., Torre, M. L., Perteghella, S., & Grolli, S. (2021). Canine mesenchymal cell lyosecretome production

and safety evaluation after allogenic intraarticular injection in osteoarthritic dogs. *Animals: An Open Access Journal from MDPI*, *11*(11), 3271. https://doi.org/10.3390/ani11113271

Pagano, T. B., Wojcik, S., Costagliola, A., De Biase, D., Iovino, S., Iovane, V., Russo, V., Papparella, S., & Paciello, O. (2015). Age related skeletal muscle atrophy and upregulation of autophagy in dogs. *Veterinary Journal*, *206*(1), 54–60. https://doi.org/10.1016/j.tvjl.2015.07.005

Sharun, K., Muthu, S., Mankuzhy, P. D., Pawde, A. M., Chandra, V., Lorenzo, J. M., Dhama, K., Amarpal, & Sharma, G. T. (2022). Cell-free therapy for canine osteoarthritis: Current evidence and prospects. *The Veterinary Quarterly*, *42*(1), 224–230. https://doi.org/10.1080/01652176.2022.2145620

Steenkamp, W., Rachuene, P. A., Dey, R., Mzayiya, N. L., & Ramasuvha, B. E. (2022). The correlation between clinical and radiological severity of osteoarthritis of the knee. *SICOT-J*, *8*, 14. https://doi.org/10.1051/sicotj/2022014

Takahashi, K., & Yamanaka, S. (2006). Induction of pluripotent stem cells from mouse embryonic and adult fibroblast cultures by defined factors. *Cell*, *126*(4), 663–676. https://doi.org/10.1016/j.cell.2006.07.024

Vetmetrica™ Health related quality of life questionnaire https://www.newmetrica.com/vetmetrica-hrql/

Walton, M. B., Cowderoy, E., Lascelles, D., & Innes, J. F. (2013). Evaluation of construct and criterion validity for the "Liverpool osteoarthritis in Dogs" (LOAD) clinical metrology instrument and comparison to two other instruments. *PLOS ONE*, *8*(3), e58125. https://doi.org/10.1371/journal.pone.0058125

Wessely, M., Brühschwein, A., & Schnabl-Feichter, E. (2017). Evaluation of intra- and inter-observer measurement variability of a radiographic stifle osteoarthritis scoring system in dogs. *Veterinary and Comparative Orthopaedics and Traumatology*, *30*(6), 377–384. https://doi.org/10.3415/VCOT-16-09-0134

WSAVA body condition score. https://wsava.org/wp-content/uploads/2020/01/Body-Condition-Score-Dog.pdf

WSAVA muscle condition score. https://wsava.org/wp-content/uploads/2020/01/Muscle-Condition-Score-Chart-for-Dogs.pdf

Chapter 15

Current best practice in veterinary regenerative medicine (VRM)

Best practice and evidence-based veterinary regenerative medicine (VRM)

Establishing best practice in VRM is a challenge, and there are numerous choices available to clinicians, which can be bewildering. It is important, wherever possible, to have a firm foundation in science and scientific literature so that any VRM undertaken can be consistent and evidence-based; however, this can prove challenging in a rapidly developing discipline such as VRM. Acknowledgement of the 'art' as well as the science may engender enough flexibility to allow the field to advance without being held back by excessive constraints. A balance between the pursuit of evidence-based VRM and the need to advance the discipline of VRM is necessary. The principles of *primum non nocere* and *nonmaleficence* remain non-negotiable underpinning principles of all veterinary interventions.

What is the ideal candidate for VRM?

Clinical cases of small animals affected by MSK conditions represent a wide range of possible combinations of the multiple variables that exist in VRM. These include patient characteristics, disease type, acuteness or chronicity of the condition, and its severity. Other factors are the materials and facilities that may be accessible and finally the budget for veterinary care that is available.

Patient factors

- Species
- Breed
- Age
- Physique
- Activity level
- Temperament

Disease factors

- Accuracy of diagnosis
- Specifics of condition
- Number of areas affected by the condition
- Time frame of disease
- Reversibility of pathology
- Comorbidities

Facilities, equipment, and materials available

- Standard of veterinary premises, such as access to operating theatres
- Presence of laboratory equipment, such as centrifuges
- Clinician skill, expertise, and experience

Patient factors for veterinary regenerative medicine (VRM)

Species

In this book, the discussion has mainly centred on pet animals, and especially dogs. Cats are also amenable to both PRP and MSC therapies, as are other species. Rabbits have been used as an experimental model for the PRP effects on cartilage grafts (Manafi et al., 2012), PRP, hyaluronic acid, and the MSC effects on knee (stifle) OA (Chen et al., 2018). The author has no personal experience of VRM in clinical rabbit cases.

Breed

Very small dog breeds may present challenges with the collection of sufficient blood volume for PRP production. The same is true in feline patients. Extra-lean breeds, such as sight hounds, have less available adipose tissue than other breeds, which may be significant when harvesting adipose tissue for MSC manufacture.

Age

Younger MSCs are more biologically active than their aged counterparts. As patients are often in the senior age bracket, so are their MSCs. In this situation, MSCs from a younger patient (such as allogeneic MSCs, where these are available and licensed) would be expected to be more efficacious than their autologous equivalents. Continuing with this point, the younger the cells, the more biologically useful they would be after transplant. Therefore, cells from the fetal adnexa, such as umbilical cord MSCs, would be the most desirable, always bearing in mind that these will be either allogeneic or xenogeneic. Another possibility is the cryopreservation and banking of MSCs from the young patient for potential use later in life when the need arises. Adipose tissue can be collected at the time of neutering of male and female dogs, and after laboratory processing, the MSCs are cryo-stored until they are required. This service may be offered in certain locations, such as Cell Therapy Sciences in Coventry, UK; and VetStem Biopharma Inc. in Poway, California, USA.

Physique

Having overweight or obesity is generally detrimental to MSK diseases, especially OA. Additionally, venepuncture, to collect the volume of blood required for PRP, typically collected from the jugular vein, may also be more challenging. On the positive side, the presence of adiposity may be beneficial for adipose tissue availability for the harvesting of MSCs.

Activity level

Owners of more active dogs, such as those involved in sports or working, may be more inclined to request VRM at an early stage to regain optimal function for their dogs.

Temperament

As with most veterinary care, VRM will be greatly facilitated by patient cooperation. Excessively nervous or aggressive patients may not lend themselves well to the procedures required for good practice in VRM, especially regarding the extended follow-up that is ideal.

Disease factors for veterinary regenerative medicine (VRM)

Accuracy of diagnosis

Speculatively applying VRM without a verifiable diagnosis is neither appropriate nor justifiable and is outside the realm of evidence-based veterinary medicine. Unlike systemically administered pharmaceuticals, orthobiologics are targeted, locally acting 'medicines'. In contrast to, for example, an NSAID, which may be administered, and often is, based on a presumptive diagnosis of OA, beneficial effects may be observed when the actual focus of pathology has not been accurately pinpointed. Injecting orthobiologics into the wrong location could be expected to yield disappointing results and is not advisable.

Specific features of the condition

Selecting the correct combination of treatments for any given MSK condition will depend on the exact nature of the problem. In cases of joint instability, such as CCL rupture, surgery is usually the treatment of choice. This can be supplemented by VRM; however, VRM on its own would not be considered best practice for full CCL rupture.

Number of areas affected by the condition

Multiple MSK problems can be present simultaneously or subsequently develop during the course of the primary condition. All of these may need to be addressed. Using a VRM that lends itself to multiple injections in different anatomical locations can be beneficial. To this end, PRP, autologous MSCs, and micro-fragmented adipose tissue could each be considered.

Time frame of disease

In broad terms, the earlier in the course of disease VRM is used, the more effective it is likely to be. With increased chronicity comes a lower expectation of clinical improvement. That being stated, in the paper by Armitage et al. (2023), all 245 cases managed by VRM had previously failed to respond to 'conventional' medical management, indicating that even very chronic cases may benefit from VRM.

Reversibility of pathology

Many acute injuries, such as a muscle strain or a joint sprain, may have pathologies that are largely reversible. In such situations, it is possible that recovery can be aided by, for example, PRP. The tissue regeneration may be complete with minimal long-term implications. Degenerative conditions such as OA, on the other hand, are notoriously resistant to disease modification. Moderate to severe OA cases generally have marked physical changes in the joint tissues. It is not a reasonable expectation for such lesions to be reduced or resolved by VRM. That is not to say that clinical improvements will not be observed after orthobiologics such as MSCs have been injected into chronic and severely affected joints; it is still common to see the beneficial effects of the anti-inflammatory and immunomodulatory properties of VRM. In a review conducted by Ip et al. (2020) on human knee OA, the authors concluded that PRP was more effective in milder cases, while MSC injections demonstrated efficacy in moderately severe cases. Neither treatment showed more than minimal impact in cohorts with severe OA.

Comorbidities

Patients with MSK conditions often have concurrent MSK or non-MSK comorbidities that the clinician should account for when formulating a therapeutic plan. These comorbidities may impact the effectiveness of the VRM or even contra-indicate it. VRM is commonly integrated as one component of a multimodal treatment plan. Taking OA as an example, it would be inappropriate to avoid or jettison all other treatment modalities and administer VRM alone. Almost invariably, the multimodal osteoarthritis management (MMOAM) will include analgesic medication, adiposity management, and physical therapy. The drawback of an MMOAM approach is identifying which treatment mode is having the most effect and subsequently, which treatment may be safely withdrawn without compromising the patient's condition. Additionally, CMI data can become obscured by the interplay of multiple therapies.

Recording orthobiologic characteristics

It is recommended that, whenever possible, detailed information about the orthobiologic being injected is meticulously recorded. This will facilitate comparison between treatments and identify desirable and perhaps less desirable features.

In the case of PRP, it is best practice to perform haematological examinations, such as a full blood count, before PRP preparation. This will provide measures of erythrocyte parameters, counts of various leukocytes, and platelet numbers. After PRP preparation, the PRP can be similarly analysed so that all parameters can be compared. In so doing, each case will receive PRP of a known composition. This applies not only to the platelet concentration, which should be four to six times the starting concentration in the blood, but also the erythrocytes and leukocytes. Thus, it will be known whether the PRP is leukocyte-rich, or leukocyte-poor, and which leukocyte subtype level (neutrophils, agranulocytes) have been altered and to what degree. Additionally, this will verify that the PRP system apparatus has produced PRP with the desired components in the desired proportions before it is injected.

Autologous cultured and expanded MSCs are manufactured by licensed laboratories that adhere to GMP. Each vial of MSCs for injection needs to be accompanied by a certificate from the laboratory. This document should state the number of MSCs, the cell viability percentage, the cell morphology, and the batch sterility.

Off-the-shelf MSC products, such as EUC-MSCs (DogStem®, Dômes Pharma), are produced in batches that are strictly controlled and monitored, meaning that clinician can be confident in the quality of the orthobiologic products.

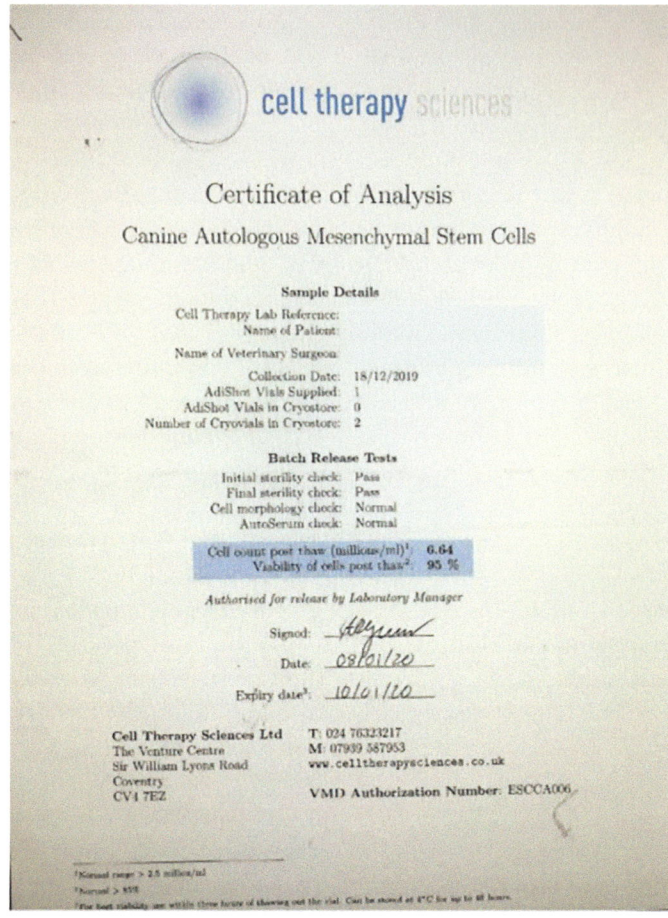

Fig. 15.1 A typical certificate that accompanies shipped cultured and expanded autologous MSCs (Courtesy of Cell Therapy Sciences, Coventry, UK).

Facilities, equipment, and materials available for veterinary regenerative medicine (VRM)

Aseptic techniques are essential for performing VRM, and IA injections should be avoided in environments where an aseptic field cannot be maintained.

Availability of centrifuges

PRP usually necessitates the minimum investment in a centrifuge. Certain centrifuges have been developed and marketed specifically for PRP preparation. Many of these have been adapted from those used in human medicine. Acquiring a validated veterinary PRP system is advisable (Carr et al., 2015) and consistent with evidence-based veterinary medicine. Standard centrifuges, if the physical parameters are appropriate, can be used to prepare PRP 'in-house', though these may not, strictly speaking, be validated. The Centrifuga Microhematocrito Premiere XC-3012 (Vetefarma), for example, is a 'standard' centrifuge that has been used to perform centrifugation for PRP processing (Dr Priscilla Berni, University of Parma, Italy, personal communication, 2023). A strict aseptic technique is mandatory when producing PRP 'in-house', so laboratory facilities such as laminar flow hoods are required.

Clinician skill, expertise, and experience

The clinical techniques required for commencing VRM in practice are not especially challenging *per se*. Veterinarians can readily acquire the required aptitudes for IA injections. Competence in MSK ultrasound is desirable though not currently widely practised in small animals. Establishing competence in this imaging modality will undoubtedly enhance any clinician's ability to offer more targeted and, therefore, effective VRM.

Monitoring patients after veterinary regenerative medicine (VRM)

Accurate patient assessment before, during, and following VRM application is considered best practice. The more care and attention devoted to this aspect, the more the patient and potentially all future patients receiving VRM stand to benefit.

Clinical metrology instruments (CMIs) and veterinary regenerative medicine (VRM)

VRM is a relatively recent addition to veterinary medicine in small animals. As with all developing specialities, there is a learning curve for the clinicians and scientists involved. The greater the communication and collaboration between individuals and organisations, the more rapidly and safely the field will progress. When all those involved understand and 'speak the same language' regarding the clinical assessment of patients, more meaningful conclusions can be reached. One of the frustrations of comparing studies in VRM, for example, is the heterogeneity of the outcome measures adopted by different researchers in different studies. How much easier would comparisons be if a standard set of outcome measures was adopted universally? An ideal panel of outcome measures would include objective methods such as force plate data. However, since these are often unavailable in practice, the next best option is CMIs. Even among CMIs, several are in common use, so standardisation of the ones used would be desirable for different studies to become comparable. The author currently uses the Liverpool Osteoarthritis in Dogs (LOAD) owner questionnaire for all canine OA cases receiving VRM (Walton et al., 2013).

Co-administration of orthobiologics with pharmaceuticals

Orthobiologics are commonly used as an integral part of a multimodal therapeutic approach to the management of the presenting MSK condition. This raises the question of how pharmaceutical products may affect orthobiologic activity. Potential adverse effects on the platelets or the MSCs, either administered or resident in the target tissue, may arise from the pH of the injected substance or its chemical or biological effects. The following are common medicines that may be considered for co-administration with orthobiologics.

Steroids

Locally injected depot corticosteroid has long been a mainstay in human sports medicine. Steroid products can be injected IA or intra-lesionally into various MSK structures. These are powerful agents that can have widespread on-target and off-target effects. Not all their actions are positive. In many conditions, steroids act as an alternative to orthobiologics such as PRP. Triamcinolone, administered via IA injection, has been demonstrated to be effective in dogs with OA (Alves et al., 2020). While the anti-inflammatory action of steroids is profound, PRP has the advantage of being markedly 'trophic' to the tissues, thereby promoting repair. It is generally not recommended for orthobiologics to be co-injected with steroids. On the contrary, a laboratory study on tenocytes suggested that the combination of PRP with steroids could be indicated for rotator cuff problems in the human shoulder (Jo et al., 2017). Regarding MSCs co-administered with steroids, the picture may be different. A laboratory study using a mouse hepatic fibrosis model found that MSCs could ameliorate liver pathology (Chen et al., 2014). Co-administration with dexamethasone blocked the action of the MSCs, resulting in no positive effect on the disease. The authors concluded that the profound anti-inflammatory effects of the steroid negated the MSC effects since inflammation is a key requirement for these cells to influence the tissue repair process. In summary, whether using PRP or MSCs, the best recommendation currently is to avoid co-administration with corticosteroids.

NSAIDs

The theoretical contra-indication of concurrent NSAID administration with PRP has already been discussed. The current practice for MSK conditions, and especially OA, is a multimodal approach. The author continues to provide NSAIDs as one of the pillars of an MMOAM when using orthobiologics. However, it is often observed that the requirement for NSAIDs are reduced, or even eliminated, after orthobiologic administration.

Local analgesics

Local analgesics (local anaesthetics) are useful for IA injection during procedures that may result in pain, including the administration of orthobiologics. The local analgesics available vary in the severity of their deleterious effects on the transplanted cells. In human RM, there appears to be a hierarchy of cell toxicity where ropivacaine is considered safer than lignocaine, and bupivacaine is the least desirable (Kubrova et

al., 2021). Both cell viability and gene expression profiles may be affected. Consequently, the author currently avoids the co-administration of local analgesics with orthobiologics.

Antimicrobials

Parenterally administered antibiotics and antibacterials may be considered alongside orthobiologics in some situations; however, orthobiologics are rarely indicated in the face of an active bacterial infection. At certain stages of the MSC culture and expansion process, antibiotics are integral to the methodology. This indicates that these antibiotics, at least in the concentrations used, and in an *in vitro* context, are safe for MSCs to survive and flourish. It is therefore unlikely that systemically administered antibiotics will have adverse effects on transplanted orthobiologics *in vivo*. Should highly concentrated formulations of antibiotics be co-administered with orthobiologics, by IA injection, for example, it seems logical that the pharmaceutical would be detrimental to the transplanted MSCs or platelets. While outside the scope of this book, it is interesting that studies such as that by Johnson et al. (2017) have demonstrated a synergistic effect of IV-administered MSCs along with antibiotics in managing bacterial infections associated with biofilm formation.

Monoclonal antibodies

The advent of systemically administered specific anti-nerve growth factor monoclonal antibodies in both dogs (Librela®, Zoetis) and cats (Solensia®, Zoetis) for OA has ushered in a new era of MMOAM. However, the possible interactions with the commonly co-administered medicine categories and these anti-nerve growth factor monoclonal antibodies, may not yet be fully elucidated. It is certainly the case that a question mark hangs over the use of bedinvetmab (Librela®, Zoetis) with NSAIDs

(Pye et al., 2022). Clinicians are advised to seek up-to-date, locally applicable information regarding the combination of anti-nerve growth factor monoclonal antibodies, NSAIDs, and orthobiologics.

Viscosupplements

Hyaluronic acid is the best-known IA viscosupplement used in human and equine sports medicine, though it is less commonly reported in the canine and feline field. Hyaluronic acid can be combined with PRP during processing, such as in the Regen Lab SA® system, where the Cellular Matrix® blood collection tube contains hyaluronic acid, or it may be co-administered separately. To the author's knowledge, no detrimental effects on either PRP or MSCs are attributed to hyaluronic acid. Zhao et al. (2020) reported no difference in adverse events in human knee OA cases between PRP administered alone and PRP combined with hyaluronic acid. The synergistic effects of hyaluronic acid with allogeneic BM-derived MSCs were demonstrated in a canine model of cartilage damage; the combination outperformed hyaluronic acid alone and in the control group (Li, 2018).

Polyacrylamide gels

Polyacrylamide gels are available for IA injection in humans, horses, and, more recently, dogs. One example is a 2.5% cross-linked polyacrylamide hydrogel (marketed as ArthramidVet®, ConturaVet). Once injected into a damaged or diseased joint, the polyacrylamide gel adheres to the synovium. Over a period of approximately two weeks, the gel integrates into the synovial tissues, where it forms a long-lasting 'cushion'. Cells migrate into the 'membrane' that forms, making it hypercellular, and angiogenesis furnishes it with capillaries.

To the author's knowledge, using a combination of polyacrylamide gels, PRP, and MSCs is not common practice in small animal medicine. However, a recent *in vitro* study by Nasircilar et al., (2022) on a synthetic three-dimensional cross-linked polyacrylamide hydrogel (Noltrex™) suggested that polyacrylamide gels may have beneficial effects on MSC proliferation. Additionally, the study noted positive effects of polyacrylamide gels on cultured human osteoblasts.

A logical approach toward choosing which IA therapy to inject in any given situation is to be encouraged. Clinicians may deem it necessary or desirable to provide joint lubrication, in which case hyaluronic acid or a polyacrylamide gel may be chosen. If acute inflammation is present, then an IA depot steroid could be more suitable, or, alternatively, where a trophic stimulus is indicated, an orthobiologic may be the preferred option.

Single or multiple orthobiologic administration

Regarding the frequency of orthobiologic administration, it is possible to provide a single treatment or to follow up with repeat injections. Logically, additional 'topping up' of the orthobiologic would intuitively improve the effectiveness of the therapy. This was found to be the case in a review of human knee OA by Ip et al. (2020) where it was concluded that repeated orthobiologic injection and more concentrated doses are more efficacious than a single administration. In the author's experience, a single administration is often sufficient to result in enough patient improvement that repeat administrations are difficult to justify. Severe, chronic, and refractory cases, however, are likely to require a regime of multiple orthobiologic administrations. Counselling of animal owners at an early stage is important in this regard so they are made aware that a 'course of VRM' is often indicated, and to allow them to prepare for the additional procedures and especially the associated costs involved.

Summary of best practice when performing veterinary regenerative medicine (VRM)

For optimal integration of VRM into clinical practice, clinicians are encouraged to consider the following recommendations:

- Ensure an **accurate diagnosis** has been established.

In the author's opinion, there is no substitute for accurately diagnosing the clinical problem. VRMs are generally unsuited to speculative use or application without a solid empirical foundation.

- Gain sufficient **theoretical knowledge** of VRM.

It is hoped that a book such as this will arm veterinarians with sufficient information to safely and appropriately implement VRM. Clinicians are also advised to stay informed about current developments in this rapidly evolving field.

- Gain the **technical skills** necessary for VRM.

Skills such as IA injection techniques and MSK ultrasound can be acquired on practical courses. Administering IA injections is an essential skill in VRM.

- Establish **baseline CMI values** before undertaking VRM.

How effective the VRM turns out to be can only be judged if appropriate baseline values are meticulously recorded before the treatment, then compared with those same values after the treatment. An obvious caveat to bear in mind is the placebo effect, which is relevant for both owners, caregivers, and clinicians alike (Conzemius & Evans, 2012).

- Continue to **monitor CMI values** during the post-VRM administration period.

Regularly tracking CMI values during this period provides valuable data for evaluating treatment outcomes. The more data points collected, the more informative the analysis becomes. A suggested timeline could be as follows: CMI and any other measurements at day zero (the day of VRM administration), followed by one, two, and three months, then six, nine, and twelve months, and continuing every three months as required.

- Critically **evaluate each case**, and preferably a series of cases.

Assessing which VRM cases benefit, and which do not, allows clinicians to refine VRM protocols to improve outcomes in future cases.

- Publish **case reports** whenever possible.

Real-world case reports and series of cases add considerable weight to the pool of collective experience in VRM. However, from the perspective of scientific rigour, there are obvious drawbacks, such as the lack of placebo-controls and blinding. Despite these factors, reporting VRM outcomes remains valuable for sharing practical insights. For example, Armitage et al. (2023) provided detailed information on 245 consecutive VRM cases. Contributions from clinicians using VRM in practice in this way massively enhance our understanding of how best to apply VRM in patient care.

- **Confer with colleagues** in the VRM discipline for the benefit of all.

A relatively small but growing community of veterinarians is involved in offering VRM in practice. Clinicians are encouraged to seek appropriate local expertise to establish a mutually beneficial network. Examples of such cooperation are already in evidence at the time of writing, such as GISMvet in Italy and an international VRM collaboration centred on North Macedonia. Taking a One Health One Medicine (Cavill, 2023) approach to RM may be beneficial. Small animal veterinarians may develop relationships with clinicians and scientists in related fields such as equine and human medicine. The sharing of knowledge and experience across species in this way can improve the care for all patients.

- Consider **interaction with pharmaceuticals**.

Awareness of contra-indications and any controversies relating to the co-administration of orthobiologics alongside other medicinal products is essential. For example, while the traditional practice of avoiding NSAIDs when using PRP remains a consideration, this is now regarded as less rigid than it was previously (Carr et al., 2015).

- **Continuous improvement**.

VRM, like all branches of veterinary medicine and surgery, cannot simply be learned once without being revisited. The VRM speciality continues to develop apace, requiring all involved to continually be cognisant of current trends and developments and to critically evaluate these from an evidence-based veterinary medicine point of view.

Possible ways to promote further improvements in the field of veterinary regenerative medicine (VRM)

The more meaningful data available to clinicians, the better we can select the most appropriate orthobiologics and apply them most effectively. To this end, a worthwhile endeavour would be the creation of an *MSCs for Canine OA Registry*. This could be set up at a national or international level. Patients could be anonymously registered and followed up using standardised measurements such as CMIs. An example of a clinical registry is the Cruciate Registry in the United Kingdom administered by Vet Knowledge, under the auspices of the Royal College of Veterinary Surgeons. Such cooperation could massively influence best practice in orthobiologic medicine for our canine patients.

> ## Chapter 15 key points
>
> - Patient factors, disease factors, available facilities, and expertise should be considered when planning VRM.
> - Clinicians should be knowledgeable about VRM and highly skilled in IA injections.
> - Ideally, all the characteristics of the orthobiologics used should be recorded in detail.
> - Monitoring using CMIs is recommended.
> - A registry for MSCs would be helpful to further best practice.

Chapter 15 references

Alves, J. C., Santos, A., Jorge, P., Lavrador, C., & Carreira, L. M. (2020). A pilot study on the efficacy of a single intra-articular administration of triamcinolone acetonide, hyaluronan, and a combination of both for clinical management of osteoarthritis in police working dogs. *Frontiers in Veterinary Science, 7,* 512523. https://doi.org/10.3389/fvets.2020.512523

Armitage, A. J., Miller, J. M., Sparks, T. H., Georgiou, A. E., & Reid, J. (2023). Efficacy of autologous mesenchymal stromal cell treatment for chronic degenerative musculoskeletal conditions in dogs: A retrospective study. Frontiers in Veterinary Science, 9, 1014687. https://doi.org/10.3389/fvets.2022.1014687

Carr, B. J., Canapp, Jr., S. O., Mason, D. R., Cox, C., & Hess, T. (2015). Canine platelet-rich plasma systems: A prospective analysis. *Frontiers in Veterinary Science, 2,* 73. https://doi.org/10.3389/fvets.2015.00073

Cavill, K. (2023). An introduction to the interface between osteoarthritis, one health and one medicine. *Vet Edge on-line* Retrieved December 2023. https://indd.adobe.com/view/bef060ec-aef3–44b0-ad88–0e91857d6f01

Chen, X., Gan, Y., Li, W., Su, J., Zhang, Y., Huang, Y., Roberts, A. I., Han, Y., Li, J., Wang, Y., & Shi, Y. (2014). The interaction between mesenchymal stem cells and steroids during inflammation. *Cell Death and Disease*, *5*(1), e1009. https://doi.org/10.1038/cddis.2013.537

Chen, Y.-C., Hsu, Y.-M., Tan, K. P., Fang, H.-W., & Chang, C.-H. (2018). Intraarticular injection for rabbit knee osteoarthritis: Effectiveness among hyaluronic acid, platelet-rich plasma, and mesenchymal stem cells. *Journal of the Taiwan Institute of Chemical Engineers*, *91*, 138–145. https://doi.org/10.1016/j.jtice.2018.05.051

Conzemius, M. G., & Evans, R. B. (2012). Caregiver placebo effect for dogs with lameness from osteoarthritis. *Journal of the American Veterinary Medical Association*, *241*(10), 1314–1319. https://doi.org/10.2460/javma.241.10.1314

GISMvet- Gruppo Italiano Staminale Mesenchimale. https://www.gismonline.it

Ip, H. L., Nath, D. K., Sawleh, S. H., Kabir, M. H., & Jahan, N. (2020). Regenerative medicine for knee osteoarthritis–the efficacy and safety of intra-articular platelet-rich plasma and mesenchymal stem cells injections: A literature review. *Cureus*, *12*(9), e10575. https://doi.org/10.7759/cureus.10575

Jo, C. H., Lee, S. Y., Yoon, K. S., & Shin, S. (2017). Effects of platelet-rich plasma with concomitant use of a corticosteroid on tenocytes from degenerative rotator cuff tears in interleukin 1β–induced tendinopathic conditions. *The American Journal of Sports Medicine*, *45*(5), 1141–1150. https://doi.org/10.1177/0363546516681294

Johnson, V., Webb, T., Norman, A., Coy, J., Kurihara, J., Regan, D., & Dow, S. (2017). Activated mesenchymal stem cells interact with antibiotics and host innate immune responses to control chronic bacterial infections. *Scientific Reports*, *7*(1), 9575. https://doi.org/10.1038/s41598-017-08311-4

Kubrova, E., Su, M., Galeano-Garces, C., Galvan, M. L., Jerez, S., Dietz, A. B., Smith, J., Qu, W., & Van Wijnen, A. J. (2021). Differences in cytotoxicity of lidocaine, ropivacaine, and bupivacaine on the viability and metabolic activity of human adipose-derived mesenchymal stem cells. *American Journal of Physical Medicine and Rehabilitation*, *100*(1), 82–91. https://doi.org/10.1097/PHM.0000000000001529

Li, L., Duan, X., Fan, Z., Chen, L., Xing, F., Xu, Z., Chen, Q., & Xiang, Z. (2018). Mesenchymal stem cells in combination with hyaluronic acid for articular cartilage defects. *Scientific Reports*, *8*(1), 9900. https://doi.org/10.1038/s41598-018-27737-y

Manafi, A., Kaviani Far, K., Moradi, M., Manafi, A., & Manafi, F. (2012). Effects of platelet-rich plasma on cartilage grafts in rabbits as an animal model. *World Journal of Plastic Surgery*, *1*(2), 91–98.

Nasircilar, A., Bülbül, M. V., Kalender, S. M., Bozkurt, C., & Keskin, İ. (2022). Effects of polyacrylamide hydrogel used in the treatment of osteoarthritis on mesenchymal stem cells and human osteoblasts. *Journal of Surgery and Medicine*, *6*(4), 498–502. https://doi.org/10.28982/josam.1006577

Pye, C., Bruniges, N., Peffers, M., & Comerford, E. (2022). Advances in the pharmaceutical treatment options for canine osteoarthritis. *The Journal of Small Animal Practice*, *63*(10), 721–738. https://doi.org/10.1111/jsap.13495, https://knowledge.rcvs.org.uk/quality-improvement/canine-cruciate-registry/

Royal College of Veterinary Surgeons (RCVS) knowledge cruciate registry.

Walton, M. B., Cowderoy, E., Lascelles, D., & Innes, J. F. (2013). Evaluation of construct and criterion validity for the "Liverpool osteoarthritis in Dogs" (LOAD) clinical metrology instrument and comparison to two other instruments. *PLOS ONE, 8*(3), e58125. https://doi.org/10.1371/journal.pone.0058125

Zhao, J., Huang, H., Liang, G., Zeng, L.-F., Yang, W., & Liu, J. (2020). Effects and safety of the combination of platelet-rich plasma (PRP) and hyaluronic acid (HA) in the treatment of knee osteoarthritis: A systematic review and meta-analysis. *BMC Musculoskeletal Disorders*, *21*(1), 224. https://doi.org/10.1186/s12891-020-03262-w

Section VI

Chapter 16

Veterinary regenerative medicine (VRM) case studies

Suggested informed consent for veterinary regenerative medicine (VRM)

All veterinary interventions mandate that informed animal owner consent is acquired in advance. Where VRM is concerned, owners will often already have their own preconceptions about, for example, what stem cells are and what stem cell therapy is capable of. The hype surrounding the subject may have influenced their opinions and led them to seek out VRM. An accurate and balanced explanation of the current state of the art of VRM is essential *before* embarking on any therapeutic journey. It is important to choose the appropriate vocabulary for the individual client(s) while neither oversimplifying the information nor overloading them with excessive scientific or medical

jargon. Bespoke written materials (such as those included here), diagrams, and videos can be implemented to back up the veterinary consultation. There should be plenty of time allocated for questions. Where information is lacking or incomplete, such as how effective a treatment will be or how long a beneficial effect may last, honestly explaining this to owners is the best policy.

Owners should be informed on exactly what form of VRM is being applied for their animal's condition. They should be appraised of the current knowledge base on this intervention and what benefits can reasonably be expected. A discussion on adverse events should also be included. The use of clinical metrology should be encouraged at all stages of treatment.

Written consent forms are considered essential whenever veterinary procedures are proposed. Each clinician will have some version of this for surgery, which can be adapted for VRM.

Important note

There is no substitute for properly conducted clinical studies regarding VRMs, as discussed in previous chapters. However, individual case studies, while uncontrolled and anecdotal, may fulfil a different requirement: that of translating the science of VRM into a real-world setting. Clinical cases rarely fit neatly into textbook categories, and each case will have its own variations and comorbidities. The following case descriptions pertain to real-world patients, all of which are or were under the author's care. They are anonymised, and the owners have given their informed consent for the information and images to be used for educational purposes. The cases illustrate the author's progression in the field of VRM, with therapies becoming more refined as knowledge has accumulated over the years. They also reflect the apparatus and facilities that were available at the time the cases were managed. Again, innovations in equipment and technology are ongoing in VRM. None of the case descriptions have been retrospectively altered to emphasise 'ideal or perfect VRM case management'. Instead, they are all presented 'warts and all' and contain areas for discussion and have potential for improvement. Some of their limitations, for example, the lack of objective measures like CMIs, are identified in the concluding sections.

Case 1

Presentation

A one-year-old, female Rottweiler was referred for investigations and management of a long-standing, bilateral thoracic limb lameness. She weighed 42.5kg and had a body condition score of 6/9 (mildly overweight).

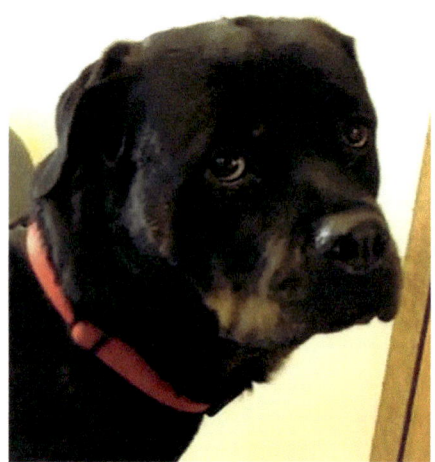

Fig. 16.1.1 Case 1

Current treatment before commencing regenerative medicine

- Paracetamol 1000mg BID (23.5mg/kg BID)
- Gabapentin 300mg SID (7mg/kg SID)
- Meloxicam 3.4mg SID (0.08mg/kg SID)
- Cannabidiol oil 4 drops BID
- Multivitamins
- Joint supplements
- Class 4 laser ('dose' unknown)
- Physiotherapy

CT studies of the elbows were requested. These revealed bilateral elbow joint incongruence and bilateral fragmented medial coronoid processes (Fig. 16.1.2).

Diagnosis

Bilateral elbow dysplasia was diagnosed, consisting of bilateral fragmented coronoid processes and incongruence.

Initial adjustments in medical management

Despite the combination of existing medication, supplements, and other modalities, the patient remained lame and had significant pain on elbow palpation. To simplify matters, a new multimodal treatment plan was proposed, which included:

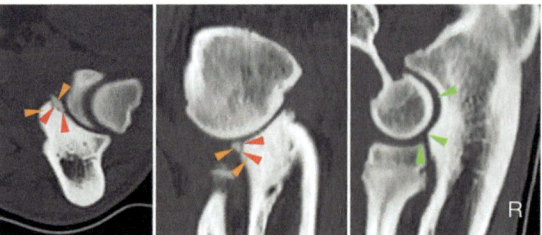

Fig. 16.1.2 CT images of Case #1. The right elbow shows a fragmented coronoid process (red and orange arrowheads), and incongruence (green arrowheads).

- Management of the adiposity.
- Reduction of the dose of paracetamol to 10mg/kg twice daily, which is lower than the current recommendation of 10–15mg three times daily (Bello & Dye, 2023).
- Phasing out all other medication.
- Collection of inguinal adipose tissue for harvesting of autologous MSCs (for the current treatment and for cryo-banking).

Rationale for VRM and decision-making

A 'conventional' MMOAM approach had thus far produced disappointing results. Both VRM and surgery (such as arthroscopic removal of the fragmented coronoid processes and/or osteotomy to improve the incongruence) were considered. A recent review has urged caution when recommending surgery for this condition (Kähn et al., 2023), while another described a common narrative of lack of evidence for the efficacy of arthroscopic surgery (Burton, 2023). VRM was chosen since it is less invasive and would not preclude surgery if the VRM proved to be ineffective.

Regenerative medicine (RM)

8×10^6 autologous AD-MSCs (AdiShot®, Cell Therapy Sciences) were injected into each elbow joint. A week's course of meloxicam at 0.1mg/kg once daily was administered.

Case progression

- At 6 months after MSC administration, no medication was necessary.
- The body condition score was 5/9, with a new, reduced weight of 38.6kg.
- The patient was sound at exercise, and only occasionally stiff on rising.
- At 18 months, there was no recurrence of lameness and still no requirement for medication.

Conclusion

The clinical response to autologous AD-MSCs injected on a single occasion into each elbow appeared to produce an excellent response, as judged by the resolution of the thoracic limb lameness despite the withdrawal of all the analgesic medication. Criticism of this case could involve the lack of CMI measurements. In hindsight, a set of CMI data would have been very useful, as is always the case in VRM. The reduction in adiposity probably contributed to the successful management of this case due to the anti-inflammatory effects of reducing the adipokine load. The size of this effect is unknown. Surgical management of elbow dysplasia has long been practised and a plethora of techniques have been described. In this case, surgery was avoided in favour of IA MSCs, and the outcome appears to endorse this decision. The future progression of OA in both elbows is inevitable. One advantage of the choice to use autologous MSCs is that cryo-banking will provide a source of future MSC aliquots that can be repeatedly administered at intervals as required.

Case 1 references

Bello, A. M., & Dye, C. (2023). Current perceptions and use of paracetamol in dogs among veterinary surgeons working in the United Kingdom. *Veterinary Medicine and Science*, *9*(2), 679–686. https://doi.org/10.1002/vms3.1058

Burton, N. J. (2023). Review of minimally invasive surgical procedures for assessment and treatment of medial coronoid process disease. *Veterinary Surgery*, *52*(6), 790–800. https://doi.org/10.1111/vsu.13986

Kähn, H. C., Zablotski, Y., & Meyer-Lindenberg, A. (2023). Therapeutic success in fragmented coronoid process disease and other canine medial elbow compartment pathology: A systematic review with meta-analyses. *Frontiers in Veterinary Science*, *10*, 1228497. https://doi.org/10.3389/fvets.2023.1228497

Case 2

Presentation

A six-year-old, spayed, female Labrador retriever was presented with a history of bilateral hock osteoarthritis dissecans (OCD) diagnosed during puppyhood. The patient had been demonstrating lameness of the pelvic limbs for more than a year. The condition was unresponsive to the standard dose of meloxicam (Metacam®, Boehringer) administered at 0.1mg/kg once daily, as well as nutraceuticals, physiotherapy, and hydrotherapy.

Clinical features

On examination, there was bilateral thickening of the hocks with reduced ranges of motion. The body weight was 23.2kg, with a body condition score of 7/9. A 2/6 lameness was ascribed to both pelvic limbs. The CMI scores showed a LOAD score of 13/52 and a COAST score at stage 4/4. (Cachon et al., 2018; Cachon et al., 2023).

Imaging

On radiography, the hocks showed similar changes. Both revealed loss of the medial ridge of the talus, consistent with juvenile OCD. The medial aspect of the joints, including the medial malleolus, had been markedly remodelled by marginal osteophytosis and enthesophyte formation (Fig. 16.2.1).

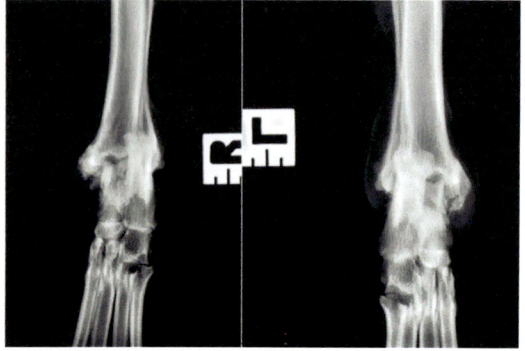

Fig. 16.2.1 Plantar-dorsal radiographs of both hocks.

Diagnosis

The clinical and radiographic information supported a diagnosis of chronic severe bilateral hock OA, as a sequel to medial talar ridge OCD.

Treatment plan

An MMOAM plan was proposed, which included:

- Adiposity management.
- Continuing with meloxicam (this may be considered somewhat controversial if used alongside PRP, albeit that current practice allows for combining these therapies (Carr, 2022)).
- RM in the form of autologous PRP and autologous AD-MSCs. On day one, autologous leukocyte-rich PRP, prepared using the V-Pet® filtration system, at 4–6x the concentration of the starting blood, was administered at 2ml per joint, plus collection of inguinal subcutaneous adipose tissue for MSC harvesting. One month later, autologous AD-MSCs were injected into both hocks at 3×10^6 cells in 1ml of suspension per joint (AdiShot®, Cell Therapy Sciences).

Rationale for VRM and decision-making

Despite being under veterinary care for over a year for management of bilateral hock OA, the condition remained refractory to the existing management combination. It therefore seemed reasonable to add VRM to the MMOAM due to its potential anti-inflammatory, immunomodulatory, and analgesic effects. PRP was administered first, since this was possible as a point-of-care orthobiologic and could improve the clinical signs rapidly. Inguinal fat for MSC culture was collected while the PRP was prepared and administered. Before the MSC injections were administered, a favourable response to the PRP was already discernible clinically and was supported by the reduction in the LOAD score down to 3/52.

Case progression

This case was followed up for a year, and during this time, the patient rapidly improved to the extent that she was not obviously lame. The LOAD scores reduced and stayed low (Fig. 16.2.2). Concurrent adiposity management resulted in achievement of an ideal target weight of 19.6kg and a body condition score of 5/9 (Fig. 16.2.2). At the one-year post-VRM examination, some meloxicam was still necessary, albeit the daily dose was 25 to 50% of the recommended dose (that is, 0.025 to 0.05mg/kg). The CMI recorded that the LOAD score was 1/52, and the COAST score remained at 4/4.

Conclusion

In this case, a positive outcome was achieved using VRM as a major part of an MMOAM plan. The success of the VRM was evidenced by the reduced lameness and improved LOAD score. The positive contribution of adiposity management is acknowledged, though this is difficult to quantify. The continued requirement for some analgesic medication, in this case a low-maintenance dose of meloxicam, is not unusual in moderate or severe OA. The decision to use PRP one month before the MSCs is unconventional. It is more usual to combine the two orthobiologics and inject them together (Armitage et al., 2023). Nonetheless, the results were favourable and long-lasting, suggesting that a synergistic effect had probably occurred. Further improvements could include, firstly, quantifying the composition of the PRP before administration. Secondly, in retrospect, requesting a more concentrated, smaller-volume MSC preparation from the laboratory may have been more suitable for the relatively confined space of the tibiotarsal joint.

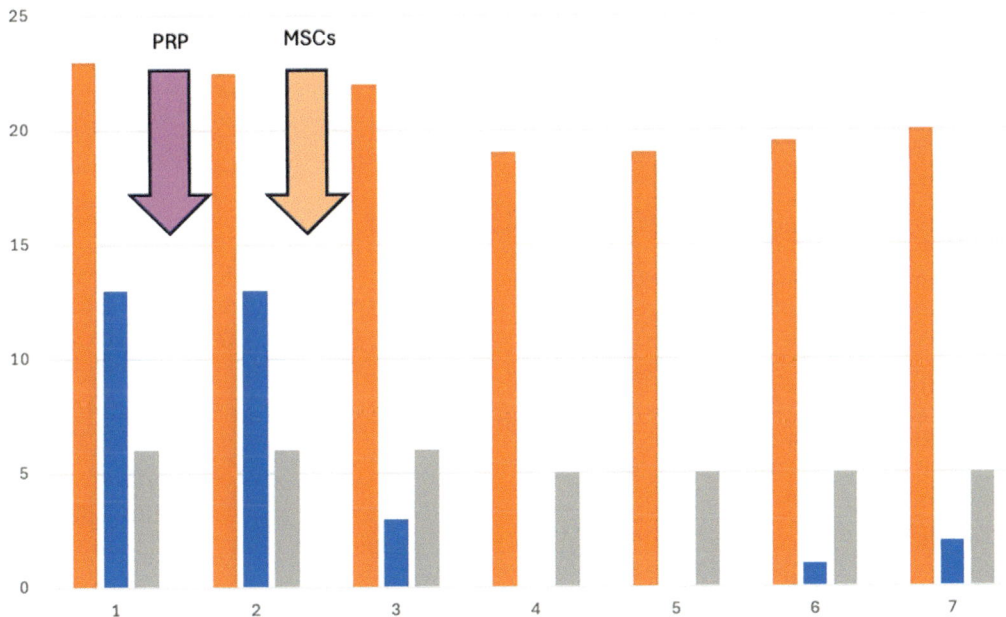

Fig. 16.2.2 Monthly progression of body weight, LOAD score, and body condition score. PRP with arrow represents the timing of the PRP administration. MSCs with the arrow depicts the time of IA injection of the MSCs. The units on the vertical scale represent body weight (orange columns), LOAD score (blue columns), and body condition score (grey columns). The units on the horizontal column are months.

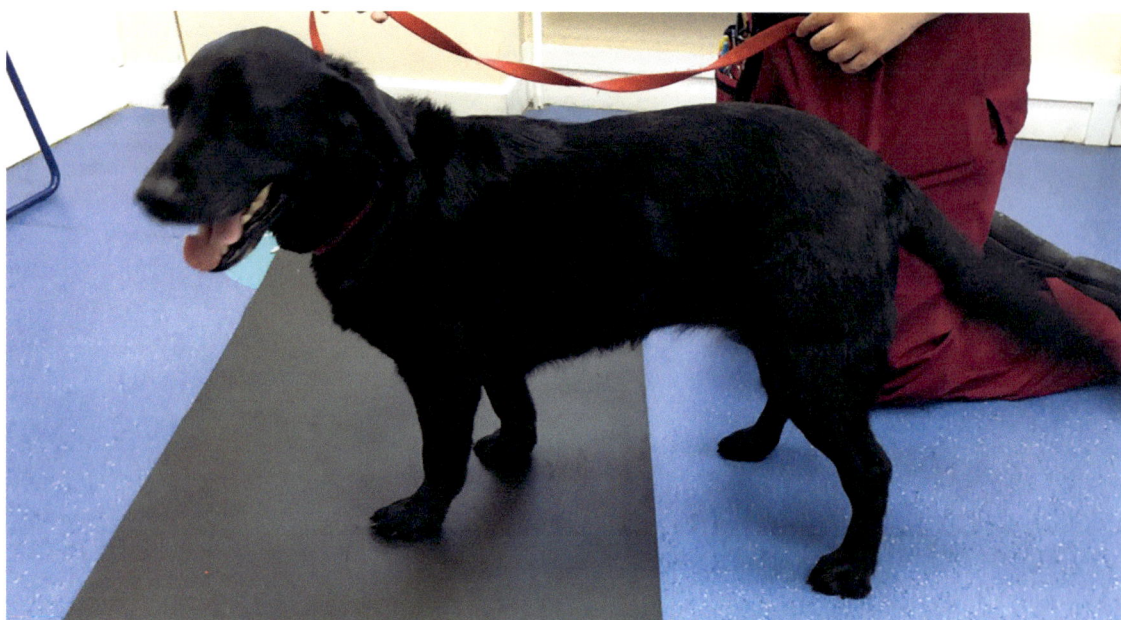

Fig. 16.2.3 Case 2 during the one-year follow-up veterinary consultation.

Case 2 references

Armitage, A. J., Miller, J. M., Sparks, T. H., Georgiou, A. E., & Reid, J. (2023). Efficacy of autologous mesenchymal stromal cell treatment for chronic degenerative musculoskeletal conditions in dogs: A retrospective study. Frontiers in Veterinary Science, 9, 1014687. https://doi.org/10.3389/fvets.2022.1014687

Cachon, T., Frykman, O., Innes, J. F., Lascelles, B. D. X., Okumura, M., Sousa, P., Staffieri, F., Steagall, P. V., Van Ryssen, B., & COAST Development Group. (2018). Face validity of a proposed tool for staging canine osteoarthritis: Canine OsteoArthritis Staging Tool (COAST). *Veterinary Journal*, *235*, 1–8. https://doi.org/10.1016/j.tvjl.2018.02.017

Cachon, T., Frykman, O., Innes, J. F., Lascelles, B. D. X., Okumura, M., Sousa, P., Staffieri, F., Steagall, P. V., & Van Ryssen, B. (2023). COAST Development Group's international consensus guidelines for the treatment of canine osteoarthritis. *Frontiers in Veterinary Science*, *10*, 1137888. https://doi.org/10.3389/fvets.2023.1137888

Carr, B. J. (2022). Platelet-rich plasma as an orthobiologic: Clinically relevant considerations. *The Veterinary Clinics of North America. Small Animal Practice*, *52*(4), 977–995. https://doi.org/10.1016/j.cvsm.2022.02.005

Case 3

Presentation

A four-year-old, neutered, male, small cross-breed dog weighing 9.9 kg with a body condition score of 5/9 was presented with intermittent lameness on the left thoracic limb following rest. This limb had an unusual morphology. The lameness had responded well to activity restriction and oral meloxicam, maintaining it at a mild level (1/6).

Clinical findings

There was a conformation typical of a chondrodystrophoid phenotype. This included 'Queen Anne' shaped thoracic limbs, carpal valgus, and external rotation (supination) of the manus (Fig. 16.3.1). Mild tenderness was noted on firm palpation of the left elbow.

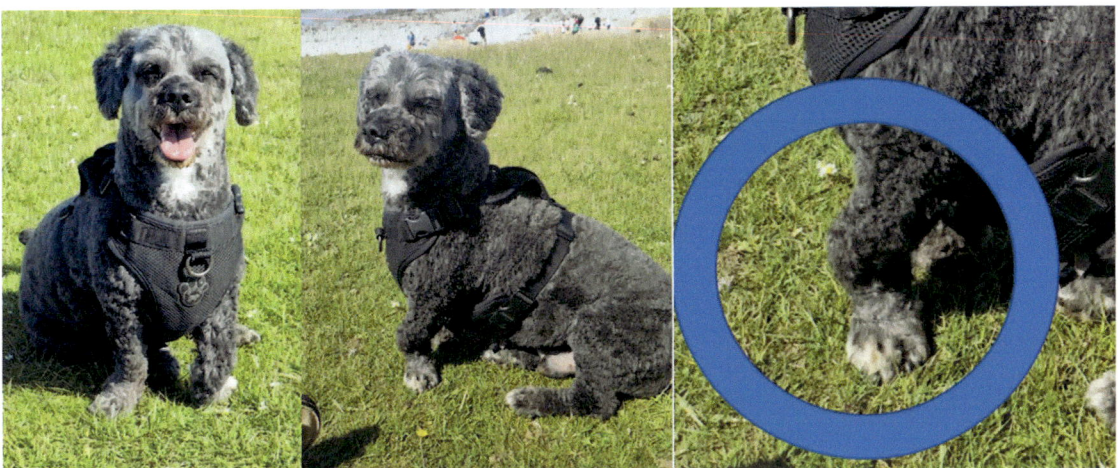

Fig. 16.3.1 Case 3 showing chondrodystrophoid conformation and severe deformity of the left thoracic limb (circled).

Imaging

Radiographic studies of the thoracic limbs were undertaken (Fig. 16.3.2, 3 & 4). CT was not available. On the radiographs, multiple anatomical abnormalities were evident. These included craniolateral bowing of the radii, relative shortening of the ulnae, humeroulnar incongruence, and external rotation with valgus deviation of the carpi.

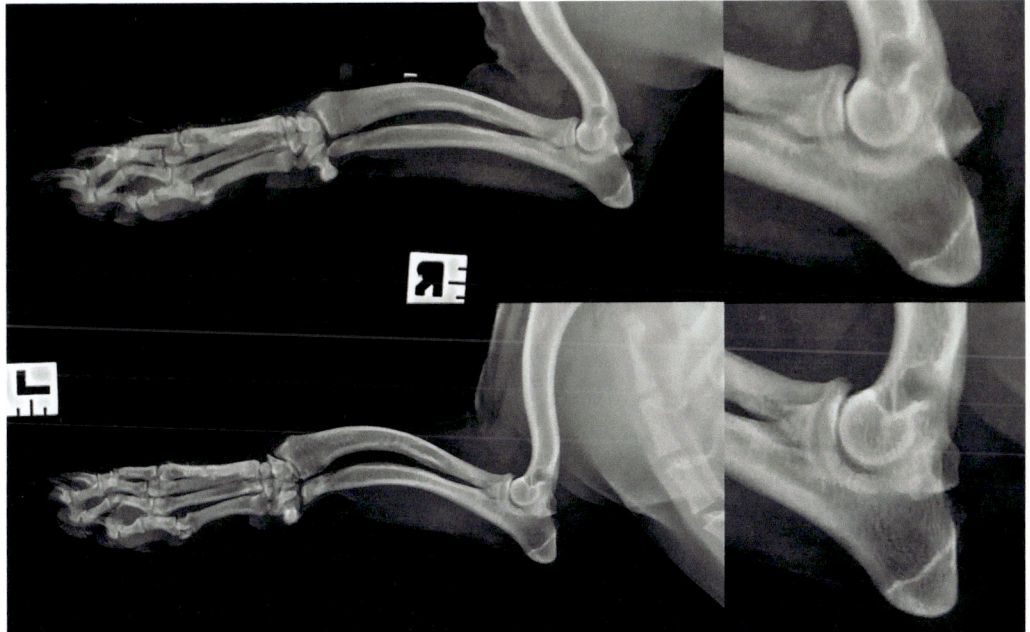

Fig. 16.3.2 Lateromedially projected radiographs of both elbows and antebrachia. There are multiple anatomical abnormalities, including cranial bowing of the radii, relative shortening of the ulnae, and humeroulnar incongruence.

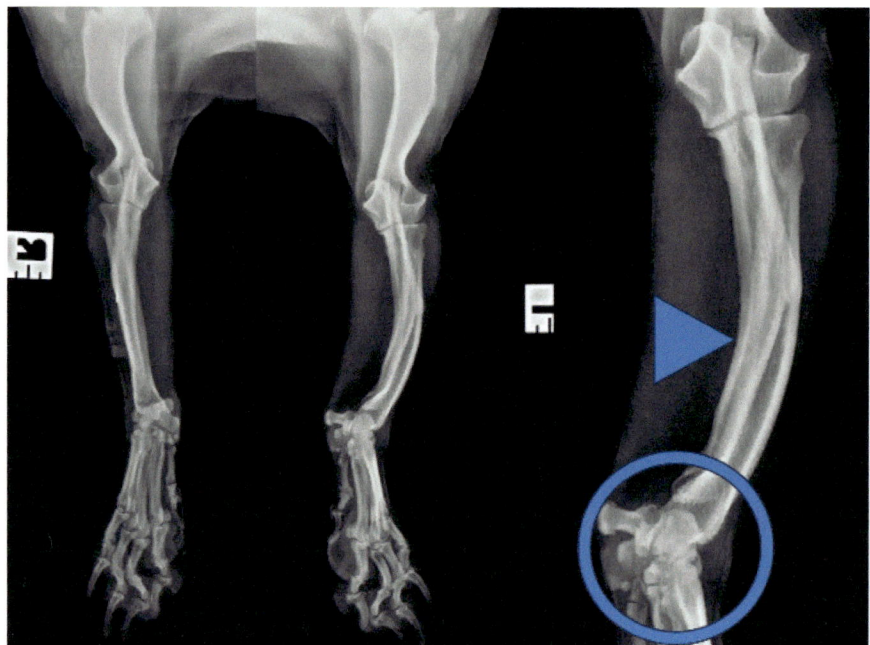

Fig. 16.3.3 Craniocaudally projected radiographs of both antebrachia. Both limbs exhibit marked deformity. The left limb is more severely affected with lateral bowing of the radius and ulna (arrowhead) and external rotation (supination) most evident at the carpus (circled).

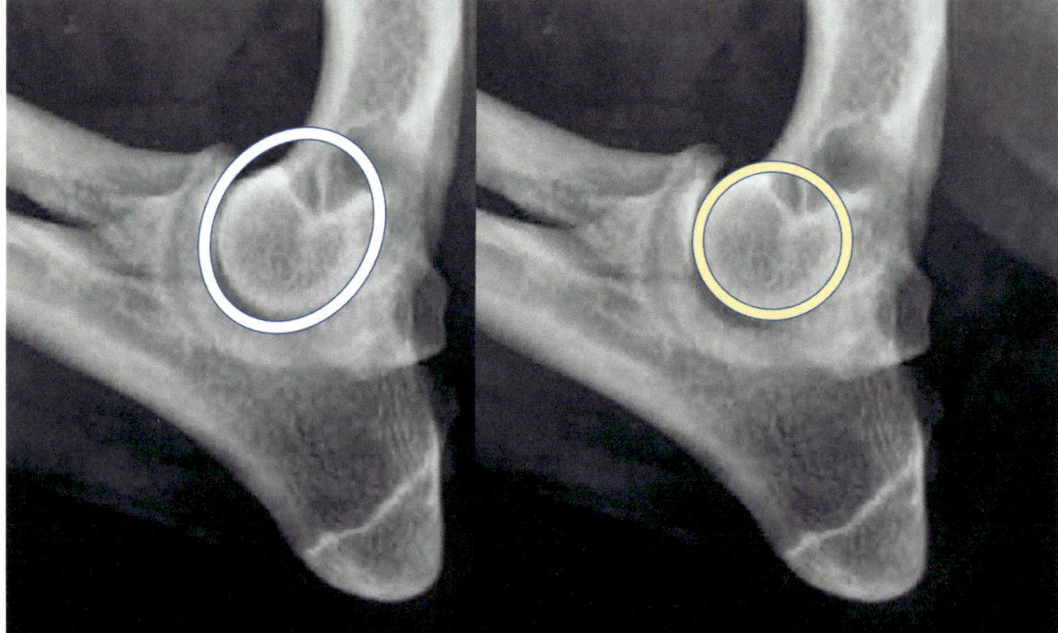

Fig. 16.3.4 Lateromedially projected radiographs of the left elbow. There is a mismatch in the articular surfaces (inferred from the subchondral bone plates) of the semilunar notch/radial head (white ellipse) and the humeral condyle (yellow circle). This is described as elbow joint incongruency.

Diagnosis

It was concluded that the cause of the observed elbow pain and lameness was left elbow joint incongruency. The resulting overloading of localised areas of the joint was likely to have led to the pain and tissue attrition, including the articular cartilage. Such changes are expected to inevitably progress to OA.

Management

All management options were considered and discussed in detail, including extensive surgery to 'correct' the deformities. Three-dimensional CT studies were suggested to characterise all the geometrical features of the skeletal components of the limbs. Subsequently, computer-assisted design/manufacture instrumentation and implants could be manufactured to facilitate corrective osteotomies in three dimensions. The relatively great expense of this approach, coupled with the surgical risks, was weighed against the relatively mild current clinical signs and the inevitability of the development of significant future OA. A simpler surgical approach, where deformity correction was not the goal, only improvement in elbow congruency, was also posited. This would involve only an oblique ulnar osteotomy to facilitate dynamic 'correction' of the humeroulnar joint 'fit'. Such surgery would be more likely effective earlier in life, before one year of age. The consensus between the owner and clinician was for a multimodal conservative medical management approach rather than surgery of any kind. This took the form of continuing to maintain a slim physique, supplementation with oral omega-3 fatty acids, and the use of NSAIDs if needed for exacerbations of pain or lameness. A referral to a veterinary physiotherapist was made to minimise the adverse effects of the observed abnormalities on the MSK system in general.

Case progression

Over the next four years, acceptable control of the developing OA was achieved. However, the expected temporary exacerbations that typify OA did occur, and overall, an acceptable outcome was observed. The problem subsequently became decompensated such that appropriate physical therapy, meloxicam, and adjunctive analgesic medication (amantadine and bedinvetmab) did not keep the lameness and joint pain under control. Reassessment at this stage revealed an increase in weight (12.7kg) and body condition score of 7/9. The adiposity was calculated to be around 2kg of excess adipose tissue.

Repeat radiography

The repeated radiographs revealed that the humeroulnar joint incongruence remained. In addition, there were, as expected, degenerative changes including marginal osteophytosis and subchondral sclerosis consistent with OA (Fig. 16.3.5).

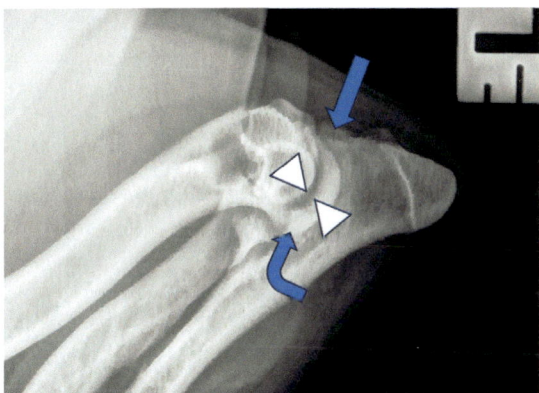

Fig. 16.3.5 Fully flexed mediolateral radiograph of left elbow. This extreme flexion may exacerbate the appearance of the incongruence (arrowheads). There are osteophytes on the anconeal process (arrow) and subcoronoid sclerosis in the ulna (bent arrow).

Management of the OA

A multimodal management of the OA was already being implemented, aligned with the current OA management paradigm (Fox, 2017). Adjustments to the existing combination of measures was proposed. This included intensifying the adiposity management, continuing the analgesic medication (meloxicam, amantadine), and maintaining physiotherapy. In addition, a course of Class IV therapeutic laser was commenced, and a sample of inguinal adipose tissue collected for MSC harvest. The LOAD questionnaire was chosen as a suitable CMI.

Regenerative medicine (RM)

Culture-expanded, autologous AD-MSCs (Adi-Shot®, Cell Therapy Sciences) were injected into both elbows and both carpi (3.64 million cells into each joint). Lead walking only was advised for three days. After the orthobiologic injections, meloxicam and amantadine were continued for one month.

Further case progression

A very rapid positive response to the injected MSCs was observed clinically. Within the first month post-administration, the lameness settled down completely, as did the pain response on elbow palpation. The analgesic medication was withdrawn. These clinical observations were borne out by the LOAD results. By eleven months after the first MSC injections, the left thoracic limb lameness was beginning to return, so the injections were repeated.

Rationale for VRM and decision-making

This case involved a similar kind of patient to that reported by Armitage et al. (2023). These dogs were generally refractory to conventional medical multimodal management. In the case described here, an argument can be made for surgical management as outlined above, to improve the joint anatomy and to aim to engender a more normal load distribution on the joint surfaces. By electing for a non-surgical

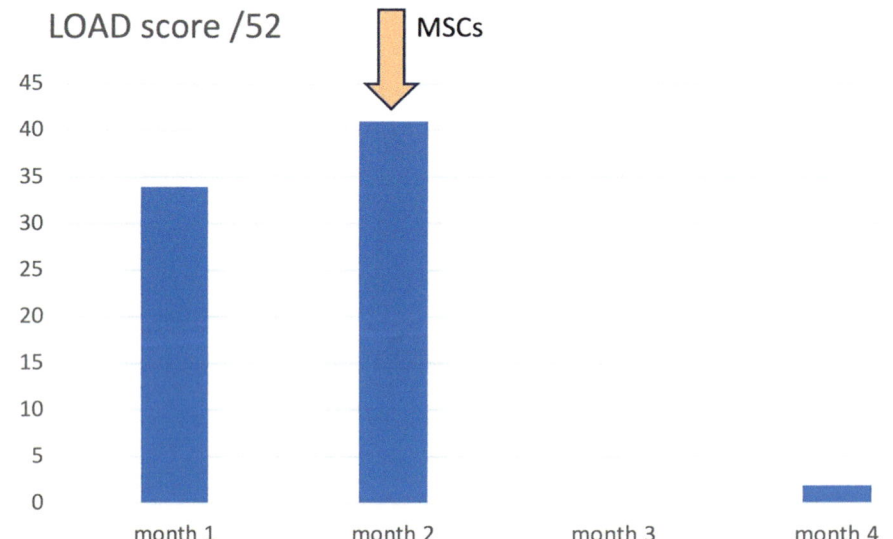

Fig. 16.3.6 Case 3 LOAD scores before and for two months following MSC administration. MSCs with arrow = the time of administration of the MSCs.

approach, the pet owner and clinician accepted that OA was inevitable and that mitigation of the impact of the OA on the patient was the aim. To this end, weight management and physical therapy are indicated with analgesic medication as needed. The choice of autologous AD-MSCs as the orthobiologic was made as there are multiple joints that are likely to require targeted IA therapy on multiple occasions. Having banked MSCs for future use is a major advantage. The interim administration of Class IV laser was chosen to augment the action of the MSCs (Armitage, 2023). In addition to the aforementioned VRM measures, PRP would have been a potentially useful addition to the treatment. The decision to administer AD-MSCs to all four of the anatomically compromised joints (both elbows and both carpi) may be controversial. Clinically it was suspected that the left elbow was the main 'seat' of the current clinical signs. Since it was not possible to determine the contributions of all joints to the problem, it was considered acceptable to inject all four joints.

Conclusion

This case exemplifies how VRM can be applied to cases of OA resulting from anatomical abnormalities. Many such cases do not have the opportunity to benefit from early surgical correction, so develop OA. While it is not claimed that orthobiologics can influence the conformational and anatomical features of the joints, targeted injection, such as performed in this case, can have rapid and long-lasting effects. The cryopreservation of the AD-MSCs in this case allows for repeated administrations, which are very likely to be necessary. Withdrawal of the analgesic medication without deterioration in the clinical signs of OA was encouraging and consistent with good orthobiologic efficacy. The adiposity management was presumably also beneficial, though it is not possible to ascertain to what degree.

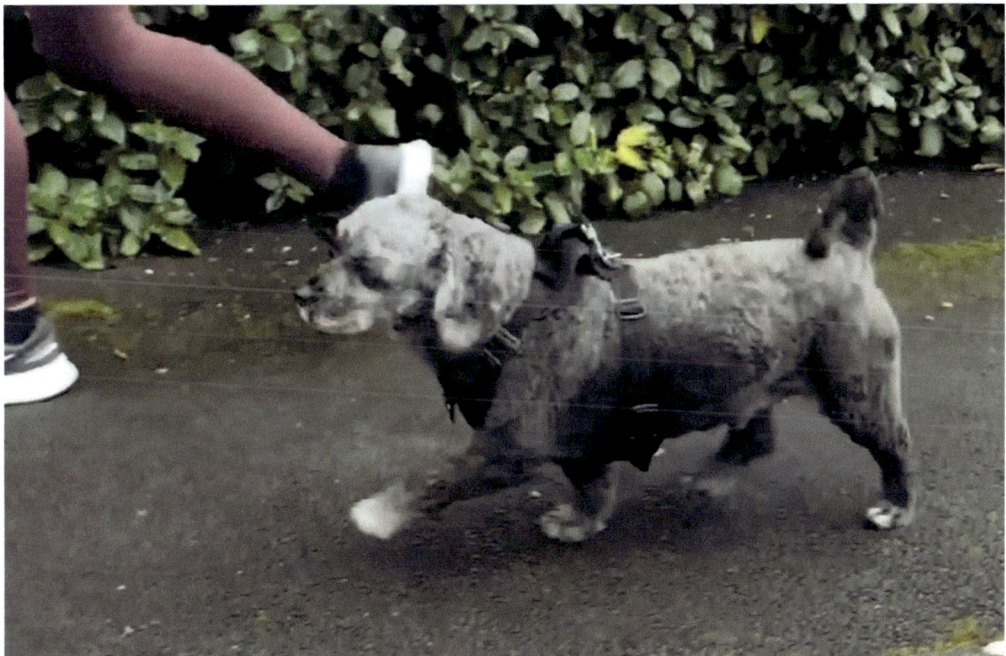

Fig. 16.3.7 Case 3 ambulating well two months after AD-MSC administration to both elbows and carpi.

Case 3 references

Armitage, A. J., Miller, J. M., Sparks, T. H., Georgiou, A. E., & Reid, J. (2023). Efficacy of autologous mesenchymal stromal cell treatment for chronic degenerative musculoskeletal conditions in dogs: A retrospective study. Frontiers in Veterinary Science, 9, 1014687. https://doi.org/10.3389/fvets.2022.1014687

Fox, S. M. (2017). *Multimodal management of canine osteoarthritis*. CRC Press. ISBN 9781840761832.

Case 4

Presentation

A six-year-old, spayed, female Labrador retriever, weighing 28kg, with a body condition score of 6/9, was presented with a two-year history of right thoracic limb lameness. The existing treatments were meloxicam (Metacam®, Boehringer) at a standard once-daily dose of 2.8mg (0.1mg/kg), bedinvetmab (Librela®, Zoetis) 15mg once monthly, paracetamol 375mg (13.4mg/kg) twice daily, and various supplements.

Imaging

The right elbow radiographs showed marked marginal osteophytosis, which is consistent with OA.

Diagnosis

Severe advanced OA of the right elbow.

Case data

CMI and staging: December LOAD 20/52, COAST 4/4, and weight 26.6kg.

Rationale for VRM and decision-making

Despite managing the right elbow OA for two years, a relatively intractable severe disability continued to be observed. The advanced joint pathology was not considered likely to be amenable to the disease-modifying effects of VRM. Despite this, clinical evidence is that even cases with severe joint disease can nonetheless

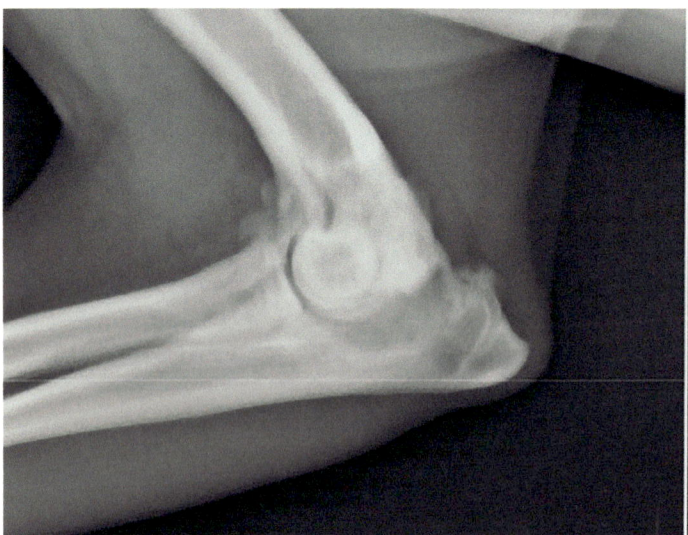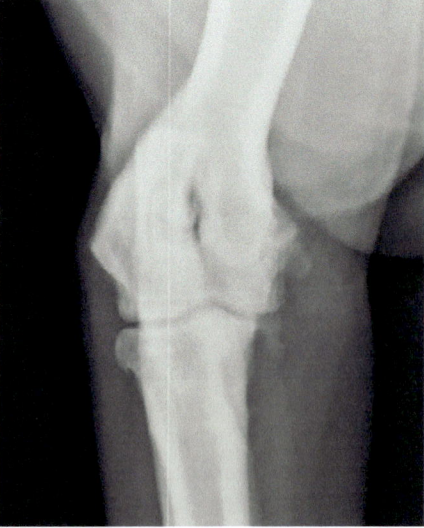

Fig. 16.4.1 Case 4: Lateromedial and craniocaudal radiographic projections of the right elbow. There is marked marginal osteophyte formation and subcoronoid sclerosis of the ulna. A large medial bone spur is present in the soft tissues at the medial coronoid area.

benefit from the anti-inflammatory and immunomodulatory effects of MSCs. Since only a single joint was affected, and a product licensed for elbow use was available, EUC-MSCs were chosen for a VRM (Dogstem®, Dômes Pharma). MSCs were chosen over PRP because of their presumed longer duration of effect. A combination of PRP and MSCs, while possible and advantageous (Armitage et al., 2023), was not possible here, as the licence for the EUC-MSCs precluded mixing it with other products.

Case progression

January: 7.5 million EUC-MSCs (Dogstem®, DÔMES PHARMA) was injected into the right elbow.

February: LOAD 12/52. The patient was still receiving bedinvetmab, meloxicam and paracetamol. Her weight had reduced to 25.2kg and her body condition score was 5/9 (ideal).

March: LOAD 20/52. The lameness had subjectively reduced (in contrast to the LOAD score) but was nonetheless 2/6. The range of motion of the right elbow was 78–148°.

June: LOAD 12/52. The range of motion in the right elbow was 64–148°.

Conclusion

A reasonable, though not spectacular, improvement was observed after VRM in this case. The LOAD score after six months was 12/52, down from 20/52. The elbow range of motion increased by 14° over a similar period. All the analgesic medication continued to be necessary at the original doses and intervals. This case in many ways typifies the observation that elbow OA is challenging to manage, even despite MMOAM including a VRM. The data collection for this patient could be improved by, for example, performing goniometry at every visit. Improvements in the VRM could be the addition

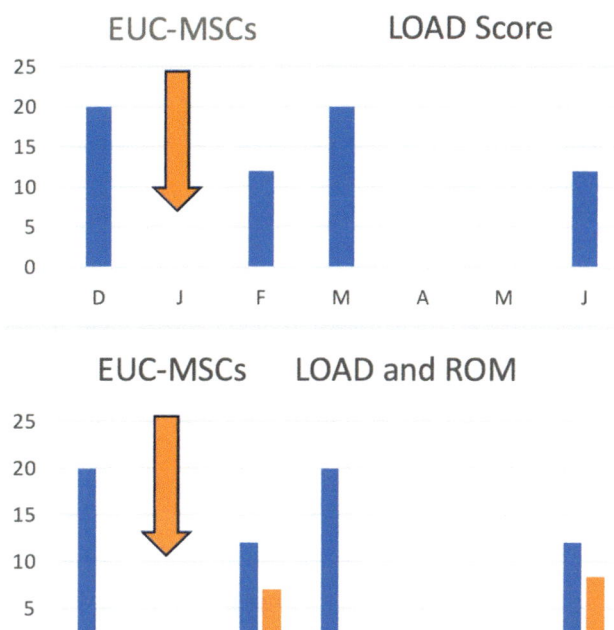

Fig. 16.4.2 Graphical depiction of LOAD scores and elbow range of motion (ROM) before and following IA injection of EUC-MSCs (orange arrow). The blue columns depict the LOAD scores. The orange columns, on the same scale, represent the change in angle of maximum elbow flexion. The horizontal axis labels represent months.

of PRP to the MSCs. For this to be undertaken, a different MSC product would need to be used, such as autologous AD-MSCs.

Case 4 references

Armitage, A. J., Miller, J. M., Sparks, T. H., Georgiou, A. E., & Reid, J. (2023). Efficacy of autologous mesenchymal stromal cell treatment for chronic degenerative musculoskeletal conditions in dogs: A retrospective study. Frontiers in Veterinary Science, 9, 1014687. https://doi.org/10.3389/fvets.2022.1014687.

Case 5

Presentation

A five-year-old, male, Labrador retriever weighing 28.7kg, with an ideal body condition score of 5/9 was presented (Fig. 16.5.1) with over a year's history of continuous lameness to one or more forelimbs. Bilateral elbow crepitus was evident. There was tenderness on medial palpation of the right elbow.

Imaging

There was mild subcoronoid sclerosis in the right elbow (see Fig. 16.5.2). The ipsilateral shoulder showed a sclerotic area in the biceps groove and an enthesophyte on the acromion (see Fig. 16.5.3).

Diagnosis

Probable OA of the right elbow and probable enthesopathies of the shoulder muscles. Further imaging, such as CT and ultrasonography were declined.

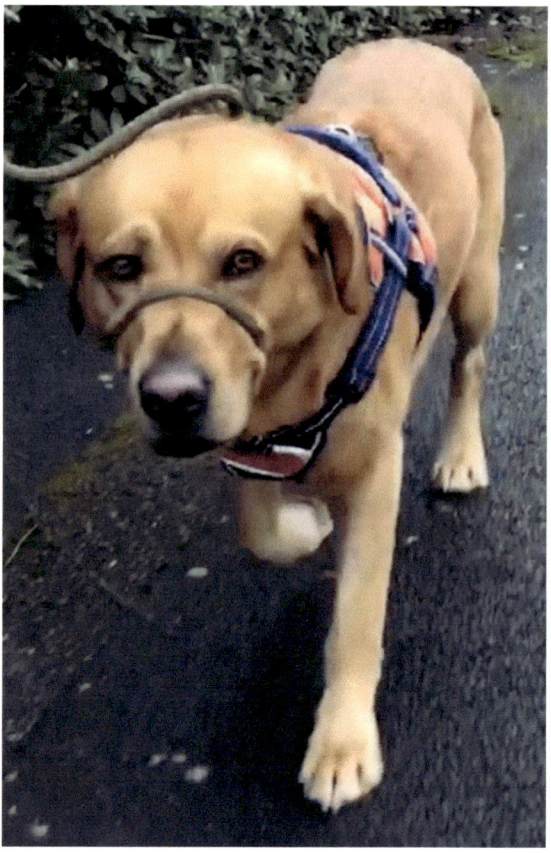

Fig. 16.5.1 Case 5 during lameness evaluation.

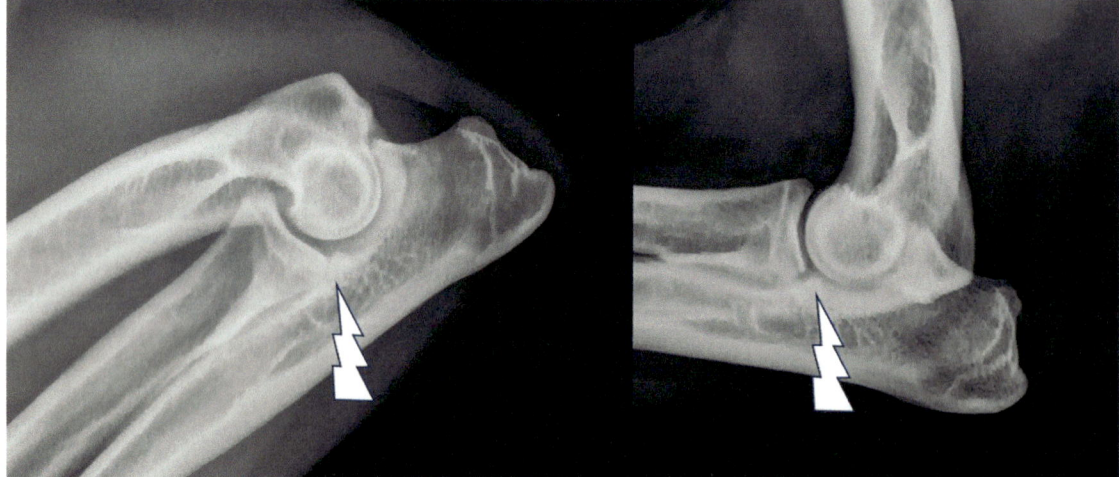

Fig. 16.5.2 Case 5: Lateromedial radiographs of the right elbow in different degrees of flexion. There is mild subcoronoid sclerosis (lightning bolts).

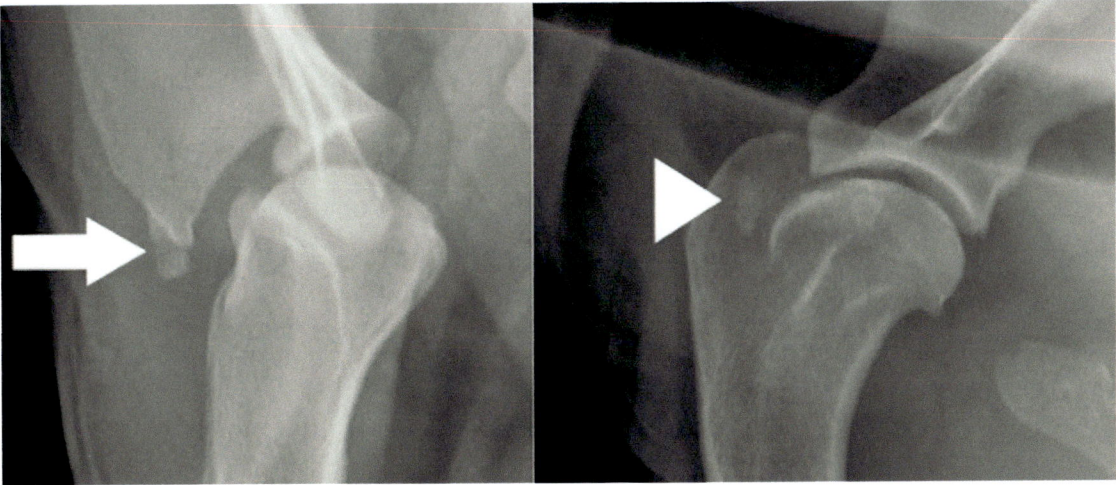

Fig. 16.5.3 Case 5: Craniocaudal and mediolateral radiographs of the right shoulder. There is a sclerotic area in the biceps groove (arrowhead) and an enthesophyte on the acromion (arrow).

Case progression

- September: LOAD 26/52. Medication with robenacoxib (Onsior®, Elanco) 40mg (1.4mg/kg) once daily. Supplement – omega-3 oil.
- October: LOAD 18/52. Continue robenacoxib and omega-3 oil. Added in Class IV laser (K-laser®) treatment.
- November: LOAD 18/52. Continue robenacoxib, omega-3 oil, and Class IV laser treatment.
- January: LOAD 18/52. Continue robenacoxib, omega-3 oil. Add in bedinvetmab (Librela®, Zoetis).
- February: LOAD 16/52. Continue all above.

Rationale for VRM and decision-making

Despite management of the problem with NSAIDs, anti-nerve growth factor monoclonal antibodies, omega-3 oil supplementation, and Class IV laser treatment, a significant disability continued as demonstrated by the LOAD score of 16/52. A different mode of management was considered to add to this hitherto only partially successful multimodal management combination. VRM was chosen for its potential for acting as a disease-modifying OA therapy. Whether to use PRP, MSCs, or both was considered. EUC-MSCs were chosen since this is licensed for use in the canine elbow, there is no requirement for tissue collection from the patient, and this can be administered under a single short sedation as an outpatient. Since the pain appeared to be localised in the right elbow only, the shoulder pathology observed on the radiographs was considered not to be clinically significant.

Further case progression (Fig. 16.5.4)

- 3 March: 7.5 million EUC-MSCs were injected into the right elbow (Dogstem®, Dômes Pharma).
- 14 March: LOAD 7/52. A significant early improvement was observed with reduced severity in lameness.
- April: LOAD 2/52. Given omega-3 oil only. By this stage, one month after EUC-MSCs, the lameness was barely detectable.
- May: LOAD 1/52. Given omega-3 oil only.
- August: LOAD 0/52. Given omega-3 oil only.

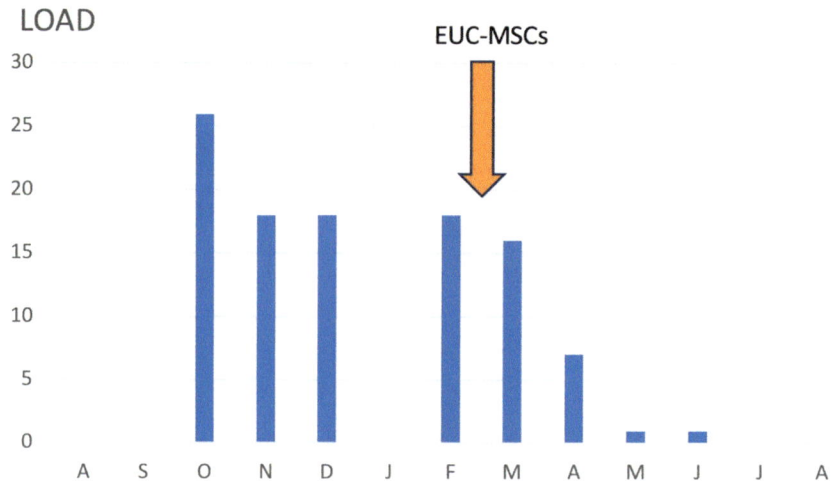

Fig. 16.5.4 Case 5: LOAD scores (columns) before and after IA injection of EUC-MSCs (arrow).

Conclusion

The long pre-VRM history of lameness typifies elbow OA in dogs. The presumptive cause is juvenile elbow dysplasia, which can be relatively clinically silent until middle age when the OA manifests and lameness is observed. This is likely to be the situation here. The shoulder pathology may be related or a separate entity. OA management is generally multimodal. In this case, a combination of modalities was implemented before using a VRM. A case such as this may benefit from VRM since, despite the chronicity of the clinical signs, relatively mild joint pathology was determined. Clearly, further investigations, such as synovial fluid analysis, arthroscopy, and CT, could have added to the diagnostic information available. However, it is debatable whether these, especially arthroscopy, an invasive procedure, could be clinically justified here. The response to the EUC-MSCs was the elimination of the lameness to the extent where the LOAD score became zero and all analgesic medication (robenacoxib, bedinvetmab) could be discontinued. It is not possible to prove a disease-modifying OA therapy effect, though the clinical response would support this notion. Alternative choices for a VRM could have been autologous MSCs, allogeneic MSCs (these were not available in the United Kingdom), and/or PRP.

Chapter 16 key points

- The cases described reflect the author's personal clinical experience with patients receiving VRM treatment.
- Although anecdotal in nature and lacking controls, the accounts demonstrate the potential for profound improvements in the application of VRM.
- The patient 'population' is notably biased, as only cases deemed likely to benefit from VRM were included in the treatment.
- It is not yet established whether autologous MSCs, allogeneic MSCs, xenogeneic MSCs, PRP, or combinations are advisable in general. The author currently makes those decisions on a case-by-case basis considering evidence-based veterinary medicine, experience, clinical acumen, plus the 'art' of veterinary medicine. Where a purely trophic action is indicated, such as for the promotion of tendon healing, PRP is most likely to be chosen. Where an immunomodulatory

effect is desired then MSCs are typically favoured.

- As the discipline evolves, today's standard practices may quickly become outdated. Clinicians should remain informed about developments in the field and be ready to adapt and refine therapeutic protocols accordingly.

Chapter 16 references

Armitage, A. J., Miller, J. M., Sparks, T. H., Georgiou, A. E., & Reid, J. (2023). Efficacy of autologous mesenchymal stromal cell treatment for chronic degenerative musculoskeletal conditions in dogs: A retrospective study. Frontiers in Veterinary Science, 9, 1014687. https://doi.org/10.3389/fvets.2022.1014687

Chen, Y.-C., Hsu, Y.-M., Tan, K. P., Fang, H.-W., & Chang, C.-H. (2018). Intraarticular injection for rabbit knee osteoarthritis: Effectiveness among hyaluronic acid, platelet-rich plasma, and mesenchymal stem cells. *Journal of the Taiwan Institute of Chemical Engineers*, *91*, 138–145. https://doi.org/10.1016/j.jtice.2018.05.051

Manafi, A., Kaviani Far, K., Moradi, M., Manafi, A., & Manafi, F. (2012). Effects of platelet-rich plasma on cartilage grafts in rabbits as an animal model. *World Journal of Plastic Surgery*, *1*(2), 91–98.

WSAVA website WSAVA body condition score. https://wsava.org/wp-content/uploads/2020/01/Body-Condition-Score-Dog.pdf

Chapter 17

The economics of veterinary regenerative medicine (VRM)

The economics of veterinary regenerative medicine (VRM): A local perspective

In common with most innovations in the medical field, VRM is moderately expensive at the point of administration. Due to inevitable owner financial constraints, many more cases could benefit from VRM than actually do. To complicate the situation, pet insurance companies in the countries where they operate may not cover a prescription of VRM.

Upfront costs for VRM can appear daunting. However, it is worthwhile viewing these costs in comparison with other therapies, for example, for OA, that may be considered alongside, or instead of, VRM. Pharmaceutical management of OA, for example, typically involves combinations of both licensed and perhaps unlicensed medication (such as the off-label use of human medication). When calculating the cost of these over, say, a year, VRM may not be, comparatively, as expensive as it appears at first glance. Furthermore, the use of VRM frequently allows other medication to be reduced or curtailed as the condition becomes controlled.

As VRM becomes more ubiquitous and mainstream, rather than occupying its current niche position, it is reasonable to expect that the cost of the products, due to economies of scale, may reduce somewhat. It seems unlikely, however, that an inexpensive cell-based product could be brought to market while maintaining quality control and necessary pathogen screening tests. One means by which a more cost-effective VRM solution may be achieved is by using products based on EVs.

Where economic constraints exist, PRP may be the most cost-effective option for VRM. Ideally, clinicians should invest in a veterinary-specific PRP centrifuge system. However, if such a system is unavailable, PRP can still be produced economically, provided the following conditions are met:

- A centrifuge is available.
- Proper technical processing protocols are followed (see Table 5.1).
- The product's composition can be verified through automated haematological cell and platelet counting.
- Strict sterility is maintained throughout the process.

In developed economies, the investment in equipment and training in VRM makes excellent sense. The primary goal is always the optimal management of the patients to alleviate their problems as effectively as possible. That said, having an economically viable therapy is also necessary. It is good veterinary practice management to ensure that new services are self-funding so that the maximum number of patients can benefit over the longer term. In the author's experience, a relatively modest investment in knowledge, training, and apparatus results in being able to offer a sustainable VRM service in practice.

Some sensible methods to increase the affordability of VRM include:

- **Cryopreservation:** Storing autologous MSCs for extended periods of three years or more allows for repeat dosing at a relatively modest cost.
- **Treat multiple sites simultaneously:** For conditions, such as OA, that can affect multiple joints, injecting several joints during the same session can reduce the overall cost of treatment.
- **Use an in-house laboratory set-up:** Using an existing centrifuge, clinicians can learn to produce autologous PRP, further reducing costs.

The economics of veterinary regenerative medicine (VRM): A global perspective

While all well-executed veterinary care provided within the private sector can be profitable, financial considerations are not the focus of this book. The author is hopeful the preceding chapters have provided a rudimentary framework for the understanding of VRM to the degree that this engenders interest in the subject. Furthermore, the possibility that an untold number of our veterinary patients may benefit from VRM now and in the near future is worthy of our attention. For context, only a small section on the global economic situation as it relates to animal stem cell medicine is included here.

Research in stem cell science has been growing steadily over the last few decades, and an enormous bank of information has accrued within the scientific literature. The challenge of turning *in vitro* studies into clinically applicable therapies for human conditions has been, on the whole, yet to be realised. The veterinary application of MSCs to MSK conditions, in particular OA, has led the RM field in horses, dogs, and cats. The successful application of these MSC technologies could serve as a proof of concept and provide a model for translational medicine. The One Medicine model should encourage advancements in both veterinary and human medicine.

Accurate data on both the veterinary and the human stem cell markets are difficult to verify. Stem cell manufacture is predominantly within the purview of private companies that own the intellectual property associated with the products and processes involved. As a result of the confidentiality that necessarily pervades this domain, estimates from different sources give rise to widely divergent ranges of monetary value for the industry.

A recent report (November 2023, Fact MR. Animal Stem Cell Therapy Market https://www.factmr.com/report/animal-stem-cell-therapy-market) estimated that the size of the veterinary stem cell market in 2024 will be USD 290.5 million. The same source forecasts that, using the observed current compound annual growth rate (CAGR) of approximately 5.2%, this market will grow to USD 474.8 million by 2034. The allogeneic component is projected to account for 63.4% of this growth. Regions where the development of stem cell sales is predicted to be especially positive include the United States, Germany, and Japan.

For comparison, in 2023, it was reported that the human stem cell therapy market was generating USD 286 million annually (December 2023, https://www.marketsandmarkets.com), and at an estimated CAGR of 16.5%, it is predicted to reach USD 615 million by 2028. The market is led by allogeneic over autologous MSCs for transplant. Adipose tissue serves as the predominant tissue source, and MSK conditions remain the leading therapeutic indication. Geographically, North America and the Asia-Pacific region dominate the market, with China emerging as the fastest-growing market within the Asia-Pacific region.

Another report, conflictingly, valued the human global stem cell therapy market an order of magnitude higher at USD 6 billion in 2020. These researchers predicted the 2028 value to be USD 12.9 billion (at a CAGR of 10.3%) (https://www.transparencymarketresearch.com/regenerative-medicines-market.html).

In conclusion, the stem cell therapy markets in both veterinary and human medicine are experiencing rapid growth, driven by the adoption of first-generation MSC-based therapies. The prospect of next-generation therapies, including, among other innovations, iPSCs and EVs, holds the potential to diversify and further expand the markets. Veterinary clinicians, however, must critically evaluate all developments to ensure that the therapies applied are both safe and effective.

Chapter 17 key points

- Both local and global factors affect the economics of VRM.
- Owner financial resources and/or lack of insurance cover often restrict VRM use.
- Both veterinary and human stem cell markets are growing rapidly.
- A One Medicine approach and a translational medicine mindset have the potential to benefit both veterinary and human patients.

Chapter 17 references

Fact MR. Animal stem cell therapy market. Retrieved January 6, 2024. https://www.factmr.com/report/animal-stem-cell-therapy-market

Markets and markets Retrieved January 6, 2024. https://www.marketsandmarkets.com/Market-Reports/stem-cell-technologies-and-global-market-

Regenerative medicine market Retrieved January 6, 2024. https://www.transparencymarketresearch.com/regenerative-medicines-market.html

Afterword

Enormous advances in the therapy and management of small animal MSK conditions continue apace. The multimodal and multidisciplinary approaches to these diseases have become firmly established in the veterinary care of pet animals. The requirement for a genuinely disease-modifying conventional therapy has hitherto remained elusive. Regenerative medicine in its present manifestations appears to be a reasonably logical approach in this respect.

The currently available therapies of PRP and MSCs are finding their place in the multimodal management paradigm. Undoubtedly, as more knowledge and experience are gained, these modalities will be refined, improved, and built upon. The discipline of veterinary regenerative medicine will become increasingly sophisticated, allowing precise targeting of various diseases with more specific orthobiologics. Later generations of regenerative medicine products may use EVs or iPSCs instead of MSCs and could involve different delivery methods such as seeded biological scaffolds.

A wide horizon of possibilities is opening up before us as clinicians involved in VRM. We need to proceed with caution in this shared endeavour to avoid, wherever possible, the adoption of unsound or unproven therapies. A collective effort should be encouraged so that, as veterinary professionals with a common purpose, including scientists, clinicians, and biopharma companies, we can move forward together in a safe and effective way.

The future of veterinary orthobiologics is bright. Even with the existing products and methods available, clinicians can readily learn to use regenerative medicines in practice. There is good evidence for efficacy, safety, and minimal risk when applying these orthobiologics. The author strongly encourages clinicians to add this powerful treatment modality to their offering.

Appendices

The following informative question and answer sheets are suggested as handouts to share with clients/owners. They can be downloaded from https://5mbooks.com/regenerative-medicine-on line-cont

Veterinary regenerative medicine

What are regenerative medicines?

Most medical treatments available to treat pets' musculoskeletal problems (those conditions affecting joints, muscles, and bones) are symptom-modifying only. That is, they may dull the pain but do not improve the condition. Regenerative veterinary medicine is a collective term for veterinary treatments that aim to affect (that is, improve) the disease process. In this way, they are very different from conventional drug treatments.

What kinds of regenerative medicines are available?

There are two main regenerative medicines widely used for pets. These are PRP and stem cells. PRP stands for platelet-rich plasma; it comes from the patient's own blood. A sample of blood is taken and then processed to concentrate small cell-like components called platelets. Platelets have the ability to release molecular messengers called growth factors. When the PRP is injected back into the pet, say into an arthritic joint, the growth factors are released to promote healing of the joint. Stem cells are capable of reducing inflammation, regulating the immune system, and promoting tissue repair. These cells can be injected on their own or mixed with PRP.

What kind of stem cells are available?

The kind of stem cells used are MSCs. MSC stands for mesenchymal stem cell. Your pet has MSCs in many parts of the body. The easiest places to harvest them from are fat or bone marrow. In the laboratory, the MSCs are extracted, purified, and expanded in number. If these MSCs are injected back into your pet, the treatment is called 'autologous MSC transplantation'.

MSCs may be harvested from a different individual of the same species. This is called 'allogeneic MSC transplantation'. If a different species provides the MSCs, then this is referred to as 'xenogeneic MSC transplantation'.

How is regenerative medicine applied?

PRP and MSCs can be injected into your pet under sedation. The most common places to do this are in arthritic joints.

How effective is regenerative medicine?

There are a large number of scientific studies on PRP and MSC treatments in dogs. These show the treatment is safe and no major harmful effects have been reported. The majority of pets benefit from the administration of regenerative medicine, and most show marked improvements in lameness, pain levels, and quality of life.

Are there any side effects of regenerative medicine?

A minority of dogs suffer swelling and tenderness of the injected area for a few days. This is easily treated using painkillers that are supplied at the time.

How long does the treatment last?

The effects of the PRP usually last for three to six months. The effects of MSCs can last longer, often up to a year or more.

Can the treatment be repeated?

Most regenerative medicines can be repeated as many times as needed.

Veterinary platelet-rich plasma therapy

Platelet-rich plasma (PRP) therapy has been recommended for your pet. PRP is an autologous treatment, which means that your pet is the donor of the PRP and the recipient.

Why are platelets used?

Platelets are small cell-like structures in the circulating blood of all mammals, including humans and our pets. Platelets are rich in protein molecules called growth factors. These are contained in granules that are released when the need arises. Platelets are plentiful in the blood, so some can be collected and used to promote tissue healing.

How is PRP prepared?

A sample of your pet's blood is collected from a vein. The blood is then placed in a centrifuge to separate the cells from the plasma. The layer containing the platelets is removed along with some of the plasma. The resulting suspension is PRP. In the PRP, there is a greater concentration of platelets than in the blood.

How is PRP injected?

With your pet under sedation, the site of the injury or disease is identified, and the PRP is injected directly. This may be into a joint, tendon, ligament, or muscle, for example.

Are there any side effects of PRP therapy?

A short-term worsening of the problem for a few days may be seen, as PRP may induce some inflammation at the injection site. Your vet will provide any necessary treatment to help this settle down.

What beneficial effects can be expected after PRP injection?

The platelets, after injection, release their growth factors, which stimulate the healing process in the tissues. The expected effects are a reduction in pain, improved limb function, and a faster recovery.

How long do the effects last?

The positive effects seen after PRP therapy typically last for three to nine months.

Can the PRP injections be repeated?

Yes. As a rule, repeating PRP injections is possible as many times as is required, as long as beneficial effects are observed.

Can other treatments be used alongside PRP therapy?

Yes. There is another regenerative medicine that may be combined with PRP, namely stem cells. Injecting both together is likely to result in these treatments having a cooperative action, increasing the effectiveness of the treatment.

Where can I go for my pet to have PRP therapy?

PRP therapy can only be administered by a veterinarian. This service may be available at your pet's local practice. If not, your vet may refer your pet to another practice where the facilities, experience, and expertise are available for PRP therapy.

Is the therapy licensed and authorised for my pet?

As the PRP is usually derived from your own pet, then legally this is more like a clinical procedure than a pharmaceutical medicine. As such, the usual legislative and licensing controls required for medicines do not apply. An exception to this is a newly developed allogeneic PRP product for dogs that is available in the USA. In this case, as the PRP comes from dogs other than the recipient, medicine licensing is required.

Veterinary autologous stem cell therapy

Stem cell therapy has been recommended for your pet. This information relates to autologous stem cells, which means that your pet is the donor of the cells and the recipient.

Why are stem cells used?

Stem cells can have multiple beneficial effects in the body in conditions such as arthritis (medically known as osteoarthritis). The main effects are anti-inflammatory, regulation of the immune system within the affected area, and the promotion of healing. Owners typically observe a reduction in pain and lameness, better function, and improvements in their pet's quality of life.

What kind of stem cells are used?

The cells we use are called MSCs. This stands for mesenchymal stem cells. MSCs have been widely studied and have been used for many years in dogs and horses. MSCs are usually collected from fatty tissue or bone marrow.

How are the stem cells collected?

The most common place tissue is collected for MSC extraction is the body fat. A small operation is needed to take this sample of fatty tissue from either the lower abdomen, the side of the chest, or just in front of the navel (inside the abdomen). The surgical wound generally heals well within two weeks.

What happens in the laboratory?

The tissue is sent to a laboratory specialising in stem cell work. Here, the tissue is processed, and the MSCs are extracted and cultured; they are then expanded by encouraging them to divide and multiply. Each treatment requires several million cells. Before leaving the laboratory, a list of quality control tests is performed to make sure the cell product is safe and effective. The MSCs are then transported back to the clinic.

How are the stem cells injected?

Your pet will be sedated for the stem cell injection. Under sterile conditions, the MSCs are injected into the target location, such as an arthritic joint.

Are there any side effects after stem cell treatment?

MSC injection is extremely safe. A small number of pets may experience a temporary worsening of the symptoms of the condition being treated. For example, if an arthritic joint is injected, then there may be some swelling and perhaps an increase in lameness for a few days. Your vet will provide painkillers and anti-inflammatory medication, which will help the situation to settle down.

What beneficial effects can be expected after stem cell injection?

The majority of pets experience noticeable improvements during the first month after injection with MSCs. The observed benefits include a reduction in pain and lameness, an increase in activity, and positive effects on quality of life.

How long do the effects last?

Autologous MSC beneficial effects are long-lasting. This ranges from around six to eighteen months in some pets.

Can the injections be repeated?

Autologous MSCs can be banked in cryo-storage (frozen at very low temperatures) in the laboratory. This means that repeat doses of MSCs can be obtained when needed for several years and repeat injections can be given.

Can other treatments be used alongside stem cell therapy?

Yes. Stem cell therapy generally forms one part of your pet's treatment. Medicines such as painkillers and anti-inflammatories are often still helpful. Other treatments that may be used alongside MSCs include platelet-rich plasma (PRP), laser therapy, physiotherapy, and surgery.

Where can I go for my pet to have stem cell therapy?

Stem cell therapy can only be administered by a veterinarian. This service may be available at your pet's local practice. If not, your vet may refer your pet to another practice where the facilities, experience, and expertise are available for stem cell therapy.

Is the treatment licensed and authorised for my pet?

The laboratory chosen performs its work under a licence from the relevant authority. In the UK, this is the Veterinary Medicines Directorate. Since the MSCs injected originated from your pet, this is not subject to the same legal regulations that a conventional medicine would be.

Veterinary xenogeneic stem cell therapy

Stem cell therapy has been recommended for your pet. This information relates to xenogeneic stem cells, which means that your pet may receive stem cells from another species of animal.

Why are stem cells used?

Stem cells can have multiple beneficial effects in the body in conditions such as osteoarthritis. The main effects are anti-inflammatory, regulation of the immune system within the affected area, and the promotion of healing. Owners typically observe a reduction in pain and lameness, increased function, and improvement in quality of life.

What kind of stem cells are used?

The cells that we use are called MSCs. This stands for mesenchymal stem cells. MSCs have been very widely studied and have been used for many years in dogs and horses. Xenogeneic MSCs are from another species, such as a horse. The umbilical cord, following birth, is usually a waste product. This can be collected instead of being discarded, and the MSCs removed as a source of stem cells for the treatment of dogs.

What happens in the laboratory?

The tissue is sent to a laboratory specialising in stem cell work. Here, the tissue is processed, and the MSCs are extracted and cultured; they are then expanded by encouraging them to divide and multiply. Master banks of cells are produced. Each treatment requires several million cells. Before leaving the laboratory, a list of quality control tests is performed to make sure that the cell product is safe and effective. The MSCs are then transported to the clinic where they can be administered to pets requiring stem cell therapy.

How are the stem cells injected?

Your pet will be sedated for the stem cell injection. Under sterile conditions, the MSCs are injected into the target location, such as an arthritic joint.

Are there any side effects after stem cell treatment?

MSC injection is extremely safe. A small number of pets may experience a temporary worsening of the symptoms of the condition being treated. For example, if an arthritic joint is injected, then there may be some swelling and perhaps an increase in the lameness for a few days. Your vet will provide painkillers and anti-inflammatory medication, which will help the situation to settle down.

What beneficial effects can be expected after stem cell injection?

The majority of pets experience noticeable improvements during the first month after injection with MSCs. The observed benefits include a reduction in pain and lameness, an increase in activity, and positive effects on quality of life.

How long do the effects last?

The beneficial effects of MSCs are long-lasting. This can range from around six to eighteen months in some pets.

Can the injections be repeated?

This depends on the licence of the MSC being used.

Can other treatments be used alongside stem cell therapy?

This depends on regulatory guidelines, which may not permit combining MSCs with other injectable products in the same joint. However, stem cell therapy frequently forms one part of your pet's treatment, and medicines such as painkillers and anti-inflammatories can be given. Other treatments that can be used alongside MSCs include laser therapy, physiotherapy, and surgery.

Where can I go for my pet to have stem cell therapy?

Stem cell therapy can only be administered by a veterinarian. This service may be available at your pet's local practice. If not, your vet may refer your pet to another practice where the facilities, experience, and expertise are available for stem cell therapy.

Is the treatment licensed and authorised for my pet?

The xenogeneic MSC product used is licensed for use in the UK under a regulatory body called the Veterinary Medicines Directorate (or VMD) and in the EU, under a regulatory body called the European Medicines Agency (or EMA).

About the author

Dr Russell Chandler is a British veterinary surgeon working in small animal private practice. He graduated from Bristol Veterinary School with a BVSc in 1987. Russell has worked in practices in the UK, Hong Kong, and Singapore. He holds the following postgraduate qualifications: RCVS Certificate in Small Animal Orthopaedics, RCVS Advanced Practitioner status in Small Animal Orthopaedics, MSc in Orthopaedic Engineering (Cardiff University), MSc in Stem Cells and Regeneration (University of Bristol), and is a member of the Royal College of Veterinary Surgeons. Dr Chandler continues to practice as a veterinary surgeon. His main clinical interests are orthopaedic surgery, osteoarthritis care, analgesia, veterinary science communication, and regenerative medicine.

Acknowledgements

The author acknowledges the generous help and inspiration afforded by colleagues including, in alphabetical order: Ross Allan, Andrew Armitage, Stephen Barabas, Priscilla Berni, Frank Barry, Stuart Carmichael, Nichi Cockburn, Stefano Grolli, Emma Hancox, Helen Harrison, Ksenjia Ilieska, Ana Ivanovska, Oscar Cordero Llana, Jamie McClement, Greg McGarrell, Jo Miller, Mary Murphy, Len Nokes, Almudena Pradera, Christine Standen, Drew Tootal, Kate Whittington, and Offer Ziera.

Credits for images

All photographs used are the property of the author and publisher unless stated otherwise. Some have been kindly provided by colleagues, in which case their courtesy is acknowledged. The graphical images were designed by the author using BioRender® and Microsoft PowerPoint®. Many of these have been modified from or inspired by previous authors' work. Where this is the case, the relevant authors are referenced.

Further reading

The preceding chapters have cited relevant information sources at the end of each chapter, with many appearing at the end of more than one chapter. This section provides a combined list of all these sources, plus other useful references, to provide a bibliography for further study of the subject. Although comprehensive, this list includes only a tiny sample of the vast body of published work available in the field, offering a glimpse into the breadth and depth of veterinary regenerative medicine. Given the rapid rate of advancement in this discipline, the author acknowledges that some materials may quickly become outdated and replaced by more relevant information. Readers are strongly encouraged, once again, to keep their knowledge as updated as possible.

Books

Fox, S. M. (2017). *Multimodal management of canine osteoarthritis*. CRC Press. ISBN 9781840761832.

Gugjoo, M. B. (2022). Therapeutic applications of mesenchymal stem cells in veterinary medicine. *Springer nature*.

Scientific papers, published articles, and other sources

Abdelrazik, H., Giordano, E., Barbanti Brodano, G., Griffoni, C., De Falco, E., & Pelagalli, A. (2019). Substantial overview on mesenchymal stem cell biological and physical properties as an opportunity in translational medicine. *International Journal of Molecular Sciences*, *20*(21), 5386. https://doi.org/10.3390/ijms20215386

Aggarwal, S., & Pittenger, M. F. (2005). Human mesenchymal stem cells modulate allogeneic immune cell responses. *Blood*, *105*(4), 1815–1822. https://doi.org/10.1182/blood-2004-04-1559

Aleksiewicz, R., Lutnicki, K., & Marcinek, T. (2023). Ultrasound monitoring of the regenerative treatment of biceps tendonitis and tenosynovitis in dogs by stem cells injections. *Medycyna Weterynaryjna*, *79*(10), 525–529.

Alves, J. C., Santos, A., & Carreira, L. M. (2023). A preliminary report on the combined effect of intra-articular platelet-rich plasma injections and photobiomodulation in canine osteoarthritis. *Animals: An Open Access Journal from MDPI*, *13*(20), 3247. https://doi.org/10.3390/ani13203247

Alves, J. C., Santos, A., Jorge, P., & Carreira, L. M. (2022). A first report on the efficacy of a single intra-articular administration of blood cell secretome, triamcinolone acetonide, and the combination of both in dogs with osteoarthritis. *BMC Veterinary Research*, *18*(1), 309. https://doi.org/10.1186/s12917-022-03413-2

Alves, J. C., Santos, A., Jorge, P., Lavrador, C., & Carreira, L. M. (2020). A pilot study on the efficacy of a single intra-articular administration of triamcinolone acetonide, hyaluronan, and a combination of both for clinical management of osteoarthritis in police working dogs. *Frontiers in Veterinary Science*, *7*, 512523. https://doi.org/10.3389/fvets.2020.512523

Alves, R., & Grimalt, R. (2018). A review of platelet-rich plasma: History, biology, mechanism of action, and classification. *Skin Appendage Disorders*, *4*(1), 18–24. https://doi.org/10.1159/000477353

Aragon, C. L., & Budsberg, S. C. (2005). Applications of evidence-based medicine: Cranial cruciate ligament injury repair in the dog. *Veterinary Surgery*, *34*(2), 93–98. https://doi.org/10.1111/j.1532-950X.2005.00016.x

Arican, M., Üney, K., Parlak, K., Uzunlu, E. O., & Sönmez, G. (2022). Proteases and collagenase enzymes activity after autologous platelet-rich plasma, bio-physically activated PRP and stem cells for the treatment of osteoarthritis in dogs. *Kafkas Universitesi Veteriner Fakultesi Dergisi*, *28*(4), 437–445, Art. no. KVFD-2022-27357.

Armitage, A. J., Miller, J. M., Sparks, T. H., Georgiou, A. E., & Reid, J. (2023). Efficacy of autologous mesenchymal stromal cell treatment for chronic degenerative musculoskeletal conditions in dogs: A retrospective study. Frontiers in Veterinary Science, 9, 1014687. https://doi.org/10.3389/fvets.2022.1014687

Arnoczky, S. P., & Sheibani-Rad, S. (2013). The basic science of platelet-rich plasma (PRP): What clinicians need to know. *Sports Medicine and Arthroscopy Review*, *21*(4), 180–185. https://doi.org/10.1097/JSA.0b013e3182999712

Aryazand, Y., Buote, N. J., Hsieh, Y., Hayashi, K., & Rosselli, D. (2023). Multifactorial assessment of leukocyte reduced platelet rich plasma injection in dogs undergoing tibial plateau leveling osteotomy: A retrospective study. *PLOS ONE*, *18*(6), e0287922. https://doi.org/10.1371/journal.pone.0287922

Astor, D. E., Hoelzler, M. G., Harman, R., & Bastian, R. P. (2013). Patient factors influencing the concentration of stromal vascular fraction (SVF) for adipose-derived stromal cell (ASC) therapy in dogs. *Canadian Journal of Veterinary Research*, *77*(3), 177–182.

Bárdos, T., Kamath, R. V., Mikecz, K., & Glant, T. T. (2001). Anti-inflammatory and chondroprotective effect of TSG-6 (tumor necrosis factor-α-stimulated gene-6) in murine models of experimental arthritis. *The American Journal of Pathology*, *159*(5), 1711–1721. https://doi.org/10.1016/s0002-9440(10)63018-0

Barfod, K. W., & Blønd, L. (2019). Treatment of osteoarthritis with autologous and microfragmented adipose tissue. *Danish Medical Journal*, *66*(10), A5565.

Barrachina, L., Arshaghi, T. E., O'Brien, A., Ivanovska, A., & Barry, F. (2023). Induced pluripotent stem cells in companion animals: How can we move the field forward? *Frontiers in Veterinary Science*, *10*, 1176772. https://doi.org/10.3389/fvets.2023.1176772

Barry, F. (2023). *Lecture from second international regenerative medicine, Skopje, Northern Macedonia.*

Bello, A. M., & Dye, C. (2023). Current perceptions and use of paracetamol in dogs among veterinary surgeons working in the United Kingdom. *Veterinary Medicine and Science*, *9*(2), 679–686. https://doi.org/10.1002/vms3.1058

Biobridge Foundation. (2020). Standardized Platelet-rich Plasma for musculoskeletal disorders. http://www.biobridge-event.com/knowledge

Black, L. L., Gaynor, J., Adams, C., Dhupa, S., Sams, A. E., Taylor, R., Harman, S., Gingerich, D. A., & Harman, R. (2008). Effect of intraarticular injection of autologous adipose-derived mesenchymal stem and regenerative cells on clinical signs of chronic osteoarthritis of the elbow joint in dogs. *Veterinary Therapeutics: Research in Applied Veterinary Medicine*, *9*(3), 192–200.

Black, L. L., Gaynor, J., Gahring, D., Adams, C., Aron, D., Harman, S., Gingerich, D. A., & Harman, R. (2007). Effect of adipose-derived mesenchymal stem and regenerative cells on lameness in dogs with chronic osteoarthritis of the coxofemoral joints: A randomized, double-blinded, multicenter controlled trial. *Veterinary Therapeutics: Research in Applied Veterinary Medicine*, *8*(4), 272–284.

Block, G. J., Ohkouchi, S., Fung, F., Frenkel, J., Gregory, C., Pochampally, R., DiMattia, G., Sullivan, D. E., & Prockop, D. J. (2009). Multipotent stromal cells are activated to reduce apoptosis in part by upregulation and secretion of stanniocalcin-1. *Stem Cells*, *27*(3), 670–681. https://doi.org/10.1002/stem.20080742

Bogers, S. H. (2018). Cell-based therapies for joint disease in veterinary medicine: What we have learned and what we need to know. *Frontiers in Veterinary Science*, *5*, 70. https://doi.org/10.3389/fvets.2018.00070

Bosch, G., van Schie, H. T. M., de Groot, M. W., Cadby, J. A., van de Lest, C. H. A., Barneveld, A., & van Weeren, P. R. (2010). Effects of platelet-rich plasma on the quality of repair of mechanically induced core lesions in equine superficial digital flexor tendons: A placebo-controlled experimental study.

Journal of Orthopaedic Research, *28*(2), 211–217. https://doi.org/10.1002/jor.20980

Braun, H. J., Kim, H. J., Chu, C. R., & Dragoo, J. L. (2014). The effect of platelet-rich plasma formulations and blood products on human synoviocytes: Implications for intra-articular injury and therapy. *The American Journal of Sports Medicine*, *42*(5), 1204–1210. https://doi.org/10.1177/0363546514525593

Brennan, M. L., Arlt, S. P., Belshaw, Z., Buckley, L., Corah, L., Doit, H., Fajt, V. R., Grindlay, D. J. C., Moberly, H. K., Morrow, L. D., Stavisky, J., & White, C. (2020). Critically appraised topics (CATs) in veterinary medicine: Applying evidence in clinical practice. *Frontiers in Veterinary Science*, *7*, 314. https://doi.org/10.3389/fvets.2020.00314

Brondeel, C., Pauwelyn, G., de Bakker, E., Saunders, J., Samoy, Y., & Spaas, J. H. (2021, May 19). Review: Mesenchymal stem cell therapy in canine osteoarthritis research: "experientia docet" (experience will teach us). *Frontiers in Veterinary Science*, *8*, 668881. https://doi.org/10.3389/fvets.2021.668881, PubMed: 34095280, PubMed Central: PMC8169969

Brown, D. C. (2014). The canine orthopedic index. Step 1: Devising the items. *Veterinary Surgery*, *43*(3), 232–240. https://doi.org/10.1111/j.1532-950X.2014.12142.x

Brown, D. C., Boston, R. C., Coyne, J. C., & Farrar, J. T. (2007). Development and psychometric testing of an instrument designed to measure chronic pain in dogs with osteoarthritis. *American Journal of Veterinary Research*, *68*(6), 631–637. https://doi.org/10.2460/ajvr.68.6.631

Budoni, M., Fierabracci, A., Luciano, R., Petrini, S., Di Ciommo, V., & Muraca, M. (2013). The immunosuppressive effect of mesenchymal stromal cells on B lymphocytes is mediated by membrane vesicles. *Cell Transplantation*, *22*(2), 369–379. https://doi.org/10.3727/096368911X582769

Buote, N. J. (2022). Laparoscopic adipose-derived stem cell harvest technique with bipolar sealing device: Outcome in 12 dogs. *Veterinary Medicine and Science*, *8*(4), 1421–1428. https://doi.org/10.1002/vms3.816

Burton, N. J. (2023). Review of minimally invasive surgical procedures for assessment and treatment of medial coronoid process disease. *Veterinary Surgery*, *52*(6), 790–800. https://doi.org/10.1111/vsu.13986

Bwalya, E. C., Kim, S., Fang, J., Wijekoon, H. M. S., Hosoya, K., & Okumura, M. (2017). Effects of pentosan polysulfate and polysulfated glycosaminoglycan on chondrogenesis of canine bone marrow-derived mesenchymal stem cells in alginate and Micromass culture. *The Journal of Veterinary Medical Science*, *79*(7), 1182–1190. https://doi.org/10.1292/jvms.17-0084

Bwalya, E. C., Kim, S., Fang, J., Wijekoon, H. M. S., Hosoya, K., & Okumura, M. (2017). Pentosan polysulfate inhibits IL-1β-induced iNOS, c-Jun and HIF-1α upregulation in canine articular chondrocytes. *PLOS ONE*, *12*(5), e0177144. https://doi.org/10.1371/journal.pone.0177144

Cabon, Q., Febre, M., Gomez, N., Cachon, T., Pillard, P., Carozzo, C., Saulnier, N., Robert, C., Livet, V., Rakic, R., Plantier, N., Saas, P., Maddens, S., & Viguier, E. (2019). Long-term safety and efficacy of single or repeated intra-articular injection of allogeneic neonatal mesenchymal stromal cells for managing pain and lameness in moderate to severe canine osteoarthritis without anti-inflammatory pharmacological support: Pilot clinical study. *Frontiers in Veterinary Science*. FEB, *6*, Art. no. 10. https://doi.org/10.3389/fvets.2019.00010

Cachon, T., Frykman, O., Innes, J. F., Lascelles, B. D. X., Okumura, M., Sousa, P., Staffieri, F., Steagall, P. V., Van Ryssen, B., & COAST Development Group. (2018). Face validity of a proposed tool for staging canine osteoarthritis: Canine OsteoArthritis Staging Tool (COAST). *Veterinary Journal*, *235*, 1–8. https://doi.org/10.1016/j.tvjl.2018.02.017

Cachon, T., Frykman, O., Innes, J. F., Lascelles, B. D. X., Okumura, M., Sousa, P., Staffieri, F., Steagall, P. V., & Van Ryssen, B. (2023). COAST Development Group's international consensus guidelines for the treatment of canine osteoarthritis. *Frontiers in Veterinary Science*, *10*, 1137888. https://doi.org/10.3389/fvets.2023.1137888

Canapp, Jr., S. O., & Carr, B. J. (2017). Regenerative medicine in the canine: A translational model. *Regenerative Treatments in Sports and Orthopedic Medicine*, *43*.

Canapp Jr, S. O., Canapp, D. A., Ibrahim, V., Carr, B. J., Cox, C., & Barrett, J. G. (2016). The use of adipose-derived progenitor cells and platelet-rich plasma combination for the treatment of supraspinatus tendinopathy in 55 dogs: a retrospective study. *Frontiers in Veterinary Science*, 61.

Canapp, Jr., S. O., Leasure, C. S., Cox, C., Ibrahim, V., & Carr, B. J. (2016). Partial cranial cruciate ligament tears treated with stem cell and platelet-rich plasma combination therapy in 36 dogs: A retrospective study. *Frontiers in Veterinary Science*, 3, 112. https://doi.org/10.3389/fvets.2016.00112

Canapp, S. (n.d.). *How to incorporate stem cell therapy into your practice.*

Canapp, S. O. (2018). Conservative treatment options for partial and complete CCL tears in dogs. *Veterinary practice news.*

Caplan, A. I. (1991). Mesenchymal stem cells. *Journal of Orthopaedic Research*, 9(5), 641–650. https://doi.org/10.1002/jor.1100090504

Caplan, A. I. (2008). All MSCs are pericytes? *Cell Stem Cell*, 3(3), 229–230. https://doi.org/10.1016/j.stem.2008.08.008

Caplan, A. I. (2017). Mesenchymal stem cells: Time to change the name! *Stem Cells Translational Medicine*, 6(6), 1445–1451. https://doi.org/10.1002/sctm.17-0051

Caplan, A. I., & Correa, D. (2011). The MSC: An injury drugstore. *Cell Stem Cell*, 9(1), 11–15. https://doi.org/10.1016/j.stem.2011.06.008

Carr, B. J. (2022). Platelet-rich plasma as an orthobiologic: Clinically relevant considerations. *The Veterinary Clinics of North America. Small Animal Practice*, 52(4), 977–995. https://doi.org/10.1016/j.cvsm.2022.02.005

Carr, B. J. (2023). Regenerative medicine and rehabilitation therapy in the canine. *The Veterinary Clinics of North America. Small Animal Practice*, 53(4), 801–827. https://doi.org/10.1016/j.cvsm.2023.02.011

Carr, B. J., Canapp, Jr., S. O., Mason, D. R., Cox, C., & Hess, T. (2015). Canine platelet-rich plasma systems: A prospective analysis. *Frontiers in Veterinary Science*, 2, 73. https://doi.org/10.3389/fvets.2015.00073

Carr, B. J., & Dycus, D. L. (2016). Canine gait analysis. *Recovery & Rehab*, 6(2), 93–100.

Cassano, J. M., Kennedy, J. G., Ross, K. A., Fraser, E. J., Goodale, M. B., & Fortier, L. A. (2018). Bone marrow concentrate and platelet-rich plasma differ in cell distribution and interleukin 1 receptor antagonist protein concentration. *Knee Surgery, Sports Traumatology, Arthroscopy*, 26(1), 333–342. https://doi.org/10.1007/s00167-016-3981-9

Catarino, J., Carvalho, P., Santos, S., Martins, Â., & Requicha, J. (2020). Treatment of canine osteoarthritis with allogeneic platelet-rich plasma: Review of five cases. *Open Veterinary Journal*, 10(2), 226–231. https://doi.org/10.4314/ovj.v10i2.12

Catarino, J., Carvalho, P., Santos, S., Martins, Â., & Requicha, J. (2020, August). Treatment of canine osteoarthritis with allogeneic platelet-rich plasma: Review of five cases. *Open Veterinary Journal*, 10(2), 226–231. https://doi.org/10.4314/ovj.v10i2.12

Caviglia, H., Daffunchio, C., Galatro, G., Cambiaggi, G., Oneto, P., Douglas Price, A. L., Landro, M. E., & Etulain, J. (2020). Inhibition of Fenton reaction is a novel mechanism to explain the therapeutic effect of intra-articular injection of PRP in patients with chronic haemophilic synovitis. *Haemophilia*, 26(4), e187–e193. https://doi.org/10.1111/hae.14075

Cavill, K. (2023). An introduction to the interface between osteoarthritis, one health and one medicine. *Vet Edge on-line* Retrieved December 2023. https://indd.adobe.com/view/bef060ec-aef3-44b0-ad88-0e91857d6f01

Chen, X., Gan, Y., Li, W., Su, J., Zhang, Y., Huang, Y., Roberts, A. I., Han, Y., Li, J., Wang, Y., & Shi, Y. (2014). The interaction between mesenchymal stem cells and steroids during inflammation. *Cell Death and Disease*, 5(1), e1009. https://doi.org/10.1038/cddis.2013.537

Chen, Y.-C., Hsu, Y.-M., Tan, K. P., Fang, H.-W., & Chang, C.-H. (2018). Intraarticular injection for rabbit knee osteoarthritis: Effectiveness among hyaluronic acid, platelet-rich plasma, and mesenchymal stem cells. *Journal of the Taiwan Institute of Chemical Engineers*, 91, 138–145. https://doi.org/10.1016/j.jtice.2018.05.051

Chiavaras, M. M., & Jacobson, J. A. (2013, February). Ultrasound-guided tendon fenestration. In *Seminars in Musculoskeletal Radiology* (Vol. 17, No. 01, pp. 085–090). Thieme Medical Publishers, 17(1), 85–90. https://doi.org/10.1055/s-0033-1333942

Collins, T., Alexander, D., & Barkatali, B. (2021). Platelet-rich plasma: A narrative review. *EFORT Open Reviews*, 6(4), 225–235. https://doi.org/10.1302/2058-5241.6.200017

Committee for medicinal products for veterinary use (CMPV) of the European Medicine Agency (EMA) (87).

Conzemius, M. G., & Evans, R. B. (2012). Caregiver placebo effect for dogs with lameness from osteoarthritis. *Journal of the American Veterinary Medical Association*, *241*(10), 1314–1319. https://doi.org/10.2460/javma.241.10.1314

Cooper, B. (2005, October). Osler's role in defining the third corpuscle, or "blood plates". In *University Medical Centre Proceedings* (Vol. 18, No. 4, pp. 376–378). Taylor & Francis, 18(4), 376–378. https://doi.org/10.1080/08998280.2005.11928097

Cosenza, S., Ruiz, M., Toupet, K., Jorgensen, C., & Noël, D. (2017). Mesenchymal stem cells derived exosomes and microparticles protect cartilage and bone from degradation in osteoarthritis. *Scientific Reports*, *7*(1), 16214. https://doi.org/10.1038/s41598-017-15376-8

Crisan, M., Yap, S., Casteilla, L., Chen, C.-W., Corselli, M., Park, T. S., Andriolo, G., Sun, B., Zheng, B., Zhang, L., Norotte, C., Teng, P.-N., Traas, J., Schugar, R., Deasy, B. M., Badylak, S., Buhring, H.-J., Giacobino, J.-P., Lazzari, L., . . . & Péault, B. (2008). A perivascular origin for mesenchymal stem cells in multiple human organs. *Cell Stem Cell*, *3*(3), 301–313. https://doi.org/10.1016/j.stem.2008.07.003

Csaki, C., Matis, U., Mobasheri, A., Putz, R., Ye, H., & Shakibaei, M. (2007). Chondrogenesis in coculture: An intensive interaction between mesenchymal stem cells and primary chondrocytes. *Journal of Stem Cells and Regenerative Medicine*, *2*(1), 117–118.

Cuervo, B., Rubio, M., Chicharro, D., Damiá, E., Santana, A., Carrillo, J. M., Romero, A. D., Vilar, J. M., Cerón, J. J., & Sopena, J. J. (2020). Objective comparison between platelet rich plasma alone and in combination with physical therapy in dogs with osteoarthritis caused by hip dysplasia. *Animals: An Open Access Journal from MDPI*, *10*(2), 175. https://doi.org/10.3390/ani10020175

Cuervo, B., Rubio, M., Sopena, J., Dominguez, J. M., Vilar, J., Morales, M., Cugat, R., & Carrillo, J. M. (2014). Hip osteoarthritis in dogs: A randomized study using mesenchymal stem cells from adipose tissue and plasma rich in growth factors. *International Journal of Molecular Sciences*, *15*(8), 13437–13460. https://doi.org/10.3390/ijms150813437

Daems, R., Van Hecke, L. V., Schwarzkopf, I., Depuydt, E., Broeckx, S. Y., David, M., Beerts, C., Vandekerckhove, P., & Spaas, J. H. (2019).

A Feasibility study on the use of equine chondrogenic induced mesenchymal stem cells as a treatment for natural occurring osteoarthritis in dogs. *Stem Cells International*, *2019*, Art. no. 4587594. https://doi.org/10.1155/2019/4587594

Dias, I. E., Cardoso, D. F., Soares, C. S., Barros, L. C., Viegas, C. A., Carvalho, P. P., & Dias, I. R. (2021). Clinical application of mesenchymal stem cells therapy in musculoskeletal injuries in dogs—A review of the scientific literature. *Open Veterinary Journal*, *11*(2), 188–202. https://doi.org/10.5455/OVJ.2021.v11.i2.2

Dias, I. E., Pinto, P. O., Barros, L. C., Viegas, C. A., Dias, I. R., & Carvalho, P. P. (2019). Mesenchymal stem cells therapy in companion animals: Useful for immune-mediated diseases? *BMC Veterinary Research*, *15*(1), 358. https://doi.org/10.1186/s12917-019-2087-2

DiMarino, A. M., Caplan, A. I., & Bonfield, T. L. (2013). Mesenchymal stem cells in tissue repair. *Frontiers in Immunology*, *4*, 201. https://doi.org/10.3389/fimmu.2013.00201

Dominici, M. L. B. K., Le Blanc, K., Mueller, I., Slaper-Cortenbach, I., Marini, F. C., Krause, D. S., Deans, R., Keating, A., Prockop, Dj., & Horwitz, E. M. (2006). Minimal criteria for defining multipotent mesenchymal stromal cells. The International Society for Cellular Therapy position statement. *Cytotherapy*, *8*(4), 315–317. https://doi.org/10.1080/14653240600855905

Dos Santos, R. G., Santos, G. S., Alkass, N., Chiesa, T. L., Azzini, G. O., da Fonseca, L. F., Dos Santos, A. F., Rodrigues, B. L., Mosaner, T., & Lana, J. F. (2021). The regenerative mechanisms of platelet-rich plasma: A review. *Cytokine*, *144*, 155560. https://doi.org/10.1016/j.cyto.2021.155560

Doss, M. X., & Sachinidis, A. (2019). Current challenges of iPSC-based disease modeling and therapeutic implications. *Cells*, *8*(5), 403. https://doi.org/10.3390/cells8050403

Enomoto, M., de Castro, N., Hash, J., Thomson, A., Nakanishi-Hester, A., Perry, E., Aker, S., Haupt, E., Opperman, L., Roe, S., Cole, T., Thompson, N. A., Innes, J. F., & Lascelles, B. D. X. (2024). Prevalence of radiographic appendicular osteoarthritis and associated clinical signs in young dogs. *Scientific Reports*, *14*(1), 2827. https://doi.org/10.1038/s41598-024-52324-9

Erol, O. D., Pervin, B., Seker, M. E., & Aerts-Kaya, F. (2021). Effects of storage media, supplements, and cryopreservation methods on quality of stem cells. *World Journal of Stem Cells*, *13*(9), 1197–1214. https://doi.org/10.4252/wjsc.v13.i9.1197

Estes, B. T., Enomoto, M., Moutos, F. T., Carson, M. A., Toth, J. M., Eggert, P., Stallrich, J., Willard, V. P., Veis, D. J., Little, D., Guilak, F., & Lascelles, B. D. X. (2021). Biological resurfacing in a canine model of hip osteoarthritis. *Science Advances*, *7*(38), Art. no. eabi5918. https://doi.org/10.1126/sciadv.abi5918

European Medicines Agency Reflection on stem cell-based medicinal products. (January 2011). https://www.ema.europa.eu/en/documents/scientific-guideline/reflection-paper-stem-cell-based-medicinal-products_en.pdf

Everts, P., Onishi, K., Jayaram, P., Lana, J. F., & Mautner, K. (2020). Platelet-rich plasma: New performance understandings and therapeutic considerations in 2020. *International Journal of Molecular Sciences*, *21*(20), 7794. https://doi.org/10.3390/ijms21207794

Fang, W. H., Chen, X. T., Vangsness, C. T., Jr., & Knee, U.-G. (2021, June 26). Ultrasound-Guided Knee Injections are more accurate than blind injections: A systematic review of randomized controlled trials. *Arthroscopy, Sports Medicine, and Rehabilitation*, *3*(4), e1177–e1187. https://doi.org/10.1016/j.asmr.2021.01.028

Farghali, H. A., AbdElKader, N. A., Khattab, M. S., & AbuBakr, H. O. (2017). Evaluation of subcutaneous infiltration of autologous platelet-rich plasma on skin-wound healing in dogs. *Bioscience Reports*, *37*(2). https://doi.org/10.1042/BSR20160503

Fitch-Tewfik, J. L., & Flaumenhaft, R. (2013). Platelet granule exocytosis: A comparison with chromaffin cells. *Frontiers in Endocrinology*, *4*, 77. https://doi.org/10.3389/fendo.2013.00077

Fitzpatrick, J., Bulsara, M., & Zheng, M. H. (2017). The effectiveness of platelet-rich plasma in the treatment of tendinopathy: A meta-analysis of randomized controlled clinical trials. *The American Journal of Sports Medicine*, *45*(1), 226–233. https://doi.org/10.1177/0363546516643716

Franini, A., Entani, M. G., Colosio, E., Melotti, L., & Patruno, M. (2023). Case report: Flexor carpi ulnaris tendinopathy in a lure-coursing dog treated with three platelet-rich plasma and platelet lysate injections. *Frontiers in Veterinary Science*, *10*, 1003993. https://doi.org/10.3389/fvets.2023.1003993

Franklin, S. P., Stoker, A. M., Bozynski, C. C., Kuroki, K., Clarke, K. M., Johnson, J. K., & Cook, J. L. (2018). Comparison of platelet-rich plasma, stromal vascular fraction (SVF), or SVF with an injectable PLGA nanofiber scaffold for the treatment of osteochondral injury in dogs. *The Journal of Knee Surgery*, *31*(7), 686–697. https://doi.org/10.1055/s-0037-1606575

Frey, C., Yeh, P. C., & Jayaram, P. (2020). Effects of antiplatelet and nonsteroidal anti-inflammatory medications on platelet-rich plasma: A systematic review. *Orthopaedic Journal of Sports Medicine*, *8*(4), 2325967120912841. https://doi.org/10.1177/2325967120912841

Friedenstein, A. J., Chailakhyan, R. K., Latsinik, N. V., Panasyuk, A. F., & Keiliss-Borok, I. V. (1974). Stromal cells responsible for transferring the microenvironment of the hemopoietic tissues: Cloning in vitro and retransplantation in vivo. *Transplantation*, *17*(4), 331–340. https://doi.org/10.1097/00007890-197404000-00001

Friedenstein, A. J., Deriglasova, U. F., Kulagina, N. N., Panasuk, A. F., Rudakowa, S. F., Luriá, E. A., & Ruadkow, I. A. (1974). Precursors for fibroblasts in different populations of hematopoietic cells as detected by the in vitro colony assay method. Experimental Hematology, 2(2), 83–92. https://doi.org/10.3389/fcell.2022.982199.

Friedenstein, A. J., Piatetzky-Shapiro, I. I., & Petrakova, K. V. (1966). Osteogenesis in transplants of bone marrow cells. *Journal of Embryology and Experimental Morphology*, *16*(3), 381–390. https://doi.org/10.1242/dev.16.3.381

Furuoka, H., Endo, K., & Sekiya, I. (2023). Mesenchymal stem cells in synovial fluid increase in number in response to synovitis and display more tissue-reparative phenotypes in osteoarthritis. *Stem Cell Research and Therapy*, *14*(1), 244. https://doi.org/10.1186/s13287-023-03487-1

Galipeau, J., Krampera, M., Barrett, J., Dazzi, F., Deans, R. J., DeBruijn, J., Dominici, M., Fibbe, W. E., Gee, A. P., Gimble, J. M., Hematti, P., Koh, M. B. C., LeBlanc, K., Martin, I., McNiece, I. K., Mendicino, M., Oh, S., Ortiz, L., Phinney, D. G., ... & Sensebe, L. (2016). International Society for Cellular Therapy perspective on immune functional assays for mesenchymal stromal cells as potency release criterion for advanced phase clinical trials. *Cytotherapy*, *18*(2), 151–159. https://doi.org/10.1016/j.jcyt.2015.11.008

Galipeau, J., & Sensébé, L. (2018). Mesenchymal stromal cells: Clinical challenges and therapeutic opportunities. *Cell Stem Cell*, *22*(6), 824–833. https://doi.org/10.1016/j.stem.2018.05.004

Garber, K. (2015). RIKEN suspends first clinical trial involving induced pluripotent stem cells. *Nature Biotechnology*, *33*(9), 890–891. https://doi.org/10.1038/nbt0915-890

Garcia-Pedraza, E., de Miguel, A. G., Gomez de Segura, I. A. G., & Pérez, A. P. (2022). Immunological safety assessment of a single and repeated intra-articular administration of xenogeneic equine umbilical cord mesenchymal stem cells under field conditions in young healthy dogs: A randomized double-blind placebo-controlled study. *Research in Veterinary Science and Medicine*, *2*. https://doi.org/10.25259/RVSM_3_2021

Ghadban, A. A., & Khashjoori, B. K. (2022). Biomechanical evaluation of the effect of acellular amniotic membrane loaded by autologous platelet rich plasma on bone healing in a dog model. *Teikyomedicaljournal.com.*

Gharibi, T., Ahmadi, M., Seyfizadeh, N., Jadidi-Niaragh, F., & Yousefi, M. (2015). Immunomodulatory characteristics of mesenchymal stem cells and their role in the treatment of multiple sclerosis. *Cellular Immunology*, *293*(2), 113–121. https://doi.org/10.1016/j.cellimm.2015.01.002

Gomez-Salazar, M., Gonzalez-Galofre, Z. N., Casamitjana, J., Crisan, M., James, A. W., & Péault, B. (2020). Five decades later, are mesenchymal stem cells still relevant? *Frontiers in Bioengineering and Biotechnology*, *8*, 148. https://doi.org/10.3389/fbioe.2020.00148

Gratwohl, A., Pasquini, M. C., Aljurf, M., Atsuta, Y., Baldomero, H., Foeken, L., Gratwohl, M., Bouzas, L. F., Confer, D., Frauendorfer, K., Gluckman, E., Greinix, H., Horowitz, M., Iida, M., Lipton, J., Madrigal, A., Mohty, M., Noel, L., Novitzky, N., . . . & Worldwide Network for Blood and Marrow Transplantation (WBMT). (2015). One million haemopoietic stem-cell transplants: A retrospective observational study. *The Lancet. Haematology*, *2*(3), e91–e100. https://doi.org/10.1016/S2352-3026(15)00028-9

Greenwood, H. L., Thorsteinsdóttir, H., Perry, G., Renihan, J., Singer, P. A., & Daar, A. S. (2006). Regenerative medicine: New opportunities for developing countries. *International Journal of Biotechnology*, *8*(1/2), 60–77. https://doi.org/10.1504/IJBT.2006.008964

Guercio, A., Di Marco, P., Casella, S., Cannella, V., Russotto, L., Purpari, G., Di Bella, S., & Piccione, G. (2012). Production of canine mesenchymal stem cells from adipose tissue and their application in dogs with chronic osteoarthritis of the humeroradial joints. *Cell Biology International*, *36*(2), 189–194. https://doi.org/10.1042/CBI20110304

Guest, D. J., Dudhia, J., Smith, R. K. W., Roberts, S. J., Conzemius, M., Innes, J. F., Fortier, L. A., & Meeson, R. L. (2022). Position statement: Minimal criteria for reporting veterinary and animal medicine research for mesenchymal stromal/stem cells in orthopaedic applications. *Frontiers in Veterinary Science*, *9*, 817041. https://doi.org/10.3389/fvets.2022.817041

Guilak, F., Estes, B. T., & Moutos, F. T. (2022). Functional tissue engineering of articular cartilage for biological joint resurfacing—The 2021 Elizabeth Winston Lanier Kappa Delta Award. *Journal of Orthopaedic Research*, *40*(8), 1721–1734. https://doi.org/10.1002/jor.25223

Gunaseeli, I., Doss, M. X., Antzelevitch, C., Hescheler, J., & Sachinidis, A. (2010). Induced pluripotent stem cells as a model for accelerated patient- and disease-specific drug discovery. *Current Medicinal Chemistry*, *17*(8), 759–766. https://doi.org/10.2174/092986710790514480

Gupta, S., Paliczak, A., & Delgado, D. (2021). Evidence-based indications of platelet-rich plasma therapy. *Expert Review of Hematology*, *14*(1), 97–108. https://doi.org/10.1080/17474086.2021.1860002

Harman, R., Carlson, K., Gaynor, J., Gustafson, S., Dhupa, S., Clement, K., Hoelzler, M., McCarthy, T., Schwartz, P., & Adams, C. (2016). A prospective, randomized, masked, and placebo-controlled efficacy study of intraarticular allogeneic adipose stem cells for the treatment of osteoarthritis in dogs. *Frontiers in Veterinary Science*, *3*, 81. https://doi.org/10.3389/fvets.2016.00081

Hayflick, L., & Moorhead, P. S. (1961). The serial cultivation of human diploid cell strains. *Experimental Cell Research*, *25*(3), 585–621. https://doi.org/10.1016/0014-4827(61)90192-6

Henig, I., & Zuckerman, T. (2014). Hematopoietic stem cell transplantation-50 years of evolution and future perspectives. *Rambam Maimonides Medical Journal*, *5*(4), e0028. https://doi.org/10.5041/RMMJ. 10162

Herbst, L., Groten, F., Murphy, M., Shaw, G., Nießing, B., & Schmitt, R. H. (2023). Automated production at scale of induced pluripotent stem cell-derived mesenchymal stromal cells, chondrocytes and extracellular vehicles: Towards real-time release. *Processes*, *11*(10), 2938. https://doi.org/10.3390/pr11102938

Hernigou, P. (2015). Bone transplantation and tissue engineering, part IV. Mesenchymal stem cells: History in orthopaedic surgery from Cohnheim and Goujon to the Nobel Prize of Yamanaka. *International Orthopaedics*, *39*(4), 807–817. https://doi.org/10.1007/s00264-015-2716-8

Hielm-Björkman, A. K., Rita, H., & Tulamo, R.-M. (2009). Psychometric testing of the Helsinki chronic pain index by completion of a questionnaire in Finnish by owners of dogs with chronic signs of pain caused by osteoarthritis. *American Journal of Veterinary Research*, *70*(6), 727–734. https://doi.org/10.2460/ajvr.70.6.727

Holton, J., Imam, M., Ward, J., & Snow, M. (2016). The basic science of bone marrow aspirate concentrate in chondral injuries. *Orthopedic Reviews*, *8*(3), 6659. https://doi.org/10.4081/or.2016.6659

Hu, C., & Li, L. (2019). The immunoregulation of mesenchymal stem cells plays a critical role in improving the prognosis of liver transplantation. *Journal of Translational Medicine*, *17*(1), 412. https://doi.org/10.1186/s12967-019-02167-0

Huňáková, K., Hluchý, M., Špaková, T., Matejová, J., Mudroňová, D., Kuricová, M., Rosocha, J., & Ledecký, V. (2020). Study of bilateral elbow joint osteoarthritis treatment using conditioned medium from allogeneic adipose tissue-derived MSCs in Labrador retrievers. *Research in Veterinary Science*, *132*, 513–520. https://doi.org/10.1016/j.rvsc.2020.08.004

Ip, H. L., Nath, D. K., Sawleh, S. H., Kabir, M. H., & Jahan, N. (2020). Regenerative medicine for knee osteoarthritis–the efficacy and safety of intra-articular platelet-rich plasma and mesenchymal stem cells injections: A literature review. *Cureus*, *12*(9), e10575. https://doi.org/10.7759/cureus.10575

Irmak, G., Demirtaş, T. T., & Gümüşderelioğlu, M. (2020). Sustained release of growth factors from photoactivated platelet rich plasma (PRP).

European Journal of Pharmaceutics and Biopharmaceutics, *148*, 67–76. https://doi.org/10.1016/j.ejpb. 2019.11.011

Ivanovska, A., Wang, M., Arshaghi, T. E., Shaw, G., Alves, J., Byrne, A., Butterworth, S., Chandler, R., Cuddy, L., Dunne, J., Guerin, S., Harry, R., McAlindan, A., Mullins, R. A., & Barry, F. (2022, June 10). Manufacturing mesenchymal stromal cells for the treatment of osteoarthritis in canine patients: Challenges and recommendations. *Frontiers in Veterinary Science*, *9*, 897150. https://doi.org/10.3389/fvets.2022.897150

Jacques, E., & Suuronen, E. J. (2020). The progression of regenerative medicine and its impact on therapy translation. *Clinical and Translational Science*, *13*(3), 440–450. https://doi.org/10.1111/cts.12736

Jaegger, G., Marcellin-Little, D. J., & Levine, D. (2002). Reliability of goniometry in Labrador Retrievers. *American Journal of Veterinary Research*, *63*(7), 979–986. https://doi.org/10.2460/ajvr.2002.63.979

Jankowski, M., Kaczmarek, M., Wąsiatycz, G., Konwerska, A., Dompe, C., Bukowska, D., Antosik, P., Mozdziak, P., & Kempisty, B. (2022, September 16). Expression profile of new gene markers involved in differentiation of canine adipose-derived stem cells into chondrocytes. *Genes*, *13*(9), 1664. https://doi.org/10.3390/genes13091664

Jeffery, N. D., & Granger, N. (2012). Is' stem cell therapy' becoming 21st century snake oil? *Veterinary Surgery*, *41*(2), 189–190. https://doi.org/10.1111/j.1532-950X.2011.00956.x

Jeong, S. Y., Ha, J., Lee, M., Jin, H. J., Kim, D. H., Choi, S. J., Oh, W., Yang, Y. S., Kim, J.-S., Kim, B.-G., Chang, J. H., Cho, D.-H., & Jeon, H. B. (2015). Autocrine action of thrombospondin-2 determines the chondrogenic differentiation potential and suppresses hypertrophic maturation of human umbilical cord blood-derived mesenchymal stem cells. *Stem Cells*, *33*(11), 3291–3303. https://doi.org/10.1002/stem.2120

Jeong, S. Y., Kim, D. H., Ha, J., Jin, H. J., Kwon, S.-J., Chang, J. W., Choi, S. J., Oh, W., Yang, Y. S., Kim, G., Kim, J. S., Yoon, J.-R., Cho, D. H., & Jeon, H. B. (2013). Thrombospondin-2 secreted by human umbilical cord blood-derived mesenchymal stem cells promotes chondrogenic differentiation. *Stem Cells*, *31*(10), 2136–2148. https://doi.org/10.1002/stem.1471

Jeske, R., Yuan, X., Fu, Q., Bunnell, B. A., Logan, T. M., & Li, Y. (2021). In vitro culture expansion shifts the immune phenotype of human adipose-derived mesenchymal stem cells. *Frontiers in Immunology*, *12*, 621744. https://doi.org/10.3389/fimmu.2021.621744

Jeyaraman, M., Muthu, S., Jeyaraman, N., & Gupta, A. (2022). Photoactivated platelet-rich plasma: Is it the future of platelet-rich plasma? *Regenerative Medicine*, *17*(9), 607–609. https://doi.org/10.2217/rme-2022-0063

Jifcovici, A., Solano, M. A., Fitzpatrick, N., Findji, L., Blunn, G., & Sanghani-Kerai, A. (2021). Comparison of Fat harvested from flank and falciform regions for stem cell therapy in dogs. *Veterinary Sciences*, *8*(2), 19. https://doi.org/10.3390/vetsci8020019

Jo, C. H., Lee, S. Y., Yoon, K. S., & Shin, S. (2017). Effects of platelet-rich plasma with concomitant use of a corticosteroid on tenocytes from degenerative rotator cuff tears in interleukin 1β–induced tendinopathic conditions. *The American Journal of Sports Medicine*, *45*(5), 1141–1150. https://doi.org/10.1177/0363546516681294

Johal, H., Khan, M., Yung, S. P., Dhillon, M. S., Fu, F. H., Bedi, A., & Bhandari, M. (2019). Impact of platelet-rich plasma use on pain in orthopaedic surgery: A systematic review and meta-analysis. *Sports Health*, *11*(4), 355–366. https://doi.org/10.1177/1941738119834972

Johnson, V., Webb, T., Norman, A., Coy, J., Kurihara, J., Regan, D., & Dow, S. (2017). Activated mesenchymal stem cells interact with antibiotics and host innate immune responses to control chronic bacterial infections. *Scientific Reports*, *7*(1), 9575. https://doi.org/10.1038/s41598-017-08311-4

Jovic, D., Yu, Y., Wang, D., Wang, K., Li, H., Xu, F., Liu, C., Liu, J., & Luo, Y. (2022). A brief overview of global trends in MSC-based cell therapy. *Stem Cell Reviews and Reports*, *18*(5), 1525–1545. https://doi.org/10.1007/s12015-022-10369-1

Kähn, H. C., Zablotski, Y., & Meyer-Lindenberg, A. (2023). Therapeutic success in fragmented coronoid process disease and other canine medial elbow compartment pathology: A systematic review with meta-analyses. *Frontiers in Veterinary Science*, *10*, 1228497. https://doi.org/10.3389/fvets.2023.1228497

Kemilew, J., Sobczyńska-Rak, A., Żylińska, B., Szponder, T., Nowicka, B., & Urban, B. (2019). The use of allogenic stromal vascular fraction (SVF) cells in degenerative joint disease of the spine in dogs. *In Vivo*, *33*(4), 1109–1117. https://doi.org/10.21873/invivo.11580

Khurana, A., Goyal, A., Kirubakaran, P., Akhand, G., Gupta, R., & Goel, N. (2021). Efficacy of autologous conditioned serum (ACS), platelet-rich plasma (PRP), hyaluronic acid (HA) and steroid for early osteoarthritis knee: A comparative analysis. *Indian Journal of Orthopaedics*, *55* Suppl. 1, 217–227. https://doi.org/10.1007/s43465-020-00274-5

Kiefer, K. M., O'Brien, T. D., Pluhar, E. G., & Conzemius, M. (2015). Canine adipose-derived stromal cell viability following exposure to synovial fluid from osteoarthritic joints. *Veterinary Record Open*, *2*(1), e000063. https://doi.org/10.1136/vetreco-2014-000063

Kim, A. Y., Elam, L. H., Lambrechts, N. E., Salman, M. D., & Duerr, F. M. (2022). Appendicular skeletal muscle mass assessment in dogs: A scoping literature review. *BMC Veterinary Research*, *18*(1), 280. https://doi.org/10.1186/s12917-022-03367-5

Kim, J.-H., Park, C., & Park, H.-M. (2009). Curative effect of autologous platelet-rich plasma on a large cutaneous lesion in a dog. *Veterinary Dermatology*, *20*(2), 123–126. https://doi.org/10.1111/j.1365-3164.2008.00711.x

Kim, S., Elam, L., Johnson, V., Hess, A., Webb, T., Dow, S., & Duerr, F. (2022). Intra-articular injections of allogeneic mesenchymal stromal cells vs. high molecular weight hyaluronic acid in dogs with osteoarthritis: Exploratory data from a double-blind, randomized, prospective clinical trial. *Frontiers in Veterinary Science*, *9*, 890704. https://doi.org/10.3389/fvets.2022.890704

Kim, S. E., Pozzi, A., Yeh, J.-C., Lopez-Velazquez, M., Au Yong, J. A., Townsend, S., Dunlap, A. E., Christopher, S. A., Lewis, D. D., Johnson, M. D., & Petrucci, K. (2019). Intra-articular umbilical cord derived mesenchymal stem cell therapy for chronic elbow osteoarthritis in dogs: A double-blinded, placebo-controlled clinical trial. *Frontiers in Veterinary Science*, *6*, 474. https://doi.org/10.3389/fvets.2019.00474

Kim, Y. S., Kim, Y. I., & Koh, Y. G. (2021). Intra-articular injection of human synovium-derived mesenchymal stem cells in beagles with surgery-induced osteoarthritis. *The Knee*, *28*, 159–168. https://doi.org/10.1016/j.knee.2020.11.021

Kirkby, K. A., & Lewis, D. D. (2012). Canine hip dysplasia: Reviewing the evidence for nonsurgical management. *Veterinary Surgery*, *41*(1), 2–9. https://doi.org/10.1111/j.1532-950X.2011.00928.x

Knighton, D. R., Hunt, T. K., Thakral, K. K., & Goodson 3rd, W. H. (1982). Role of platelets and fibrin in the healing sequence: An in vivo study of angiogenesis and collagen synthesis. *Annals of Surgery*, *196*(4), 379–388. https://doi.org/10.1097/00000658-198210000-00001

Koç, O. N., & Lazarus, H. M. (2001). Mesenchymal stem cells: Heading into the clinic. *Bone Marrow Transplantation*, *27*(3), 235–239. https://doi.org/10.1038/sj.bmt.1702791

Koike, M., Nojiri, H., Kanazawa, H., Yamaguchi, H., Miyagawa, K., Nagura, N., Banno, S., Iwase, Y., Kurosawa, H., & Kaneko, K. (2018). Superoxide dismutase activity is significantly lower in end-stage osteoarthritic cartilage than non-osteoarthritic cartilage. *PLOS ONE*, *13*(9), e0203944. https://doi.org/10.1371/journal.pone.0203944

Kon, E., Buda, R., Filardo, G., Di Martino, A., Timoncini, A., Cenacchi, A., Fornasari, P. M., Giannini, S., & Marcacci, M. (2010). Platelet-rich plasma: Intra-articular knee injections produced favourable results on degenerative cartilage lesions. *Knee Surgery, Sports Traumatology, Arthroscopy*, *18*(4), 472–479. https://doi.org/10.1007/s00167-009-0940-8

Krampera, M. (2011). Mesenchymal stromal cell "licensing": A multistep process. *Leukemia*, *25*(9), 1408–1414. https://doi.org/10.1038/leu.2011.108

Kriston-Pál, É., Czibula, Á., Gyuris, Z., Balka, G., Seregi, A., Sükösd, F., Süth, M., Kiss-Tóth, E., Haracska, L., Uher, F., & Monostori, É. (2017). Characterization and therapeutic application of canine adipose mesenchymal stem cells to treat elbow osteoarthritis. *Canadian Journal of Veterinary Research*, *81*(1), 73–78.

Kriston-Pál, É., Haracska, L., Cooper, P., Kiss-Tóth, E., Szukacsov, V., & Monostori, É. (2020). A regenerative approach to canine osteoarthritis using allogeneic, adipose-derived mesenchymal stem cells. Safety results of a long-term follow-up. *Frontiers in Veterinary Science*, *7*, 510. https://doi.org/10.3389/fvets.2020.00510

Kubrova, E., Su, M., Galeano-Garces, C., Galvan, M. L., Jerez, S., Dietz, A. B., Smith, J., Qu, W., & Van Wijnen, A. J. (2021). Differences in cytotoxicity of lidocaine, ropivacaine, and bupivacaine on the viability and metabolic activity of human adipose-derived mesenchymal stem cells. *American Journal of Physical Medicine and Rehabilitation*, *100*(1), 82–91. https://doi.org/10.1097/PHM.0000000000001529

Kuroki, K., Cook, J. L., Stoker, A. M., Turnquist, S. E., Kreeger, J. M., & Tomlinson, J. L. (2005). Characterizing osteochondrosis in the dog: Potential roles for matrix metalloproteinases and mechanical load in pathogenesis and disease progression. *Osteoarthritis and Cartilage*, *13*(3), 225–234. https://doi.org/10.1016/j.joca.2004.11.005

Landesberg, R., Roy, M., & Glickman, R. S. (2000). Quantification of growth factor levels using a simplified method of platelet-rich plasma gel preparation. *Journal of Oral and Maxillofacial Surgery*, *58*(3), 297–300; discussion 300. https://doi.org/10.1016/s0278-2391(00)90058-2

Lebkowski, J. (2011). GRNOPC1: The world's first embryonic stem cell-derived therapy. Interview with Jane Lebkowski. *Regenerative Medicine*, *6*(6) Suppl., 11–13. https://doi.org/10.2217/rme.11.77

Lee, R. H., Pulin, A. A., Seo, M. J., Kota, D. J., Ylostalo, J., Larson, B. L., Semprun-Prieto, L., Delafontaine, P., & Prockop, D. J. (2009). Intravenous hMSCs improve myocardial infarction in mice because cells embolized in lung are activated to secrete the anti-inflammatory protein TSG-6. *Cell Stem Cell*, *5*(1), 54–63. https://doi.org/10.1016/j.stem.2009.05.003

Levoux, J., Prola, A., Lafuste, P., Gervais, M., Chevallier, N., Koumaiha, Z., Kefi, K., Braud, L., Schmitt, A., Yacia, A., Schirmann, A., Hersant, B., Sid-Ahmed, M., Ben Larbi, S., Komrskova, K., Rohlena, J., Relaix, F., Neuzil, J., & Rodriguez, A.-M. (2021). Platelets facilitate the wound-healing capability of mesenchymal stem cells by mitochondrial transfer and metabolic reprogramming. *Cell Metabolism*, *33*(2), 283–299.e9. https://doi.org/10.1016/j.cmet.2020.12.006

Li, J. J., Hosseini-Beheshti, E., Grau, G. E., Zreiqat, H., & Little, C. B. (2019). Stem cell-derived extracellular vesicles for treating joint injury and osteoarthritis. *Nanomaterials*, *9*(2), 261. https://doi.org/10.3390/nano9020261

Li, J. S. Z., & Denchi, E. L. (2018, March–April). How stem cells keep telomeres in check. *Differentiation; Research in Biological Diversity*, *100*, 21–25. https://doi.org/10.1016/j.diff.2018.01.004. Epub February

2, 2018. PubMed: 29413749, PubMed Central: PMC5889314

Li, L., Duan, X., Fan, Z., Chen, L., Xing, F., Xu, Z., Chen, Q., & Xiang, Z. (2018). Mesenchymal stem cells in combination with hyaluronic acid for articular cartilage defects. *Scientific Reports*, *8*(1), 9900. https://doi.org/10.1038/s41598-018-27737-y

Li, L., Zhang, S., Zhang, Y., Yu, B., Xu, Y., & Guan, Z. (2009). Paracrine action mediates the antifibrotic effect of transplanted mesenchymal stem cells in a rat model of global heart failure. *Molecular Biology Reports*, *36*(4), 725–731. https://doi.org/10.1007/s11033-008-9235-2

Li, Y., Wu, Q., Wang, Y., Li, L., Bu, H., & Bao, J. (2017). Senescence of mesenchymal stem cells (Review). *International Journal of Molecular Medicine*, *39*(4), 775–782. https://doi.org/10.3892/ijmm.2017.2912

Lima, V. P., Tobin, G. C., de Jesus Pereira, M. R., Silveira, M. D., Witz, M. I., & Nardi, N. B. (2019). Chondrogenic effect of liquid and gelled platelet lysate on canine adipose-derived mesenchymal stromal cells. *Research in Veterinary Science*, *124*, 393–398. https://doi.org/10.1016/j.rvsc.2019.04.022

Lin, W., Xie, L., Zhou, L., Zheng, J., Zhai, W., & Lin, D. (2023). Effects of platelet-rich plasma on subchondral bone marrow edema and biomarkers in synovial fluid of knee osteoarthritis. *The Knee*, *42*, 161–169. https://doi.org/10.1016/j.knee.2023.03.002

Liu, J., Ding, Y., Liu, Z., & Liang, X. (2020). Senescence in mesenchymal stem cells: Functional alterations, molecular mechanisms, and rejuvenation strategies. *Frontiers in Cell and Developmental Biology*, *8*, 258. https://doi.org/10.3389/fcell.2020.00258

Liu, T. P., Ha, P., Xiao, C. Y., Kim, S. Y., Jensen, A. R., Easley, J., Yao, Q., & Zhang, X. (2022). Updates on mesenchymal stem cell therapies for articular cartilage regeneration in large animal models. *Frontiers in Cell and Developmental Biology*, 10, 982199. https://doi.org/10.3389/fcell.2022.982199

Liu, Y., Lin, L., Zou, R., Wen, C., Wang, Z., & Lin, F. (2018[a]). MSC-derived exosomes promote proliferation and inhibit apoptosis of chondrocytes via lncRNA-KLF3-AS1/miR-206/GIT1 axis in osteoarthritis. *Cell Cycle*, *17*(21–22), 2411–2422. https://doi.org/10.1080/15384101.2018.1526603

Liu, Y., Zou, R., Wang, Z., Wen, C., Zhang, F., & Lin, F. (2018[b]). Exosomal KLF3-AS1 from hMSCs promoted

cartilage repair and chondrocyte proliferation in osteoarthritis. *The Biochemical Journal*, *475*(22), 3629–3638. https://doi.org/10.1042/BCJ20180675

Lozito, T. P., & Tuan, R. S. (2011). Mesenchymal stem cells inhibit both endogenous and exogenous MMPs via secreted TIMPs. *Journal of Cellular Physiology*, *226*(2), 385–396. https://doi.org/10.1002/jcp.22344

Lutter, M., Rudolf, H., Lenz, R., Hotfiel, T., & Tischer, T. (2023). What makes an orthopaedic paper highly citable? A bibliometric analysis of top orthopaedic journals with 10-year follow up. *Journal of Experimental Orthopaedics*, *10*(1), 78. https://doi.org/10.1186/s40634-023-00631-x

Maged, G., Abdelsamed, M. A., Wang, H., & Lotfy, A. (2024). The potency of mesenchymal stem/stromal cells: Does donor sex matter? *Stem Cell Research and Therapy*, *15*(1), 112. https://doi.org/10.1186/s13287-024-03722-3

Mager, F. W. (2000). *Zur Kniegelenksarthrose des Hundes nach vorderer Kreuzbandruptur – Ein retrospektiver Vergleich dreier Operationsmethoden* [Unpublished dissertation]. Ludwig-Maximilians University.

Magruder, M., & Rodeo, S. A. (2021). Is antiplatelet therapy contraindicated after platelet-rich plasma treatment? A narrative review. *Orthopaedic Journal of Sports Medicine*. CB, *9*(6).

Maki, C. B., Beck, A., Wallis, C. B. C. C., Choo, J., Ramos, T., Tong, R., ... & Izadyar, F. (2020). Intra-articular administration of allogeneic adipose derived MSCs reduces pain and lameness in dogs with hip osteoarthritis: a double blinded, randomized, placebo-controlled pilot study. *Frontiers in Veterinary Science*, 570

Manafi, A., Kaviani Far, K., Moradi, M., Manafi, A., & Manafi, F. (2012). Effects of platelet-rich plasma on cartilage grafts in rabbits as an animal model. *World Journal of Plastic Surgery*, *1*(2), 91–98.

Mancuso, P., Raman, S., Glynn, A., Barry, F., & Murphy, J. M. (2019). Mesenchymal stem cell therapy for osteoarthritis: The critical role of the cell secretome. *Frontiers in Bioengineering and Biotechnology*, *7*, 9. https://doi.org/10.3389/fbioe.2019.00009

Martin, G. R. (1981). Isolation of a pluripotent cell line from early mouse embryos cultured in medium conditioned by teratocarcinoma stem cells. *Proceedings of the National Academy of Sciences of the United States of America*, *78*(12), 7634–7638. https://doi.org/10.1073/pnas.78.12.7634

Martinet, L., Fleury-Cappellesso, S., Gadelorge, M., Dietrich, G., Bourin, P., Fournié, J.-J., & Poupot, R. (2009). A regulatory cross-talk between Vγ9Vδ2 T lymphocytes and mesenchymal stem cells. *European Journal of Immunology*, *39*(3), 752–762. https://doi.org/10.1002/eji.200838812

Marx, C., Silveira, M. D., Selbach, I., da Silva, A. S., Braga, L. M. G. M., Camassola, M., & Nardi, N. B. (2014). Acupoint injection of autologous stromal vascular fraction and allogeneic adipose-derived stem cells to treat hip dysplasia in dogs. *Stem Cells International*, *2014*, 391274. https://doi.org/10.1155/2014/391274

Marx, R. E., Carlson, E. R., Eichstaedt, R. M., Schimmele, S. R., Strauss, J. E., & Georgeff, K. R. (1998). Platelet-rich plasma: Growth factor enhancement for bone grafts. *Oral Surgery, Oral Medicine, Oral Pathology, Oral Radiology, and Endodontics*, *85*(6), 638–646. https://doi.org/10.1016/s1079-2104(98)90029-4

Matis, U., Brahm-Jorda, T., Jorda, C. et al. (2005). Radiographic evaluation of the progression of osteoarthritis after tibial plateau levelling osteotomy in 93 dogs. *Veterinary and Comparative Orthopaedics and Traumatology*, *18*, A32.

Maumus, M., Manferdini, C., Toupet, K., Peyrafitte, J.-A., Ferreira, R., Facchini, A., Gabusi, E., Bourin, P., Jorgensen, C., Lisignoli, G., & Noël, D. (2013). Adipose mesenchymal stem cells protect chondrocytes from degeneration associated with osteoarthritis. *Stem Cell Research*, *11*(2), 834–844. https://doi.org/10.1016/j.scr.2013.05.008

Mazzucco, L., Balbo, V., Cattana, E., Guaschino, R., & Borzini, P. (2009). Not every PRP-gel is born equal Evaluation of growth factor availability for tissues through four PRP–gel preparations: Fibrinet®, RegenPRP–Kit®, Plateltex® and one manual procedure. *Vox Sanguinis*, *97*(2), 110–118. https://doi.org/10.1111/j.1423-0410.2009.01188.x

McDougall, R. A., Canapp, S. O., & Canapp, D. A. (2018). Ultrasonographic findings in 41 dogs treated with bone marrow aspirate concentrate and platelet-rich plasma for a supraspinatus tendinopathy: A retrospective study. *Frontiers in Veterinary Science*, *5*, 98. https://doi.org/10.3389/fvets.2018.00098

Meeson, R. L., Todhunter, R. J., Blunn, G., Nuki, G., & Pitsillides, A. A. (2019). Spontaneous dog osteoarthritis—A One Medicine vision. *Nature Reviews. Rheumatology*, *15*(5), 273–287. https://doi.org/10.1038/s41584-019-0202-1

Merlo, B., & Iacono, E. (2023, November 19). Beyond canine adipose tissue-derived mesenchymal stem/stromal cells transplantation: An update on their secretome characterization and applications. *Animals (Basel)*, *13*(22), 3571. https://doi.org/10.3390/ani13223571

Meyer-Lindenberg, A., & Kilchling, T. (2018). Use of mesenchymal stem cells in dogs. *Tierarztliche Praxis. Ausgabe K, Kleintiere/Heimtiere*, *46*(6), 416–425. https://doi.org/10.1055/s-0038-1677407

Millis, D., & Levine, D. (2013). *Canine rehabilitation and physical therapy*. Elsevier Health Sciences.

Mindrescu, C., Thorbecke, G. J., Klein, M. J., Vilček, J., & Wisniewski, H. G. (2000). Amelioration of collagen-induced arthritis in DBA/1J mice by recombinant TSG–6, a tumor necrosis factor/interleukin–1–inducible protein. *Arthritis and Rheumatism*, *43*(12), 2668–2677. https://doi.org/10.1002/1529-0131(200012)43:12<2668::AID-ANR6>3.0.CO;2-E

Minteer, D. M., Marra, K. G., & Rubin, J. P. (2015). Adipose stem cells: Biology, safety, regulation, and regenerative potential. *Clinics in Plastic Surgery*, *42*(2), 169–179. https://doi.org/10.1016/j.cps.2014.12.007

Mocchi, M., Bari, E., Dotti, S., Villa, R., Berni, P., Conti, V., Del Bue, M., Squassino, G. P., Segale, L., Ramoni, R., Torre, M. L., Perteghella, S., & Grolli, S. (2021). Canine mesenchymal cell lyosecretome production and safety evaluation after allogenic intraarticular injection in osteoarthritic dogs. *Animals: An Open Access Journal from MDPI*, *11*(11), Art. no. 3271. https://doi.org/10.3390/ani11113271

Mocchi, M., Dotti, S., Del Bue, M. D., Villa, R., Bari, E., Perteghella, S., Torre, M. L., & Grolli, S. (2020). Veterinary regenerative medicine for musculoskeletal disorders: Can mesenchymal stem/stromal cells and their secretome be the new frontier? *Cells*, *9*(6), 1453. https://doi.org/10.3390/cells9061453

Mohiuddin, A., Lewis, P., Choudhury, K., & Sadiq, B. (2019). Clinical outcome of photoactivated platelet-rich plasma in the treatment of knee osteoarthritis. *Rheumatol. Orthop. Med*, *4*(1), 1–4.

Mokarizadeh, A., Delirezh, N., Morshedi, A., Mosayebi, G., Farshid, A.-A., & Mardani, K. (2012). Microvesicles derived from mesenchymal stem cells: Potent organelles for induction of tolerogenic signaling. *Immunology Letters*, *147*(1–2), 47–54. https://doi.org/10.1016/j.imlet.2012.06.001

Monteleone, K., Marx, R., & Ghurani, R. (2000, September). Wound repair/cosmetic surgery healing enhancement of skin graft donor sites with platelet-rich plasma. In 82nd Annual Meeting of the American Association of Oral and Maxillofacial Surgeons, San Francisco, CA.

Mościcka, P., & Przylipiak, A. (2021). History of autologous platelet-rich plasma: A short review. *Journal of Cosmetic Dermatology*, *20*(9), 2712–2714. https://doi.org/10.1111/jocd.14326

Mrkovački, J., Srzentić Dražilov, S., Spasovski, V., Fazlagić, A., Pavlović, S., & Nikčević, G. (2021). Case report: Successful therapy of spontaneously occurring canine degenerative lumbosacral stenosis using autologous adipose tissue-derived mesenchymal stem cells. *Frontiers in Veterinary Science*, *8*, 732073. https://doi.org/10.3389/fvets.2021.732073

Muir, P., Hans, E. C., Racette, M., Volstad, N., Sample, S. J., Heaton, C., Holzman, G., Schaefer, S. L., Bloom, D. D., Bleedorn, J. A., Hao, Z., Amene, E., Suresh, M., & Hematti, P. (2016). Autologous bone marrow-derived mesenchymal stem cells modulate molecular markers of inflammation in dogs with cruciate ligament rupture. *PLOS ONE*, *11*(8), e0159095. https://doi.org/10.1371/journal.pone.0159095

Naldini, A., Morena, E., Fimiani, M., Campoccia, G., Fossombroni, V., & Carraro, F. (2008). The effects of autologous platelet gel on inflammatory cytokine response in human peripheral blood mononuclear cells. *Platelets*, *19*(4), 268–274. https://doi.org/10.1080/09537100801947426

Narayanaswamy, R., Patro, B. P., Jeyaraman, N., Gangadaran, P., Rajendran, R. L., Nallakumarasamy, A., Jeyaraman, M., Ramani, P., & Ahn, B.-C. (2023). Evolution and clinical advances of platelet-rich fibrin in musculoskeletal regeneration. *Bioengineering*, *10*(1), 58. https://doi.org/10.3390/bioengineering10010058

Nasircilar, A., Bülbül, M. V., Kalender, S. M., Bozkurt, C., & Keskin, İ. (2022). Effects of polyacrylamide hydrogel used in the treatment of osteoarthritis on mesenchymal stem cells and human osteoblasts. *Journal of Surgery and Medicine*, *6*(4), 498–502. https://doi.org/10.28982/josam.1006577

Neupane, M., Chang, C.-C., Kiupel, M., & Yuzbasiyan-Gurkan, V. (2008). Isolation and characterization of canine adipose–derived mesenchymal stem cells. *Tissue Engineering. Part A*, *14*(6), 1007–1015. https://doi.org/10.1089/ten.tea.2007.0207

Nicpoń, J., Marycz, K., Grzesiak, J., Śmieszek, A., & Toker, Z. Y. (2014). The advantages of autologous adipose derived mesenchymal stem cells (AdMSCs) over the non-steroidal anti-inflammatory drugs (NSAIDs) application for degenerative elbow joint disease treatment in dogs-Twelve cases. *Kafkas Üniversitesi Veteriner Fakültesi Dergisi*, *20*(3), 345–350.

Oh, J., Son, Y. S., Kim, W. H., Kwon, O. K., & Kang, B. J. (2021). Mesenchymal stem cells genetically engineered to express platelet-derived growth factor and heme oxygenase-1 ameliorate osteoarthritis in a canine model. *Journal of Orthopaedic Surgery and Research*, *16*(1), 1–16.

Okamoto-Okubo, C. E., Cassu, R. N., Joaquim, J. G. F., dos Reis Mesquita, L. D., Rahal, S. C., Oliveira, H. S. S., Takahira, R., Arruda, I., Maia, L., Cruz Landim, F. D., & Luna, S. P. L. (2021). Chronic pain and gait analysis in dogs with degenerative hip joint disease treated with repeated intra-articular injections of platelet-rich plasma or allogeneic adipose-derived stem cells. *The Journal of Veterinary Medical Science*, *83*(5), 881–888. https://doi.org/10.1292/jvms.20-0730

Olsen, A., Johnson, V., Webb, T., Santangelo, K. S., Dow, S., & Duerr, F. M. (2019). Evaluation of intravenously delivered allogeneic mesenchymal stem cells for treatment of elbow osteoarthritis in dogs: A pilot study. *Veterinary and Comparative Orthopaedics and Traumatology*, *32*(3), 173–181. https://doi.org/10.1055/s-0039-1678547

Olsson, D. C., Teixeira, B. L., Jeremias, T. D. S., Réus, J. C., De Luca Canto, G. D. L., Porporatti, A. L., & Trentin, A. G. (2021). Administration of mesenchymal stem cells from adipose tissue at the hip joint of dogs with osteoarthritis: A systematic review. *Research in Veterinary Science*, *135*, 495–503. https://doi.org/10.1016/j.rvsc.2020.11.014

Opneja, A., Kapoor, S., & Stavrou, E. X. (2019). Contribution of platelets, the coagulation, and fibrinolytic systems to cutaneous wound healing. *Thrombosis Research*, *179*, 56–63. https://doi.org/10.1016/j.thromres.2019.05.001

Ortolano, G. A., & Wenz, B. (2014). A review of the pathogenesis of osteoarthritis and the use of intra-articular platelet therapy for joint disease in animals and humans. *Bone and Tissue Regeneration Insights*, *5*. https://doi.org/10.4137/BTRI.S14578

Owen, M. (1988). Marrow stromal stem cells. *Journal of Cell Science. Supplement*(Supplement_10), 10, 63–76. https://doi.org/10.1242/jcs.1988.supplement_10.5

Owen, M., & Friedenstein, A. J. (2007, September). Stromal stem cells: Marrow–derived osteogenic precursors. In *Ciba Foundation Symposium 136–Cell and Molecular Biology of Vertebrate Hard Tissues: Cell and Molecular Biology of Vertebrate Hard Tissues: Ciba Foundation Symposium 136*. John Wiley & Sons, Ltd, (42–60).

Pagano, T. B., Wojcik, S., Costagliola, A., De Biase, D., Iovino, S., Iovane, V., Russo, V., Papparella, S., & Paciello, O. (2015). Age related skeletal muscle atrophy and upregulation of autophagy in dogs. *Veterinary Journal*, *206*(1), 54–60. https://doi.org/10.1016/j.tvjl.2015.07.005

Pandey, S., Hickey, D. U., Drum, M., Millis, D. L., & Cekanova, M. (2019). Platelet-rich plasma affects the proliferation of canine bone marrow-derived mesenchymal stromal cells in vitro. *BMC Veterinary Research*, *15*(1), 269. https://doi.org/10.1186/s12917-019-2010-x

Park, S. A., Reilly, C. M., Wood, J. A., Chung, D. J., Carrade, D. D., Deremer, S. L., Seraphin, R. L., Clark, K. C., Zwingenberger, A. L., Borjesson, D. L., Hayashi, K., Russell, P., & Murphy, C. J. (2013). Safety and immunomodulatory effects of allogeneic canine adipose-derived mesenchymal stromal cells transplanted into the region of the lacrimal gland, the gland of the third eyelid and the knee joint. *Cytotherapy*, 15(12), 1498–1510. https://doi.org/10.1016/j.jcyt.2013.06.009

Parlak, K., Üney, K., Uzunlu, E. O., Yalçın, M., & Arican, M. (2022). The effect of intra-articular platelet-rich plasma bio-physically activated PRP and mesenchymal stem cell administration for interleukins in dogs with osteoarthritis. *Veterinarski Arhiv*, *92*(4), 459–468. https://doi.org/10.24099/vet.arhiv.1695

Paterson, K. L., Nicholls, M., Bennell, K. L., & Bates, D. (2016). Intra-articular injection of photo-activated platelet-rich plasma in patients with knee osteoarthritis: A double-blind, randomized controlled pilot study. *BMC Musculoskeletal Disorders*, *17*, 67. https://doi.org/10.1186/s12891-016-0920-3

Perry, A. R., & Linch, D. C. (1996). The history of bone-marrow transplantation. *Blood Reviews*, *10*(4), 215–219. https://doi.org/10.1016/s0268-960x(96)90004-1

Phillips, B. (2014). The crumbling of the pyramid of evidence. *BMJ blogs*.

Pinheiro, L. L., de Lima, A. R., & Branco, É. (2019). Is stem cell commerce in small animal therapies scientifically and morally justified? *Stem Cell Reviews and Reports*, *15*(4), 506–518. https://doi.org/10.1007/s12015-019-09898-z

Pintore, A., Notarfrancesco, D., Zara, A., Oliviero, A., Migliorini, F., Oliva, F., & Maffulli, N. (2023, May). Intra-articular injection of bone marrow aspirate concentrate (BMAC) or adipose-derived stem cells (ADSCs) for knee osteoarthritis: A prospective comparative clinical trial. *Journal of Orthopaedic Surgery and Research*, *18*(1), 350. https://doi.org/10.1186/s13018-023-03841-2

Pittenger, M. F., Discher, D. E., Péault, B. M., Phinney, D. G., Hare, J. M., & Caplan, A. I. (2019). Mesenchymal stem cell perspective: Cell biology to clinical progress. *npj Regenerative Medicine*, *4*(1), 22. https://doi.org/10.1038/s41536-019-0083-6

Pittenger, M. F., Mackay, A. M., Beck, S. C., Jaiswal, R. K., Douglas, R., Mosca, J. D., Moorman, M. A., Simonetti, D. W., Craig, S., & Marshak, D. R. (1999). Multilineage potential of adult human mesenchymal stem cells. *Science*, *284*(5411), 143–147. https://doi.org/10.1126/science.284.5411.143

Pond, M. J., & Nuki, G. (1973). Experimentally induced osteoarthritis in the dog. *Annals of the Rheumatic Diseases*, *32*(4), 387–388. https://doi.org/10.1136/ard.32.4.387

Prišlin, M., Vlahović, D., Kostešic, P., Ljolje, I., Brnić, D., Turk, N., Lojkić, I., Kunić, V., Karadjole, T., & Krešic, N. (2022). An outstanding role of adipose tissue in canine stem cell therapy. *Animals: An Open Access Journal from MDPI*, *12*(9). *Stem Cells in Domestic Animals*, 191. https://doi.org/10.3390/ani12091088

Punzón, E., García-Castillo, M., Rico, M. A., Padilla, L., & Pradera, A. (2023, May 17). Local, systemic, and immunologic safety comparison between xenogeneic equine umbilical cord mesenchymal stem cells, allogeneic canine adipose mesenchymal stem cells and placebo: A randomized controlled trial. *Frontiers in Veterinary Science*, *10*, 1098029. https://doi.org/10.3389/fvets.2023.1098029, PubMed: 372 66387, PubMed Central: PMC10229832

Punzón, E., Salgüero, R., Totusaus, X., Mesa-Sánchez, C., Badiella, L., García-Castillo, M., & Pradera, A. (2022). Equine umbilical cord mesenchymal stem cells demonstrate safety and efficacy in the treatment of canine osteoarthritis: A randomized placebo-controlled trial. Journal of the American Veterinary Medical Association, 260(15), 1947–1955. https://doi.org/10.2460/javma.22.06.0237

Pye, C., Bruniges, N., Peffers, M., & Comerford, E. (2022). Advances in the pharmaceutical treatment options for canine osteoarthritis. *The Journal of Small Animal Practice*, *63*(10), 721–738. https://doi.org/10.1111/jsap.13495

Ramalho-Santos, M., & Willenbring, H. (2007). On the origin of the term "stem cell". *Cell Stem Cell*, *1*(1), 35–38. https://doi.org/10.1016/j.stem.2007.05.013

Rehman, J., Traktuev, D., Li, J., Merfeld-Clauss, S., Temm-Grove, C. J., Bovenkerk, J. E., Pell, C. L., Johnstone, B. H., Considine, R. V., & March, K. L. (2004). Secretion of angiogenic and antiapoptotic factors by human adipose stromal cells. *Circulation*, *109*(10), 1292–1298. https://doi.org/10.1161/01.CIR.0000121425.42966.F1

Reich, C. M., Raabe, O., Wenisch, S., Bridger, P. S., Kramer, M., & Arnhold, S. (2012). Isolation, culture and chondrogenic differentiation of canine adipose tissue-and bone marrow-derived mesenchymal stem cells–a comparative study. *Veterinary Research Communications*, *36*(2), 139–148. https://doi.org/10.1007/s11259-012-9523-0

Ribatti, D., & Crivellato, E. (2007). Giulio Bizzozero and the discovery of platelets. *Leukemia Research*, *31*(10), 1339–1341. https://doi.org/10.1016/j.leukres.2007.02.008

Ryan, J. M., Barry, F. P., Murphy, J. M., & Mahon, B. P. (2005). Mesenchymal stem cells avoid allogeneic rejection. *Journal of Inflammation*, *2*, 8. https://doi.org/10.1186/1476-9255-2-8

Sack, D., Canapp, D., Canapp, S., Majeski, S., Curry, J., Sutton, A., & Cullen, R. (2023). Iliopsoas strain demographics, concurrent injuries, and grade determined by musculoskeletal ultrasound in 72 agility dogs. *Canadian Journal of Veterinary Research*, *87*(3), 196–201.

Sanghani-Kerai, A., Black, C., Cheng, S. O., Collins, L., Schneider, N., Blunn, G., Watson, F., & Fitzpatrick, N. (2021). Clinical outcomes following intraarticular injection of autologous adipose-derived mesenchymal stem cells for the treatment of osteoarthritis in dogs characterized by weight-bearing asymmetry. *Bone and Joint Research*, *10*(10), 650–658. https://doi.org/10.1302/2046-3758.1010.BJR-2020-0540.R1

Santavanond, J. P., Rutter, S. F., Atkin-Smith, G. K., & Poon, I. K. H. (2021). Apoptotic bodies: Mechanism of formation, isolation and functional relevance. *Sub-Cellular Biochemistry*, *97*, 61–88. https://doi.org/10.1007/978-3-030-67171-6_4

Sasaki, A., Mizuno, M., Mochizuki, M., & Sekiya, I. (2019). Mesenchymal stem cells for cartilage regeneration in dogs. *World Journal of Stem Cells*, *11*(5), 254–269. https://doi.org/10.4252/wjsc.v11.i5.254

Sasaki, A., Mizuno, M., Ozeki, N., Katano, H., Otabe, K., Tsuji, K., Koga, H., Mochizuki, M., & Sekiya, I. (2018). Canine mesenchymal stem cells from synovium have a higher chondrogenic potential than those from infrapatellar fat pad, adipose tissue, and bone marrow. *PLOS ONE*, *13*(8), Art. no. e0202922. https://doi.org/10.1371/journal.pone.0202922

Sawyere, D. M., Lanz, O. I., Dahlgren, L. A., Barry, S. L., Nichols, A. C., & Werre, S. R. (2016). Cytokine and growth factor concentrations in canine autologous conditioned serum. *Veterinary Surgery*, *45*(5), 582–586. https://doi.org/10.1111/vsu.12506

Scattini, G., Pellegrini, M., Severi, G., Cagiola, M., & Pascucci, L. (2023). The stromal vascular fraction from canine adipose tissue contains mesenchymal stromal cell subpopulations that show time-dependent adhesion to cell culture plastic vessels. *Animals: An Open Access Journal from MDPI*, *13*(7), 1175. https://doi.org/10.3390/ani13071175

Sembronio, S., Tel, A., Tremolada, C., Lazzarotto, A., Isola, M., & Robiony, M. (2021). Temporomandibular joint arthrocentesis and microfragmented adipose tissue injection for the treatment of internal derangement and osteoarthritis: A randomized clinical trial. *Journal of Oral and Maxillofacial Surgery*, *79*(7), 1447–1456. https://doi.org/10.1016/j.joms.2021.01.038

Sen, A., Sooryadas, S., Dinesh, P. T., Varghese, R., & Pratheesh, M. D. Preparation of platelet rich plasma in dogs–standardisation of double centrifugation method. https://www.researchgate.net/profile/Dine sh-Parathazhathayil/publication/364343325_ Preparation_of_Platelet_Rich_Plasma_in_Dogs__ Standardisation_of_Double_Centrifugation_Meth od/links/634cf9bd76e39959d6c8bf92/Preparation-of-Platelet-Rich-Plasma-in-Dogs-Standardisation-of-Double-Centrifugation-Method.pdf

Sethe, S., Scutt, A., & Stolzing, A. (2006). Aging of mesenchymal stem cells. *Ageing Research Reviews*, *5*(1), 91–116. https://doi.org/10.1016/j.arr.2005.10.001

Shah, K., Drury, T., Roic, I., Hansen, P., Malin, M., Boyd, R., Sumer, H., & Ferguson, R. (2018). Outcome of allogeneic adult stem cell therapy in dogs suffering from osteoarthritis and other joint defects. *Stem Cells International*, *2018*, 7309201. https://doi.org/10.1155/2018/7309201

Sharun, K., Jambagi, K., Dhama, K., Kumar, R., Pawde, A. M., & Amarpal. (2021). Therapeutic potential of platelet-rich plasma in canine medicine. *Archives of Razi Institute*, *76*(4), 721–730. https://doi.org/10.22092/ari.2021.355953.1749

Sharun, K., Muthu, S., Mankuzhy, P. D., Pawde, A. M., Chandra, V., Lorenzo, J. M., Dhama, K., Amarpal, & Sharma, G. T. (2022). Cell-free therapy for canine osteoarthritis: Current evidence and prospects. *The Veterinary Quarterly*, *42*(1), 224–230. https://doi.org/10.1080/01652176.2022.2145620

Shin, H.-S., Woo, H.-M., & Kang, B.-J. (2017). Optimisation of a double-centrifugation method for preparation of canine platelet-rich plasma. *BMC Veterinary Research*, *13*(1), 198. https://doi.org/10.1186/s12917-017-1123-3

Shotorbani, B. B., Alizadeh, E., Salehi, R., & Barzegar, A. (2017). Adhesion of mesenchymal stem cells to biomimetic polymers: A review. *Materials Science and Engineering. C, Materials for Biological Applications*, *71*, 1192–1200. https://doi.org/10.1016/j.msec.2016.10.013

Sotiropoulou, P. A., Perez, S. A., Gritzapis, A. D., Baxevanis, C. N., & Papamichail, M. (2006). Interactions between human mesenchymal stem cells and natural killer cells. *Stem Cells*, *24*(1), 74–85. https://doi.org/10.1634/stemcells.2004-0359

Spangrude, G. J., Heimfeld, S., & Weissman, I. L. (1988). Purification and characterization of mouse hematopoietic stem cells. *Science*, *241*(4861), 58–62. https://doi.org/10.1126/science.2898810

Srzentić Dražilov, S., Mrkovački, J., Spasovski, V., Fazlagić, A., Pavlović, S., & Nikčević, G. (2018). The use of canine mesenchymal stem cells for the autologous treatment of osteoarthritis. *Acta Veterinaria Hungarica*, *66*(3), 376–389. https://doi.org/10.1556/004.2018.034

Steenkamp, W., Rachuene, P. A., Dey, R., Mzayiya, N. L., & Ramasuvha, B. E. (2022). The correlation between clinical and radiological severity of osteoarthritis of the knee. *SICOT-J*, *8*, 14. https://doi.org/10.1051/sicotj/2022014

Suga, H., Eto, H., Shigeura, T., Inoue, K., Aoi, N., Kato, H., Nishimura, S., Manabe, I., Gonda, K., & Yoshimura, K. (2009). IFATS collection: Fibroblast growth factor-2-induced hepatocyte growth factor secretion by adipose-derived stromal cells inhibits postinjury fibrogenesis through a c-Jun N-terminal kinase-dependent mechanism. *Stem Cells*, *27*(1), 238–249. https://doi.org/10.1634/stem cells.2008-0261

Sullivan, M. O., Gordon-Evans, W. J., Fredericks, L. P., Kiefer, K., Conzemius, M. G., & Griffon, D. J. (2015). Comparison of mesenchymal stem cell surface markers from bone marrow aspirates and adipose stromal vascular fraction sites. *Frontiers in Veterinary Science*, *2*, 82. https://doi.org/10.3389/fvets.2015.00082

Sundman, E. A., Cole, B. J., & Fortier, L. A. (2011). Growth factor and catabolic cytokine concentrations are influenced by the cellular composition of platelet-rich plasma. *The American Journal of Sports Medicine*, *39*(10), 2135–2140. https://doi.org/10.1177/0363546511417792

Taguchi, T., Borjesson, D. L., Osmond, C., & Griffon, D. J. (2019). Influence of donor's age on immuno-modulatory properties of canine adipose tissue-derived mesenchymal stem cells. *Stem Cells and Development*, *28*(23), 1562–1571. https://doi.org/10.1089/scd.2019.0118

Takahashi, K., & Yamanaka, S. (2006). Induction of pluripotent stem cells from mouse embryonic and adult fibroblast cultures by defined factors. *Cell*, *126*(4), 663–676. https://doi.org/10.1016/j.cell.2006.07.024

Tambella, A. M., Attili, A. R., Dini, F., Palumbo Piccionello, A., Vullo, C., Serri, E., Scrollavezza, P., & Dupré, G. (2014). Autologous platelet gel to treat chronic decubital ulcers: A randomized, blind controlled clinical trial in dogs. *Veterinary Surgery*, *43*(6), 726–733. https://doi.org/10.1111/j.1532-95 0X.2014.12148.x

Teunissen, M., Verseijden, F., Riemers, F. M., van Osch, G. J. V. M., & Tryfonidou, M. A. (2014). The advantages of autologous adipose derived mesenchymal stem cells (AdMSCs) over the NSAIDs application for degenerative elbow joint disease treatment in dogs – Twelve cases. *Kafkas Universitesi Veteriner Fakultesi Dergisi*, *20*(3), 345–350.

Teunissen, M., Verseijden, F., Riemers, F. M., van Osch, G. J. V. M., & Tryfonidou, M. A. (2021). The lower in vitro chondrogenic potential of canine adipose tissue-derived mesenchymal stromal cells (MSC) compared to bone marrow-derived MSC is not improved by BMP-2 or BMP-6. *The Veterinary Journal*, *269*, Art. no. 105605. https://doi.org/10.1016/j.tvjl.2020.105605

Thomas, E. D., Lochte, Jr., H. L., Lu, W. C., & Ferrebee, J. W. (1957). Intravenous infusion of bone marrow in patients receiving radiation and chemotherapy. *The New England Journal of Medicine*, *257*(11), 491–496. https://doi.org/10.1056/NEJM19 5709122571102

Thomson, J. A., Itskovitz-Eldor, J., Shapiro, S. S., Waknitz, M. A., Swiergiel, J. J., Marshall, V. S., & Jones, J. M. (1998). Embryonic stem cell lines derived from human blastocysts. *Science*, *282*(5391), 1145–1147. https://doi.org/10.1126/science.282.5391.1145

Thornton, O. R., & Li, W. (2023). Revolutionizing arthritis treatment: The synergy of iPSCs and extracellular vesicles-based acellular therapies for joint tissue repair. *Revolutionizing arthritis treatment: The synergy of iPSCs and extracellular vesicles-based acellular therapies for joint tissue repair*, *8*, *4*, 33–38.

Till, J. E., & McCulloch, E. A. (2011). A direct measurement of the radiation sensitivity of normal mouse bone marrow cells 1. *Radiation Research*, *175*(2), 145–149. https://doi.org/10.1667/RRXX28.1

Toh, W. S., Lai, R. C., Hui, J. H. P., & Lim, S. K. (2017, July). MSC exosome as a cell-free MSC therapy for cartilage regeneration: Implications for osteoarthritis treatment. In *Seminars in Cell and Developmental Biology*. Academic Press, *67*. https://doi.org/10.1016/j.semcdb.2016.11.008

Tremolada, C. (2022). Microfractured adipose tissue graft (Lipogems®) and regenerative surgery. *J. Orthop. Re. s Ther*, *7*, 1210.

Tremolada, C., Colombo, V., & Ventura, C. (2016). Adipose tissue and mesenchymal stem cells: State of the art and Lipogems® technology development. *Current Stem Cell Reports*, *2*(3), 304–312. https://doi.org/10.1007/s40778-016-0053-5

Ullah, M., Liu, D. D., & Thakor, A. S. (2019). Mesenchymal stromal cell homing: Mechanisms and strategies for improvement. *iScience*, *15*, 421–438. https://doi.org/10.1016/j.isci.2019.05.004

Upchurch, D. A., Renberg, W. C., Roush, J. K., Milliken, G. A., & Weiss, M. L. (2016). Effects of administration of adipose-derived stromal vascular fraction and platelet-rich plasma to dogs with osteoarthritis of the hip joints. *American Journal of Veterinary Research*, *77*(9), 940–951. https://doi.org/10.2460/ajvr.77.9.940

Upchurch, D. A., Renberg, W. C., Roush, J. K., Milliken, G. A., & Weiss, M. L. (2022, December). Use of mesenchymal stem cells in dogs. *Veterinary Quarterly*, *42*(1), 224–230.

Velarde, F., Ezquerra, S., Delbruyere, X., Caicedo, A., Hidalgo, Y., & Khoury, M. (2022). Mesenchymal stem cell-mediated transfer of mitochondria: Mechanisms and functional impact. *Cellular and Molecular Life Sciences*, *79*(3), 177. https://doi.org/10.1007/s00018-022-04207-3

Venator, K. P., Frye, C. W., Gamble, L.-J., & Wakshlag, J. J. (2020). Assessment of a single intra-articular stifle injection of pure platelet rich plasma on symmetry indices in dogs with unilateral or bilateral stifle osteoarthritis from long-term medically managed cranial cruciate ligament disease. *Veterinary Medicine*, 11, 31–38. https://doi.org/10.2147/VMRR. S238598

Vilar, J. M., Batista, M., Morales, M., Santana, A., Cuervo, B., Rubio, M., Cugat, R., Sopena, J., & Carrillo, J. M. (2014). Assessment of the effect of intraarticular injection of autologous adipose-derived mesenchymal stem cells in osteoarthritic dogs using a double blinded force platform analysis. *BMC Veterinary Research*, *10*(1), Art. no. 143. https://doi.org/10.1186/1746-6148-10-143

Vilar, J. M., Cuervo, B., Rubio, M., Sopena, J., Domínguez, J. M., Santana, A., & Carrillo, J. M. (2016). Effect of intraarticular inoculation of mesenchymal stem cells in dogs with hip osteoarthritis by means of objective force platform gait analysis: Concordance with numeric subjective scoring scales. *BMC Veterinary Research*, *12*(1), Art. no. 223. https://doi.org/10.1186/s12917-016-0852-z

Vilar, J. M., Morales, M., Santana, A., Spinella, G., Rubio, M., Cuervo, B., Cugat, R., & Carrillo, J. M. (2013). Controlled, blinded force platform analysis of the effect of intraarticular injection of autologous adipose-derived mesenchymal stem cells associated to PRGF-Endoret in osteoarthritic dogs. *BMC Veterinary Research*, 9, 131. https://doi.org/10.1186/1746-6148-9-131

Vilar, J. M., Rubio, M., Spinella, G., Cuervo, B., Sopena, J., Cugat, R., Garcia-Balletbó, M., Dominguez, J. M., Granados, M., Tvarijonaviciute, A., Ceron, J. J., & Carrillo, J. M. (2016). Serum collagen type II cleavage epitope and serum hyaluronic acid as biomarkers for treatment monitoring of dogs with hip osteoarthritis. *PLOS ONE*, *11*(2), e0149472. https://doi.org/10.1371/journal.pone.0149472

Walton, M. B., Cowderoy, E., Lascelles, D., & Innes, J. F. (2013). Evaluation of construct and criterion validity for the "Liverpool osteoarthritis in Dogs" (LOAD) clinical metrology instrument and comparison to two other instruments. *PLOS ONE*, *8*(3), e58125. https://doi.org/10.1371/journal.pone.0058125

Wang, L., Huang, S., Li, S., Li, M., Shi, J., Bai, W., Wang, Q., Zheng, L., & Liu, Y. (2019). Efficacy and safety of umbilical cord mesenchymal stem cell therapy for rheumatoid arthritis patients: A prospective phase I/II study. *Drug Design, Development and Therapy*, 13, 4331–4340. https://doi.org/10.2147/DDDT.S225613

Weiss, A. R. R., & Dahlke, M. H. (2019). Immunomodulation by mesenchymal stem cells (MSCs): Mechanisms of action of living, apoptotic, and dead MSCs. *Frontiers in Immunology*, *10*, 1191. https://doi.org/10.3389/fimmu.2019.01191

Weiss, D. J., English, K., Krasnodembskaya, A., Isaza-Correa, J. M., Hawthorne, I. J., & Mahon, B. P. (2019). The necrobiology of mesenchymal stromal cells affects therapeutic efficacy. *Frontiers in Immunology*, *10*, 1228. https://doi.org/10.3389/fimmu.2019.01228

Weissman, I. L., & Shizuru, J. A. (2008). The origins of the identification and isolation of hematopoietic stem cells, and their capability to induce donor-specific transplantation tolerance and treat autoimmune diseases, *The Journal of the American Society of Hematology*. *Blood*, *112*(9), 3543–3553.

https://doi.org/10.1182/blood-2008-08-078220

Wessely, M., Brühschwein, A., & Schnabl-Feichter, E. (2017). Evaluation of intra- and inter-observer measurement variability of a radiographic stifle osteoarthritis scoring system in dogs. *Veterinary and Comparative Orthopaedics and Traumatology*, *30*(6), 377–384. https://doi.org/10.3415/VCOT-16-09-0134

Whitworth, D. J., Frith, J. E., Frith, T. J. R., Ovchinnikov, D. A., Cooper-White, J. J., & Wolvetang, E. J. (2014). Derivation of mesenchymal stromal cells from canine induced pluripotent stem cells by inhibition of the TGF-β/activin signalling pathway. *Stem Cells and Development*, *23*(24), 3021–3033. https://doi.org/10.1089/scd.2013.0634

Wong, S. C., Medrano, L. C., Hoftman, A. D., Jones, O. Y., & McCurdy, D. K. (2021). Uncharted waters: Mesenchymal stem cell treatment for pediatric refractory rheumatic diseases; a single center case series. *Pediatric Rheumatology Online Journal*, *19*(1), 87. https://doi.org/10.1186/s12969-021-00575-5

Wright, A., Snyder, L., Knights, K., He, H., Springer, N. L., Lillich, J., & Weiss, M. L. (2020). A protocol for the isolation, culture, and cryopreservation of umbilical cord-derived canine mesenchymal stromal cells: Role of cell attachment in long-term maintenance. *Stem Cells and Development*, *29*(11), 695–713. https://doi.org/10.1089/scd.2019.0145

Xie, X., Zhao, S., Wu, H., Xie, G., Huangfu, X., He, Y., & Zhao, J. (2013). Platelet-rich plasma enhances autograft revascularization and reinnervation in a dog model of anterior cruciate ligament reconstruction. *The Journal of Surgical Research*, *183*(1), 214–222, ISSN 0022-4804. https://doi.org/10.1016/j.jss.2013.01.020

Yamasaki, S., Hashimoto, Y., Takigami, J., Terai, S., Mera, H., Nakamura, H., & Wakitani, S. (2015). Effect of the direct injection of bone marrow mesenchymal stem cells in hyaluronic acid and bone marrow stimulation to treat chondral defects in the canine model. *Regenerative Therapy*, 2, 42–48. https://doi.org/10.1016/j.reth.2015.10.003

Yang, Y. K., Ogando, C. R., Wang See, C., Chang, T.-Y., & Barabino, G. A. (2018). Changes in phenotype and differentiation potential of human mesenchymal stem cells aging in vitro. *Stem Cell Research and Therapy*, *9*(1), 131. https://doi.org/10.1186/s13287-018-0876-3

Yaradilmis, Y. U., Demirkale, I., Safa Tagral, A., Caner Okkaoglu, M., Ates, A., & Altay, M. (2020). Comparison of two platelet rich plasma formulations with viscosupplementation in treatment of moderate grade gonarthrosis: A prospective randomized controlled study. *Journal of Orthopaedics*, *20*, 240–246. https://doi.org/10.1016/j.jor.2020.01.041

Yin, C., & Heit, B. (2021). Cellular responses to the efferocytosis of apoptotic cells. *Frontiers in Immunology*, *12*, 631714. https://doi.org/10.3389/fimmu.2021.631714

Yoshida, R., & Murray, M. M. (2013). Peripheral blood mononuclear cells enhance the anabolic effects of platelet–rich plasma on anterior cruciate ligament fibroblasts. *Journal of Orthopaedic Research*, *31*(1), 29–34. https://doi.org/10.1002/jor.22183

Yu, J., Vodyanik, M. A., Smuga-Otto, K., Antosiewicz-Bourget, J., Frane, J. L., Tian, S., Nie, J., Jonsdottir, G. A., Ruotti, V., Stewart, R., Slukvin, I. I., & Thomson, J. A. (2007). Induced pluripotent stem cell lines derived from human somatic cells. *Science*, *318*(5858), 1917–1920. https://doi.org/10.1126/science.1151526

Yun, S., Ku, S.-K., & Kwon, Y.-S. (2016). Adipose-derived mesenchymal stem cells and platelet-rich plasma synergistically ameliorate the surgical-induced osteoarthritis in Beagle dogs. *Journal of Orthopaedic Surgery and Research*, *11*, 9. https://doi.org/10.1186/s13018-016-0342-9

Zakrzewski, W., Dobrzyński, M., Szymonowicz, M., & Rybak, Z. (2019). Stem cells: Past, present, and future. *Stem Cell Research and Therapy*, *10*(1), 68. https://doi.org/10.1186/s13287-019-1165-5

Zaripova, L. N., Midgley, A., Christmas, S. E., Beresford, M. W., Pain, C., Baildam, E. M., & Oldershaw, R. A. (2023). Mesenchymal stem cells in the pathogenesis and therapy of autoimmune and autoinflammatory diseases. *International Journal of Molecular Sciences*, *24*(22), 16040. https://doi.org/10.3390/ijms242216040

Zeira, O., Scaccia, S., Pettinari, L., Ghezzi, E., Asiag, N., Martinelli, L., Zahirpour, D., Dumas, M. P., Konar, M., Lupi, D. M., Fiette, L., Pascucci, L., Leonardi, L., Cliff, A., Alessandri, G., Pessina, A., Spaziante, D., & Aralla, M. (2018). Intra-articular administration of autologous micro-fragmented adipose tissue in dogs with spontaneous osteoarthritis: Safety, feasibility, and clinical outcomes. *Stem Cells Translational Medicine*, *7*(11), 819–828. https://doi.org/10.1002/sctm.18-0020

Zhang, B., Yin, Y., Lai, R. C., Tan, S. S., Choo, A. B. H., & Lim, S. K. (2014). Mesenchymal stem cells secrete immunologically active exosomes. *Stem Cells and Development*, *23*(11), 1233–1244. https://doi.org/10.1089/scd.2013.0479

Zhang, B.-Y., Wang, B.-Y., Li, S.-C., Luo, D.-Z., Zhan, X., Chen, S.-F., Chen, Z.-S., Liu, C.-Y., Ji, H.-Q., Bai, Y.-S., Li, D.-S., & He, Y. (2018). Evaluation of the curative effect of umbilical cord mesenchymal stem cell therapy for knee arthritis in dogs using imaging technology. *Stem Cells International*, *2018*, 1983025. https://doi.org/10.1155/2018/1983025

Zhao, J., Huang, H., Liang, G., Zeng, L.-F., Yang, W., & Liu, J. (2020). Effects and safety of the combination of platelet-rich plasma (PRP) and hyaluronic acid (HA) in the treatment of knee osteoarthritis: A systematic review and meta-analysis. *BMC Musculoskeletal Disorders*, *21*(1), 224. https://doi.org/10.1186/s12891-020-03262-w

Zheng, G., Ge, M., Qiu, G., Shu, Q., & Xu, J. (2015). Mesenchymal stromal cells affect disease outcomes via macrophage polarization. *Stem Cells International*, 2015, 989473. https://doi.org/10.1155/2015/989473

Zhou, Y., Zhang, J., Wu, H., Hogan, M. V., & Wang, J. H.-C. (2015, September 15). The differential effects of leukocyte-containing and pure platelet-rich plasma (PRP) on tendon stem/progenitor cells – Implications of PRP application for the clinical treatment of tendon injuries. *Stem Cell Research and Therapy*, *6*(1), 173. https://doi.org/10.1186/s13287-015-0172-4

Zhu, Y., Chen, X., & Liao, Y. (2023). Mesenchymal stem cells-derived apoptotic extracellular vesicles (ApoEVs): Mechanism and application in tissue regeneration. *Stem Cells*, *41*(9), 837–849. https://doi.org/10.1093/stmcls/sxad046

Zhu, Y., Wang, Y., Zhao, B., Niu, X., Hu, B., Li, Q., Zhang, J., Ding, J., Chen, Y., & Wang, Y. (2017). Comparison of exosomes secreted by induced pluripotent stem cell-derived mesenchymal stem cells and synovial membrane-derived mesenchymal stem cells for the treatment of osteoarthritis. *Stem Cell Research and Therapy*, *8*(1), 64. https://doi.org/10.1186/s13287-017-0510-9

Zielniok, K., Burdzinska, A., Murcia Pienkowski, V., Koppolu, A., Rydzanicz, M., Zagozdzon, R., & Paczek, L. (2021, July 29). Gene expression profile of human mesenchymal stromal cells exposed to hypoxic and pseudohypoxic preconditioning-an analysis by RNA sequencing. *International Journal of Molecular Sciences*, *22*(15), 8160. https://doi.org/10.3390/ijms22158160

Zubin, E., Conti, V., Leonardi, F., Zanichelli, S., Ramoni, R., & Grolli, S. (2015). Regenerative therapy for the management of a large skin wound in a dog. *Clinical Case Reports*, *3*(7), 598–603. https://doi.org/10.1002/ccr3.253

Organisations, websites, web articles, and social media resources

British Small Animal Veterinary Association (BSAVA) for information on joint injections.

BTI Biotechnology. https://bti-biotechnologyinstitute.com/

Canine Arthritis Management (CAM). https://caninearthritis.co.uk/

Cell Therapy Sciences https://www.celltherapysciences.co.uk/

Committee for Medicinal Products for Veterinary Use. (2019). Questions and answers on allogeneic stem cell-based products for veterinary use: Specific questions on extraneous agents (Ema/Cvmp/Advent/803494/2016-Rev.1). https://www.ema.europa.eu/en/documents/scientific-guideline/questions-answers-allogenic-stem-cell-based-products-veterinary-use-specific-questions-extraneous_en-0.pdf Retrieved April 22, 2023

European Medicines Agency. Reflection paper on stem-cell based medicinal products. ema.europa.eu. https://www.ema.europa.eu/en/documents/scientific-guideline/reflection-paper-stem-cell-based-medicinal-products_en.pdf

Fact MR. Animal stem cell therapy market. https://www.factmr.com/report/animal-stem-cell-therapy-market

Food and Drug Administration (USA). Regenerative medicine advanced therapy (RMAT) designation https://www.fda.gov/vaccines-blood-biologics/cellular-gene-therapy-products/regenerative-medicine-advanced-therapy-designation

Elton 2022. Growth Factors versus Cytokines. https://qkine.com/2022/05/27/growth-factors-vs-cytokines/

Guide for intra-articular injections: Dogstem® video https://dogstem.co.uk/

Italiano Stamilani, G. *Mesenchimali (GISMVet).* https://www.gismonline.it/, https://www.legislation.gov.uk/ukpga/2008/22/contents

Kim, S., Chaudhary, P. K., & Kim, S. (2021); 5 (Suppl 2). https://abstracts.esth.org/abstract/standardization-of-the-use-in-veterinary-regenerative-medicine/. Retrieved January 8, 2024. Standardization of platelet-rich plasma preparation with optimal platelet function for the use in veterinary regenerative medicine [Abstract]. *Research and Practice in Thrombosis and Haemostasis.*

Human Fertilisation and Embryology Act 1990. https://www.legislation.gov.uk/ukpga/1990/37/contents, Schedule 2.

Markets and markets Retrieved January 6, 2024. https://www.marketsandmarkets.com/Market-Reports/stem-cell-technologies-and-global-market-

Nupsala website https://nupsala.com/

Royal College of Veterinary Surgeons (RCVS) knowledge cruciate registry. https://knowledge.rcvs.org.uk/quality-improvement/canine-cruciate-registry/

The human fertilisation and embryology act. (2008). *Remedial* Order, *2018.* https://www.stemcell.com/media/files/wallchart/WA10021-Roles_for_MSCs_as_Medicinal_Signaling_Cells.pdf

Vet stem cell hub. Educational resource on LinkedIn®.

Veterinary Osteoarthritis Alliance (VOA). https://www.vet-oa.com

Vetmetrica® Health related quality of life (HRQL) questionnaire https://www.vetmetrica.com/

WSAVA body condition score. https://wsava.org/wp-content/uploads/2020/01/Body-Condition-Score-Dog.pdf

WSAVA muscle condition score. https://wsava.org/wp-content/uploads/2020/01/Muscle-Condition-Score-Chart-for-Dogs.pdf

Index

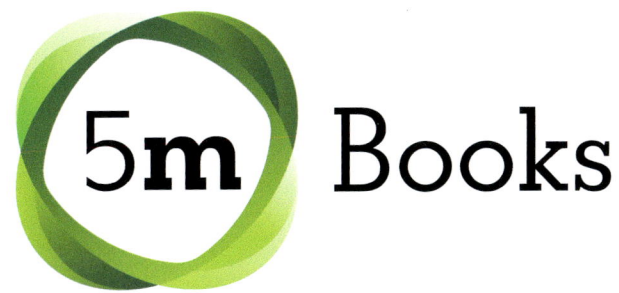

£50 FREE BOOKS?

Tell us about how you came to this book and we'll enter you in our next draw to win £50 of our books.

Scan the QR code to start or visit https://forms.office.com/e/97P5QTyZmk

We at 5m are passionate about improving the health and happiness of the animals we farm and live with and of the environment we farm in.

Our mission is to publish the highest quality books in veterinary and animal sciences, agriculture and aquaculture.

Join us at www.5mbooks.com or follow our social media channels to be part of our community and to find out more about our books and authors.

We welcome proposals for new books in the areas in which we publish. We would be delighted to hear from you, please email us: hello@5mbooks.com

www.5mbooks.com

 @5mBooks | @5m_Books | @5m_Books
 linkedin.com/company/5mbooks

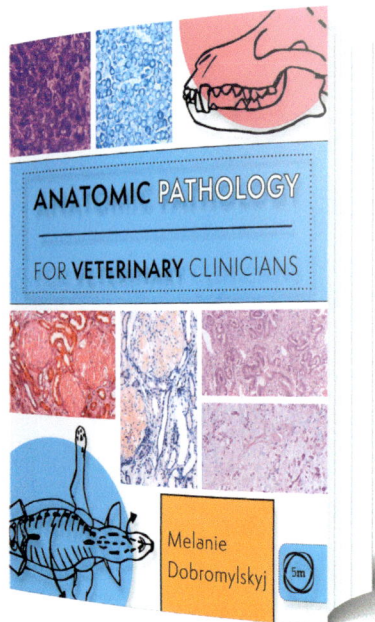

Anatomic Pathology for Veterinary Clinicians

Melanie Dobromylskyj

This book is a concise guide for practising vets on anatomic pathology that will aid the reader's understanding of pathology, thus allowing optimisation of diagnostic tests.

Anatomic Pathology for Veterinary Clinicians will teach practitioners how to:

• Take quality biopsy samples to get better results

• Understand histopathology reports

• Know when additional tests are warranted and are likely to give clinically useful information

Jul 2023 | ISBN 9781789182378
£55 | $85 | €66 | 220p PB

Diagnostic Radiology in Small Animal Practice 2nd Edition

Silke Hecht

This reference book covers using digital radiology and medical imaging procedures such as ultrasound, MRI and scintigraphy in veterinary practice. The approach is a step-by-step guide, with tips and techniques to ensure optimal X-rays and advice on how to improve radiation protection. All commonly kept pets are included: small mammals, birds, amphibians and reptiles.

Dec 2020 | ISBN 9781789180930
£150 | $235 | €180 | 532p HB

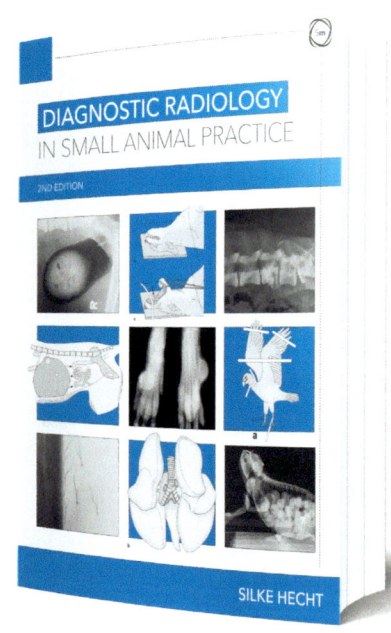